RELIGION AND MEDICINE IN THE MIDDLE AGES

This volume presents papers delivered at a conference held by the University of York's Centre of Medieval Studies at King's Manor, York, on 22 May 1999, under the title 'Medicine and Religion in the Middle Ages'. It also includes further invited papers on this theme, together with the Annual Quodlibet lecture on medieval theology, delivered by Vivian Nutton on 21 May 1999.

Joseph Ziegler's introduction sketches the varying relations between medicine and religion in the medieval west, which ranged between opposition and concord. Vivian Nutton provides a general account of the assimilation of the Galenic medical corpus into Christian medieval culture, showing how it became acceptable to Christians, Muslims, and Jews. By contrast Danielle Jacquart's examination of Jacques Despars's commentary on Avicenna's *Canon* shows a physician struggling with apparent dissonance between religious dogma and medical theory. Michael McVaugh looks closely at the particular case of Arnau de Vilanova's double career as a scholastic physician and a visionary mystic, while William Courtenay provides an updated list and a study of medical doctors (mostly from Paris in the period 1337–46) who had also studied or held degrees in theology, once again underlining the permeable disciplinary boundaries between medicine and theology. The meeting-point of ecclesiastical regulation and midwives is the subject of Kathryn Taglia's meticulous analysis of north French synodal legislation, which provides precious glimpses of the (growing?) specialisation of midwifery. Jessalynn Bird provides both a study of the personnel and patients of hospitals and *leprosaria* as they were seen by Jacques de Vitry, and also an edition of his sermons to hospitallers and a translation of his extraordinary general survey of hospitals. Peregrine Horden ventures into a hitherto unstudied domain, the use of religious chant as part of the therapeutic process in the medieval hospital. Peter Biller uses data from inquisitors' records to show the dense provision of medical care in the rural communities of Languedoc, which he uses as a backcloth for an investigation of the medical practice of two groups of heretics in that region, Cathars and Waldensians. Maaike van der Lugt traces the debate about the *incubus* from late Antiquity to the Renaissance, following both the theories of physicians and dream theorists, and the alternative demonological explanation that was upheld by theologians and lay people.

The book concludes with Joseph Ziegler's exploration of discussions of Adam's immortality in the State of Innocence, showing how medical concepts infiltrated theological debate from the twelfth century onwards.

YORK MEDIEVAL PRESS

York Medieval Press is published by the University of York's Centre for Medieval Studies in association with Boydell & Brewer Ltd. Our objective is the promotion of innovative scholarship and fresh criticism on medieval culture. We have a special commitment to interdisciplinary study, in line with the Centre's belief that the future of Medieval Studies lies in those areas in which its major constituent disciplines at once inform and challenge each other.

All inquiries of an editorial kind, including suggestions for monographs and essay collections, should be addressed to: The Director, University of York, Centre for Medieval Studies, The King's Manor, York YO1 7EP (E-mail: lah1@york.ac.uk).

Publications of York Medieval Press are listed at the back of this volume.

York Studies in Medieval Theology III

RELIGION AND MEDICINE IN THE MIDDLE AGES

Edited by
PETER BILLER and JOSEPH ZIEGLER

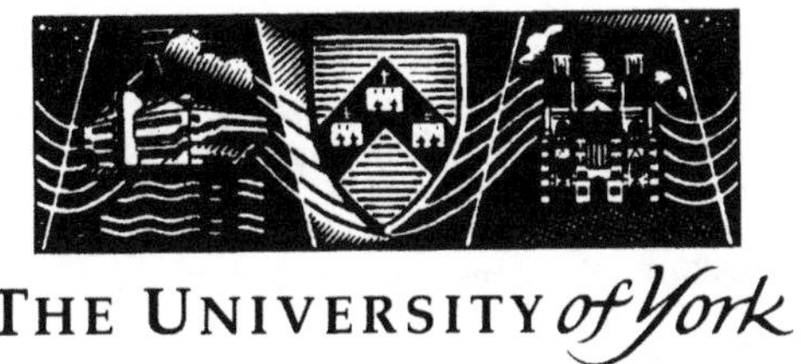

YORK MEDIEVAL PRESS

First published 2001

A York Medieval Press publication
in association with The Boydell Press
an imprint of Boydell & Brewer Ltd
PO Box 9 Woodbridge Suffolk IP12 3DF UK
and of Boydell & Brewer Inc.
PO Box 41026 Rochester NY 14604–4126 USA
website: http://www.boydell.co.uk
and with the
Centre for Medieval Studies, University of York

ISBN 1 903153 07 7

ISSN 1366–9656

A catalogue record for this book is available
from the British Library

Library of Congress Cataloging-in-Publication Data
Religion and medicine in the Middle Ages / edited by Peter Biller
and Joseph Ziegler.
p. cm. – (York studies in medieval theology, ISSN 1366–9656; 3)
Includes bibliographical references and index.
ISBN 1–903153–07–7 (alk. paper)
1. Health – Religious aspects – Catholic Church. 2. Medicine – Religious aspects – Catholic Church. 3. Medicine, Medieval. 4. Catholic Church – Doctrines. I. Biller, Peter. II. Ziegler, Joseph. III. Series.
BX1795.H4 R45 2001
261.5′61′0940902–dc21 2001035038

Typeset by Joshua Associates Ltd, Oxford

CONTENTS

CONTRIBUTORS

Peter Biller, Senior Lecturer, Department of History, University of York

Jessalynn Bird, Queen's College, Oxford

William J. Courtenay, C. H. Haskins Professor of History, Department of History, University of Wisconsin–Madison

Peregrine Horden, Wellcome Institute Lecturer in the History of Medicine, Department of History, Royal Holloway College, University of London

Danielle Jacquart, Professor at the École Pratique des Hautes Études (IVe Section), Paris

Michael R. McVaugh, William Smith Wells Professor, Department of History, University of Chapel Hill at North Carolina

Vivian Nutton, Professor of the History of Medicine, University College, London

Kathryn A. Taglia, Faculty of Arts, University of New Brunswick

Maaike van der Lugt, Maître des Conférences, Université de Paris VII

Joseph Ziegler, Lecturer, Department of General History, University of Haifa

EDITORS' NOTE

The Centre for Medieval Studies at the University of York and the editors of this volume are grateful to the Wellcome Trust for the support it gave to the original conference, to all those who took part on that occasion, and in particular to Monica Green for her contribution on the midwife in the Middle Ages. The editors are also grateful to the contributors for their patient responses to the editors; and to Pru Harrison and Pam Cope for their invaluable help in the final preparation of the text of the volume.

English translation of the Bible is given from the Douay version. We have not standardized Arabic names. These normally follow medieval conventions (for example, Avicenna), but sometimes appear in modern Western transliteration of Arabic (with Avicenna, for example, Ibn Sina). With other names we have followed the commonest modern forms.

ABBREVIATIONS

AFP	*Archivum Fratrum Praedicatorum* (Rome, 1931–)
Agrimi and Crisciani, 'Charity and Aid'	J. Agrimi and C. Crisciani, 'Charity and Aid in Medieval Christian Civilization', in *Western Medical Thought*, pp. 170–96
AHDLMA	*Archives d'histoire doctrinale et littéraire du moyen âge* (Paris, 1926–)
AL: Codices	G. Lacombe, A. Birkenmajer, M. Dulong, E. Franceschini and L. Minio-Paluello, *Aristoteles Latinus: Codices*, 3 vols. (Rome, Cambridge, Bruges and Paris, 1939–61)
Alexander of Hales, *Summa*	Alexander of Hales, *Summa theologica*, 4 vols. in 6 parts (Quaracchi, 1924–79)
AMN	Analecta Medievalia Namurcensia (Louvain, etc., 1950–)
Amundsen, *Medicine, Society, and Faith*	D. W. Amundsen, *Medicine, Society, and Faith in the Ancient and Medieval Worlds* (Baltimore and London, 1996)
Aquinas, *Summa theologiae*	Thomas Aquinas, *Summa theologiae*, Blackfriars edition, 60 vols. (London, 1964–76)
Arnau de Vilanova, *De intentione*	Arnau de Vilanova, *Tractatus de intentione medicorum*, ed. M. R. McVaugh, *AVOMO* V.1 (Barcelona, 2000)
AST	*Analecta Sacra Tarraconensia: revista de ciencias histórico-ecclesiásticas* (Barcelona, 1925–)
Augustine, *De civitate Dei*	Augustine, *La cité de Dieu*, ed. B. Dombart and A. Kalb, 5 vols., Bibliothèque Augustinienne: Oeuvres de Saint Augustin 33–7 (Paris, 1959–60)
Augustine, *De Genesi ad litteram*	Augustine, *De Genesi ad litteram libri duodecim*, ed. J. Zycha, CSEL 28 (Prague, Vienna and Leipzig, 1894)
Avicenna, *Canon*	Avicenna, *Liber canonis* (Venice, 1507; reprint, Hildesheim, 1964)
AVOMO	*Arnaldi de Villanova Opera Medica Omnia*, Seminarium Historiae Medicae Granatensis (Barcelona, 1975–)
Baldwin, *Peter the Chanter*	J. W. Baldwin, *Masters, Princes and Merchants: The Social Views of Peter the Chanter and his Circle*, 2 vols. (Princeton, 1970)
Bériac, *Lépreux*	F. Bériac, *Histoire des lépreux au moyen âge: Une société d'exclus* (Paris, 1988)
Bériou and Touati, *Voluntate dei*	N. Bériou and F.-O. Touati, *Voluntate dei leprosus: Les lépreux entre conversion et exclusion au XII*^{ème}*et*

	XIIIème *siècles*, Centro Italiano di Studi sull'Alto Medioevo (Spoleto, 1991)
Bessin	*Concilia Rotomagensis provinciae*, ed. G. Bessin, 2 vols. (Rouen, 1717), II
BFSMA	Bibliotheca Franciscana Scholastica Medii Aevi (Quaracchi and Grottaferrata, 1903–)
BGPTM	Beiträge zur Geschichte der Philosophie [from 27 (1928–30): und Theologie] des Mittelalters (Münster, 1891–)
BHM	*Bulletin of the History of Medicine* (Baltimore, 1933–)
Biblia Latina cum glossa ordinaria	*Biblia Latina cum glossa ordinaria: The Facsimile Reprint of the Editio Princeps Adolph Rusch of Strassburg 1480/81* (Turnhout, 1992)
Biller, '*Curate infirmos*'	P. Biller, '*Curate infirmos*: The Medieval Waldensian Practice of Medicine', in *The Church and Healing*, ed. W. J. Sheils, SCH 19 (Oxford, 1982), pp. 55–77
BnF	Paris, Bibliothèque nationale de France
Boeren I	P. C. Boeren, 'Les plus anciens statuts du diocèse de Cambrai (13e siècle)', *Revue de droit canonique* [de Strasbourg] 3 (1953), 1–32, 131–72, 377–415
Boeren II	P. C. Boeren, 'Les plus anciens statuts du diocèse de Cambrai (13e siècle)', *Revue de droit canonique* [de Strasbourg] 4 (1954), 131–58
Bolton, 'Hearts'	B. M. Bolton, 'Hearts not Purses? Pope Innocent III's Attitude to Social Welfare', in B. M. Bolton, *Innocent III: Studies on Papal Authority and Pastoral Care*, CS490 (Aldershot, 1995), article no. XVIII, pp. 131–44
Bonaventure, *In sententias*	Bonaventure, *Commentaria in quatuor libros sententiarum*, 4 vols. (Quaracchi, 1882–89) = *Opera omnia*, 11 vols. (Quaracchi, 1882–1902), I–IV
Bonenfant, 'Hôpitaux'	P. Bonenfant, 'Les hôpitaux en Belgique au moyen âge', *Annales de la Société Belge d'Histoire des Hôpitaux* 3 (1965), 3–44
Bonenfant-Feytmans, 'Organisations'	A. M. Bonenfant-Feytmans, 'Les organisations hospitalières vues par Jacques de Vitry (1225)', *Annales de la Société Belge d'Histoire des Hôpitaux* 28 (1980), 19–45
Brody, *Disease*	S. N. Brody, *The Disease of the Soul: Leprosy in Medieval Literature* (Ithaca and London, 1974)
BRUO	A. B. Emden, *A Biographical Register of the University of Oxford to A.D. 1500*, 3 vols. (Oxford, 1957–9)
Caesar, *Dialogus*	Caesar of Heisterbach, *Dialogus miraculorum*, ed. J. Strange, 2 vols. (Cologne, Bonn and Brussels, 1851)
Carreras Artau, '*Allocutio*'	J. Carreras Artau, 'La *Allocutio super Tetragrammaton* de Arnaldo de Vilanova', *Sefarad* 9 (1949), 75–105
CCCM	Corpus Christianorum, Continuatio Medievalis (Turnhout, 1966–)

CCSL	Corpus Christianorum, Series Latina (Turnhout, 1953–)
COD	*Conciliorum Oecumenicorum Decreta*, ed. J. Alberigo et al., 3rd edn (Bologna, 1973)
Concilia Germaniae	*Concilia Germaniae*, ed. J. F. Schannat and J. Hartzheim, 11 vols. (Cologne, 1759–90)
Crane	The Exempla *or Illustrative Stories from the* Sermones vulgares *of Jacques de Vitry*, ed. T. F. Crane (London, 1890)
CS	Variorum Collected Studies Series (London, Northampton and Aldershot, 1970–)
CSEL	Corpus Scriptorum Ecclesiasticorum Latinorum (Vienna, 1866–)
CUP	*Chartularium Universitatis Parisiensis*, ed. H. Denifle and A. Chatelain, 4 vols. (Paris, 1889–97)
de Angelis, *Innocenzo III*	P. de Angelis, *Innocenzo III (1198–1216) e la fondazione dell'Ospedale di Santo Spirito in Saxia* (Rome, 1948)
Despars	Jacques Despars, *Canon Avicenne cum explanatione Jacobi de Partibus*, 3 vols. (Lyons, 1498), unnumbered; Hain 2214
Doat	Paris, BnF, MSS Collection Doat
Dols, *Majnun*	M. W. Dols, *Majnun: The Madman in Medieval Islamic Society* (Oxford, 1992)
Eerden (van der), 'Incubus'	P. C. van der Eerden, 'Incubus: Demon, Droom of Monster', in *De betovering van het middeleeuwse christendom; Studies over ritueel en magie in de Middeleeuwen*, ed. M. Mostert and A. Demyttenaere (Hilversum, 1995), 101–28
Études, ed. Mollat	*Études sur l'histoire de la pauvreté*, ed. M. Mollat, Publications de la Sorbonne, Séries Études 8, 2 vols. (Paris, 1974)
Friedberg	*Corpus iuris canonici*, ed. E. Friedberg, 2 vols. (Leipzig, 1879)
FS	*Franciscan Studies* (New York, 1924–)
Galen: Problems	*Galen: Problems and Prospects*, ed. V. Nutton, Wellcome Institute for the History of Medicine (London, 1981)
Galen, *Usefulness of the Parts of the Body*	Galen, *On the Usefulness of the Parts of the Body*, trans. M. T. May, 2 vols., Cornell Publications in the History of Science (Ithaca, 1968)
García-Ballester, '*Artifex factivus sanitatis*'	L. García-Ballester, '*Artifex factivus sanitatis*: Health and Medical Care in Medieval Latin Galenism', in *Knowledge and the Scholarly Medical Traditions*, ed. D. Bates (Cambridge, 1995), pp. 127–50
Giles of Rome, *In sententias*	Giles of Rome, *In secundum librum sententiarum quæstiones* (Venice, 1581)
Gousset	*Les actes de la province ecclésiastique de Reims*, ed. T. M. J. Gousset, 4 vols. (Reims, 1842–4), II

Green, 'Documenting'	M. H. Green, 'Documenting Medieval Women's Medical Practice', in *Practical Medicine from Salerno to the Black Death*, ed. L. García-Ballester et al. (Cambridge, 1994), pp. 322–52; also in M. Green, *Women's Healthcare in the Medieval West: Texts and Contexts*, CS 680 (Aldershot, 2000), essay II
Greilsammer, 'Midwife'	M. Greilsammer, 'The Midwife, the Priest, and the Physician: The Subjugation of Midwives in the Low Countries at the End of the Middle Ages', *Journal of Medieval and Renaissance Studies* 21 (1991), 285–329
Gui, *Liber Sententiarum*	Bernard Gui, *Liber Sententiarum Inquisitionis Tholosanae Ab anno Christi mcccvii ad annum mcccxxiii*, ed. P. van Limborch and printed as part 2 of his *Historia Inquisitionis* (Amsterdam, 1692)
H.occ.	Jacques de Vitry, *Historia occidentalis*, ed. J. F. Hinnebusch, Spicilegium Friburgense 17 (Fribourg, 1972)
Horden, 'Discipline of Relevance'	P. Horden, 'A Discipline of Relevance: The Historiography of the Later Medieval Hospital', *SHM* 1 (1988), 359–74
Imbert (1947)	J. Imbert, *Histoire des hôpitaux français; contribution à l'étude des rapports de l'Église et l'État dans le domaine de l'assistance publique: Les hôpitaux en droit canonique (du décret du Gratien à la sécularisation de l'adminstration de l'Hôtel-Dieu de Paris en 1505)*, L'Église et l'État au Moyen Âge 7 (Paris, 1947)
Imbert (1982)	*Histoire des hôpitaux en France*, ed. J. Imbert (Toulouse, 1982)
Jacquart, *Médecine médiévale*	D. Jacquart, *La médecine médiévale dans le cadre parisien XIVe–XVe siècle*, Penser la médecine (Paris, 1998)
Jacquart, *Milieu médical*	D. Jacquart, *Le milieu médical en France du XIIe au XVe siècle: en annexe 2e supplément au «Dictionnaire» d'Ernest Wickersheimer*, Centre de Recherches d'Histoire de de Philologie de la IVe Section de l'École Pratique des Hautes Études, V, Hautes Études Médiévales et Modernes 46 (Geneva and Paris, 1981)
Jacquart, *Supplément*	D. Jacquart, *Supplément au «Dictionnaire biographique des médecins» d'Ernest Wickersheimer*, Centre de Recherches d'Histoire de de Philologie de la IVe Section de l'École Pratique des Hautes Études, V, Hautes Études Médiévales et Modernes 35 (Geneva and Paris, 1979)
Jacquart and Thomasset	D. Jacquart and C. Thomasset, *Sexuality and Medicine in the Middle Ages*, trans. A. Adamson (Princeton, 1988)

John Major, *In sententias*	John Major, *In primum [tertium] magistri sententiarum disputationes et decisiones . . .* (Paris, 1530)
Jusselin	M. Jusselin, 'Statuts synodaux et constitutions synodales du diocèse de Chartres au XIVe siècle', *Revue historique de droit français et étranger*, 4e série 8 (1929), 69–109
K	*Claudii Galeni, Opera omnia*, ed. C. G. Kuhn, 20 vols. in 22 (Leipzig, 1821–33)
Kedar, 'Twelfth-Century Description'	B. Z. Kedar, 'A Twelfth-Century Description of the Jerusalem Hospital', in *The Military Orders, Vol. 2: Welfare and Warfare*, ed. H. M. Nicholson (Aldershot, 1998), pp. 3–26
Kruger, *Dreaming*	S. F. Kruger, *Dreaming in the Middle Ages* (Cambridge, 1992)
Lee, '*Scrutamini Scripturas*'	H. Lee, '*Scrutamini Scripturas*: Joachimist Themes and *Figurae* in the Early Religious Writing of Arnold of Vilanova', *Journal of the Warburg and Courtauld Institutes* 37 (1974), 33–56
Le Grand, 'Maisons-Dieu et léproseries'	L. Le Grand, 'Les Maisons-Dieu et léproseries du diocèse de Paris au milieu du XIVe siècle', *Mémoires de la Société de l'Histoire de Paris et de l'Île-de-France* 25 (1898), 47–177
Le Grand, *Statuts*	L. Le Grand, *Statuts d'Hôtels-Dieu et de léproseries: recueil de textes du XIIe au XIVe siècle*, Collection de Textes pour servir à l'Étude et à l'Enseignement de l'Histoire (Paris, 1901)
Le Groux	*Summa statutorum synodalium cum praevia synopsi vitae episcoporum tornacensium*, ed. J. Le Groux (1726)
Lieber, 'Galen in Hebrew'	E. Lieber, 'Galen in Hebrew: The Transmission of Galen's Works in the Mediaeval Islamic World', in *Galen: Problems*, pp. 167–86
Longère, 'Pauvreté'	J. Longère, 'Pauvreté et richesse chez quelques prédicateurs durant la seconde moitié du XIIIe siècle', in *Études*, ed. Mollat, I, 255–73
Lottin, *Psychologie et morale*	O. Lottin, *Psychologie et morale aux xiie et xiiie sièles*, 6 vols. in 7 (Louvain and Gembloux, 1942–60)
McVaugh, 'Humidum Radicale'	M. R. McVaugh, 'The Humidum Radicale in Thirteenth-Century Medicine', *Traditio* 30 (1974), 259–83
Manselli, 'Religiosità'	R. Manselli, 'La religiosità d'Arnaldo da Villanova', *Bullettino dell'Istituto Storico Italiano per il Medio Evo e Archivio Muratoriano* 63 (1951), 1–100
Mansi	J. D. Mansi, *Sacrorum conciliorum nova et amplissima collectio*, 31 vols. (Florence, 1759–98)
Marangon, *Pensiero ereticale*	P. Marangon, *Il pensiero ereticale nella Marca Trevigiana e a Venezia dal 1200 al 1350* (Padua, 1984)

Mollat, *Pauvres*	M. Mollat, *Les pauvres au moyen âge: étude sociale* (Paris, 1978)
Müller (von), 'Galens Werk'	I. von Müller, 'Ueber Galens Werk vom wissenschaftlichen Beweis', *Abhandlungen der philosophisch-philologischen Classe der königlich bayerischen Akademie der Wissenschaften* 20 (1897), II, 405–78
Music as Medicine	*Music as Medicine: The History of Music Therapy since Antiquity*, ed. P. Horden (Aldershot, 2000)
Nicholas of Ockham, *Quaestiones*	Nicholas of Ockham, *Quaestiones disputatae de traductione humanae naturae a primo parente*, ed. C. Saco Alarcón (Rome, 1993)
O'Boyle, *Art of Medicine*	C. O'Boyle, *The Art of Medicine: Medical Teaching at the University of Paris, 1250–1400*, Education and Society in the Middle Ages and Renaissance 9 (Leiden, Boston and Cologne, 1998)
Olson, *Literature as Recreation*	G. Olson, *Literature as Recreation in the Later Middle Ages* (Ithaca and London, 1982)
Peden, 'Macrobius'	A. M. Peden, 'Macrobius and Medieval Dream Literature', *Medium Aevum* 54 (1985), 59–73
Peter of Tarentaise, *In sententias*	Peter of Tarentaise [Innocent V], *In IV. libros sententiarum commentaria*, 4 vols. (Toulouse, 1652; reprint, Ridgewood, NJ, 1964)
Peter the Lombard, *Sententiae*	Peter the Lombard, *Sententiae in IV libris distinctae*, ed. I. Brady, 2 vols., SB 4–5 (1971–81)
PG	*Patrologia Greca*, ed. J. P. Migne, 162 vols. (Paris, 1841–64)
Piché, *Condamnation parisinenne*	D. Piché, *La condamnation parisinenne de 1277: Texte latin, traduction, introduction et commentaire* (Paris, 1999)
Pietro d'Abano, *Conciliator*	Pietro d'Abano, *Conciliator controversiarum quae inter philosophos et medicos versantur* (Venice, 1565; reprint, Padua, 1985)
PIMS	Pontifical Institute of Medieval Studies
Pitra	*Analecta novissima spicilegii Solesmensis: Altera continuatio*, ed. J.-B. Pitra, 2 vols. (Paris, 1885–8), II
PL	*Patrologia Latina*, ed. J. P. Migne, 217 vols. (Paris, 1857–66)
Pocquet	B. Pocquet du Haut-Jussé, 'Les statuts synodaux d'Alain de la Rue, évêque de Saint-Brieuc', *Bulletin et Mémoires de la Société Archéologique du Département d'Ille-et-Vilaine* 47 (1920), 1–142
Pontal	*Les statuts synodaux français du XIIIe siècle*, vol. 1: *Les statuts de Paris et le synodal de l'ouest*, ed. and trans. O. Pontal (Paris, 1971)
Pressutti	*Regesta Honorii Papae III*, ed. P. Pressutti, 2 vols. (Rome, 1888–95)

Rawcliffe, 'Hospital Nurses'	C. Rawcliffe, 'Hospital Nurses and their Work', in *Daily Life in the Middle Ages*, ed. R. Britnell (Stroud, 1998), pp. 43–64
Rawcliffe, *Medicine for the Soul*	C. Rawcliffe, *Medicine for the Soul: The Life, Death and Resurrection of an English Hospital* (Stroud, 1999)
Rawcliffe, 'Medicine for the Soul'	C. Rawcliffe, 'Medicine for the Soul: The Medieval English Hospital and the Quest for Spiritual Health', in *Religion, Health and Suffering*, pp. 316–38
Reg. Aven.	Archivio Segreto Vaticano, Registra Avenionensia
Reg. Suppl.	Archivio Segreto Vaticano, Registra Supplicationum
Reg. Vat.	Archivio Segreto Vaticano, Registra Vaticana
Religion, Health and Suffering	*Religion, Health and Suffering*, ed. J. R. Hinnells and R. Porter (London and New York, 1999)
Reynolds, *Food and the Body*	P. L. Reynolds, *Food and the Body: Some Peculiar Questions in High Medieval Theology* (Leiden, 1999)
Ricklin, *Traum*	T. Ricklin, *Der Traum der Philosophie im 12. Jahrhundert: Traumtheorien zwischen Constantinus Africanus und Aristoteles* (Leiden, 1998)
Risse, *Mending Bodies*	G. Risse, *Mending Bodies, Saving Souls: A History of Hospitals* (New York and Oxford, 1999)
RS	Rerum Brittanicarum medii aevi scriptores, 99 vols. (London, 1858–1911) = Rolls Series
Rubin, *Charity and Community*	M. Rubin, *Charity and Community in Medieval Cambridge*, Cambridge Studies in Medieval Life and Thought, Fourth Series (Cambridge, 1987)
Saunier, *'Le pauvre malade'*	A. Saunier, *'Le pauvre malade' dans le cadre hospitalier médiéval: France du Nord vers 1300–1500* (Paris, 1993)
Saunier, 'Visiteur'	A. Saunier, 'Le visiteur, les femmes et les «obstetrices» des paroisses de l'archidiaconé de Josas de 1458 à 1470', in *Santé, médecine et assistance au Moyen Age*, Actes du 110e congrès national des sociétés savantes, Montpellier, 1985 (Paris, 1987), 43–62
SB	Spicilegium Bonaventurianum (Quaracchi, Grottaferrata and Paris, 1963–)
SCH	Studies in Church History (London/Oxford, 1964–)
SHM	*Social History of Medicine* (Oxford, 1988–)
Source Book in Medieval Science	*Source Book in Medieval Science*, ed. E. Grant (Cambridge, MA, 1974)
Sozomen, *Historia ecclesiastica*	Sozomen, *Historia ecclesiastica*, ed. J. Bidez and G. C. Hansen, Die griechischen christlichen Schriftsteller der ersten Jahrhundertn 50 (Berlin, 1960)
Spiegeler, *Hôpitaux*	P. de Spiegeler, *Les hôpitaux et l'assistance à Liège (X^{e}–XVe siècles)* (Paris, 1987)
Stegmüller, *Repertorium*	F. Stegmüller, *Repertorium commentariorum in Sententias Petri Lombardi*, 2 vols. (Würzburg, 1947), I
Synodicon, ed. Harlay	*Synodicon ecclesiae Parisiensis auctoritate*, ed. F. de Harlay (Paris, 1674)

Temkin, *Galenism*	O. Temkin, *Galenism: Rise and Decline of a Medical Philosophy*, Cornell Publications in the History of Science (Ithaca, 1973)
Temkin, *Hippocrates*	O. Temkin, *Hippocrates in a World of Pagans and Christians* (Baltimore and London, 1991)
Text and Tradition	*Text and Tradition: Studies in Ancient Medicine and its Transmission Presented to Jutta Kollesch*, ed. K.-D. Fisher, D. Nickel and P. Potter, Studies in Ancient Medicine 18 (Leiden, 1998)
The Year 1000	*The Year 1000: Medical Practice at the End of the First Millennium*, ed. P. Horden and E. Savage-Smith, *SHM* 13, special issue (2000)
Thesaurus	*Thesaurus novus anecdotorum*, ed. E. Martène and U. Durand, 5 vols. (Paris, 1717)
Touati, *Maladie*	F.-O. Touati, *Maladie et société au moyen âge: la lèpre, les lépreux et les léproseries dans la province ecclésiastique de Sens jusqu'au milieu du XIVe siècle*, Bibliothèque du Moyen Age 11 (Paris and Brussels, 1998)
Toulouse 609	Toulouse, Bibliothèque de la Ville, MS 609
VA	Peter the Chanter, *Verbum Abbreviatum*, *PL* 205
Veterum scriptorum	*Veterum scriptorum et monumentorum historicorum dogmaticorum et moralium amplissima collectio*, ed. E. Martène and U. Durand, 9 vols. (Paris, 1724)
Walzer, *Galen on Jews and Christians*	M. Walzer, *Galen on Jews and Christians* (London, 1949)
Western Medical Thought	*Western Medical Thought from Antiquity to the Middle Ages*, ed. M. D. Grmek and M. Fantini (Cambridge, MA, and London,1998)
Wickersheimer, *Dictionnaire biographique*	E. Wickersheimer, *Dictionnaire biographique des médecins en France au Moyen Age*, 2 vols. (Paris, 1936)
William of Auvergne, *Opera Omnia*	William of Auvergne, *Opera Omnia*, ed. F. Hotot and B. Le Feron, 2 vols. (Orléans and Paris, 1674; reprint Frankfurt-am-Main, 1963)
YSMT	York Studies in Medieval Theology 1– (York, 1997–)
Ziegler, *Medicine and Religion*	J. Ziegler, *Medicine and Religion c. 1300: The Case of Arnau de Vilanova* (Oxford, 1998)
Ziegler, 'Practitioners and Saints'	J. Ziegler, 'Practitioners and Saints: Medical Men in Canonization Processes in the Thirteenth to Fourteenth Centuries', *SHM* 12 (1999), 191–225
Ziegler, '*Ut dicunt medici*'	J. Ziegler, '*Ut dicunt medici*: Medical Knowledge and Theological Debates in the Second Half of the Thirteenth Century', *BHM* 73 (1999), 208–37

Introduction

Religion and Medicine in the Middle Ages

Joseph Ziegler

After its introduction this volume prints the fifth of the Annual Quodlibet Lectures on medieval theology, 'God, Galen and the depaganization of ancient medicine', delivered by Vivian Nutton on 21 May 1999. It then continues with papers delivered at a conference held by the University of York's Centre of Medieval Studies at King's Manor, York, on 22 May 1999, under the title 'Medicine and Religion in the Middle Ages', together with further invited papers on this theme, written by Jessalynn Bird, William Courtenay, Peregrine Horden and Kathryn Taglia.

*

> HONOUR the physician for the need thou hast of him: for the most High hath created him. For all healing is from God, and he shall receive gifts of the king. The skill of the physician shall lift up his head, and in the sight of great men he shall be praised. The most High hath created medicines out of the earth, and a wise man will not abhor them. Was not bitter water made sweet with wood? The virtue of these things is come to the knowledge of men, and the most High hath given knowledge to men, that he may be honoured in his wonders. By these he shall cure and shall allay their pains, and of these the apothecary shall make sweet confections, and shall make up ointments of health, and of his works there shall be no end. For the peace of God is over all the face of the earth. My son, in thy sickness neglect not thyself, but pray to the Lord, and he shall heal thee. Turn away from sin and order thy hands aright, and cleanse thy heart from all offence. Give a sweet savour, and a memorial of fine flour, and make a fat offering, and then give place to the physician. For the Lord created him: and let him not depart from thee, for his works are necessary. For there is a time when thou must fall into their hands. And they shall beseech the Lord, that he would prosper what they give for ease and remedy, for their conversation. He that sinneth in the sight of his Maker, shall fall into the hands of the physician.
> (Ecclesiasticus 38. 1–15)

The title of this collection of articles – *Religion and Medicine in the Middle Ages* – needs explanation. Although 'religion' in the medieval West principally meant monasticism or devotion, we are using it here in its broader and mainly post-medieval sense, namely a system of faith and worship and everything which relates to them.[1] We restrict our view to the Christian

[1] P. Biller, 'Words and the Medieval Notion of "Religion"', *Journal of Ecclesiastical History* 36 (1985), 351–69.

religion in Latin Christendom, not looking at other religions' encounter with medicine in this period. Comparison can be very illuminating, as can be seen, for example, in Benjamin Zeev Kedar's recent study of a description of the Hospitallers' Jerusalem hospital, possibly from the 1180s.[2] Muslims, Jews and Christians were admitted to this hospital, which supplied chicken to those who on religious grounds could not eat pork or mutton, and which had four trained physicians among its staff, far more than is known in any contemporary hospital in the Latin West. Some of the articles in this book do allude to the need to compare the results of their findings with Jewish or Islamic societies of the same period, which we hope will encourage further enquiry. But here our choice has been to focus exclusively – and therefore we hope with more depth – on the complex relationship between religion and medicine within one faith and one society.

The nature of this relationship in the medieval West has been problematic in historiography. It has been seen as dichotomous, a matter of opposition or separateness. Ecclesiastical historians have written in terms of two separate sorts of medicine, where the superior one, medicine for the soul, was provided by the ecclesiastical agents, while the body was taken care of by physicians and other medical practitioners. Medical historians have stressed the natural and religiously neutral character of the academic medicine that was developing at this period. This view is no longer satisfactory. Overlap, sometimes even ambiguity, now seems more appropriate to describe the relationship between medicine and theology, between the carers for bodies and for souls, between medical and spiritual approaches to disease. In describing the coexistence between temple medicine and Hippocratic medicine in Classical Greece, Helen King has recently shown how fused religious and secular medicine were.[3] Rather than Hippocratic medicine liberating itself from temple medicine, temple medicine occasionally copied Hippocratic medicine, Greek physicians rarely objected to temple medicine, and patients tended to cross from one sector to another in their search for proper treatment. Hippocrates and Asclepius were not perceived as incompatible alternatives. Thus the modern dichotomy between a rational and an irrational or magical approach to health care is misleading in the effort to understand the health-care systems of the ancient world. When we see, for example, physicians in the thirteenth century becoming an integral part of the judicial mechanism which led to the canonization of saints, we realize that Helen King's point applies just as powerfully to the medieval West as it does to Classical Greece.[4]

Throughout the Middle Ages physicians possessed one fundamental source upon which they could draw when asserting the legitimacy of their

[2] Kedar, 'Twelfth-Century Description'.

[3] H. King, 'Comparative Perspectives on Medicine and Religion in the Ancient World', in *Religion, Health and Suffering*, 276–94.

[4] Ziegler, 'Practitioners and Saints'.

profession, the Bible, and the translation and diffusion of Greek philosophy in the high and later Middle Ages added another source, Aristotle's anthropology. The fifteen verses of Ecclesiasticus 38 which open this introduction were fundamental for questions about the place of medicine and the physician (not to forget the apothecary) in a divinely ordained world. What is the source of medical knowledge? In what way does the physician possess the power to heal? Is medicinal cure an artificial intervention in God's plan? Who or what is responsible for the power of medicine? God? Nature? Human reason? Miracle? What is the relationship between sin and disease? What role, if any, should spiritual medicine play in procuring health?

Ecclesiasticus 38 could be (and was) used as a starting point for elaborating on the nexus sin – disease, punishment – pain and suffering. But it could also be used to supply scriptural authority to a general argument in favour of the medical profession in Christian society, which would also draw on the authority of 'The Philosopher', Aristotle.[5] Let us pause, abandoning the mountain-peak panorama and looking for a moment through a microscope, to see just how this was manifested in practice. The example I have chosen is a short treatise described as 'prologus compilatoris', which is found in London, British Library, MS Royal 12 B XXV, fols. 57r–58b. The manuscript is a fifteenth-century compilation of miscellaneous medical treatises. It is unclear whether this is a prologue for the remainder of the volume, for the following treatise, or an independent philosophical reflection by the anonymous author.[6]

The treatise is directed against the foolishness of unlearned laymen who, being entirely ignorant of the art of medicine, interfere with it and (presumably) criticize its necessity. It is impossible to say with any kind of certainty who these ignorant people were. But from the arguments in favour of medicine set forth by the anonymous author, it is possible that they had been ridiculing medicine as being a hermetic art and nothing more, denying its necessity as a science.

Ecclesiasticus 38. 1–5 is the author's starting point for discussing medicine's legitimacy.[7] In fact, he explicitly blames the critics for contradicting scripture by questioning medicine's necessity. The necessity of medicine is also evident from Aristotle's definition of man, who is composed of body and soul. Hence anyone who desires to excel in arts and studies of true wisdom must carefully weigh and choose those things which maintain and guard

[5] Cf. C. O'Boyle, 'Medicine, God, and Aristotle in the Early Universities: Prefatory Prayers in Late Medieval Medical Commentaries', *BHM* 66 (1992), 185–209.

[6] In London, British Library, MS Sloan 282, fol. 189v the treatise appears as the prologue to an ordered collection of pharmacological recipes entitled: 'Opusculum de dosis tam simplicium quam compositorum': *A Catalogue of Incipits of Medieval Scientific Writings in Latin*, ed. L. Thorndike and P. Kibre, 2nd edn (London, 1963), col. 638.

[7] For the use of Ecclesiasticus 38 by clerics and physicians see Ziegler, *Medicine and Religion*, pp. 231–7 and *passim*.

body and soul and are beneficial to man's health (*salus*) and wholeness (*integritas*). This struggle for man's health and wholeness is waged by two disciplines: theology (*diuinitatis sciencia*) which is responsible for the health of the soul (*salus anime*) and medicine (*ars phisica*) which is responsible for the health of the body (*sanitas corporis*). For the author the health of the body includes the psychological condition of the person. For when the health of the body is lost by melancholy, madness (*mania*) or frenzy (*frenesis*), and the reason of the other arts is confused and darkened, what, the author asks rhetorically, is the benefit of [theological] science? Since reasonableness cannot exist in the human person without the health of the body, which demands temperate humours that can only be regulated by the help of medicine, it is patent that the art of medicine is necessary and more dignified than all others, except theology.[8]

The necessity of medicine is evident from diseases peculiar to those studying theology. This is specifically true of members of the religious Orders (*religiosi*), who are affected by various mental conditions (*amentia, frenesis*) brought on by excessive and incessant labour of the cogitative faculty. It is therefore natural that the body follows the soul when it is disturbed, and also that the soul follows the body in its accidents.[9]

What is the character of this medicine which, together with theology, maintains the wholeness of the person? As we read further in this treatise we see that it is, in fact, a self-confident scholastic medicine, in nature essentially bookish and non-empirical.[10] The treatise goes on to portray the perfect

[8] 'Tota ista sentencia est de sancta scriptura quam quidam ydioti et ignari videntur contrariare cum dicant scienciam phisice non esse necessariam ideo in errore permittantur errare. Nos verum iter teneamus sequentes dictum philosophi dicentis: Ex quo homo constet [?] ex corpore et anima. Racionabile videtur, ut ea que conseruande corporis et anime integritati et saluti prodesse possunt, prouida consideracione perpendat et eligat quiquis vere sapiencie studiis vel artibus pollere desiderat. Inde est quod theologia, id est diuinitatis sciencia propter anime salutem et ars phisica propter corporis sanitatem [salutem: Sloan] appetenda videtur. Corporis enim salute [sanitate: Sloan] amissa siue per melancoliam vel per maniam [inaniam: Sloan] vel per frenesim ipsa eciam racione turbata et obtenebrata ceterarum arcium quid proderit sciencia? Cum enim racionabilita [racionabilitas: Sloan] in homine esse nequeat sine corporis sanitate, /57v/ sanitas vero corporis egeat humorum temperamentis, humorum temperamenta medicine expostulent adiumenta constat hanc artem omnibus esse necessariam et digniorem excepta theologia [theologia tantummodo excepta: Sloan]': London, British Library, MS Royal 12B XXV, fol. 57r–v. Cf. Ziegler, *Medicine and Religion*, pp. 121–2, for Arnau de Vilanova's perception of medicine as the most noble of all sciences.

[9] 'Videmus enim multos et eciam religiosos dum non cogitant nec inuestigant aliud nisi ut solum deum timeant et ament, subito in frenesim et amenciam et alias egritudines incidere ex assidua et nimia cogitacionum sollicitudine. Et naturale est quod corpus animam sequitur in suis perturbacionibus necnon et anima corpus in suis accidentibus': BL MS Royal 12B XXV, fol. 57v.

[10] Cf. C. Crisciani, 'Teachers and Learners in Scholastic Medicine: Some Images and Metaphors', *History of Universities* 15 (1997–9), 75–101, for how fourteenth- and

physician (*perfectus medicus*). He should have knowledge of the qualities and properties of food, simple and composite medicines, and astronomy, and the ability to unravel the causes of all diseases. These characteristics are lacking among the unqualified *laici* and women who engage in medicine and who become the target of the author's loathing.[11] Efficient cure depends on finding the causes of a disease. Hence the medical art, which is the prerequisite for theological contemplation, relies on scholastic formation, and it cannot be attained by laymen who rely on luck. Proper formation in medical art relies on books, not on experience. Here John of Damascus is confronted by Hermes, who preached adherence to individual proof via individual experiment and experience. But the determination is by Constantine the African, who preached adherence to the proofs of the ancients as they appear in the texts. Any attempt to reach a general knowledge of the whole through experience or experiments is both vain and futile.[12]

fifteenth-century physicians grasped and presented the structure of their discipline and the qualities of the good physician.

11 'Preterea ut dicit Constantinus in *Practica* [sua: Sloan] oportet medicum naturas et qualitates diuersas noscere ciborum et potuum. Oportet eciam eum omnium egritudinum omniumque causarum et accidencium naturam et noticiam scire. Congruit etiam scire quibus medicaminibus vel simplicibus vel compositis omnes egritudines curentur. Et non solum oportet medicum in hac sciencia esse eruditum verum eciam in astronomia. Unde dicit ypocras in libello *De iudiciis astrorum*: "Cuiusmodi medicus est qui astronomiam ignorat nullus homo se debet mittere in manus illius quia non est medicus perfectus." Sed mirum est de laicis et mulieribus de hac arte se intromittentibus inicii medii et finis, omnino sunt expartes et ignari qualiter audent curam alicuius sumere vel pocionem aliquam vel aliam medicinam simplicem vel compositam exhibere. Ad talium detestacionem loquitur Galenus in prologo *Experimentorum* ubi sic dicit: Non laudamus hominem ignorantem hanc artem ut habeat bonas medicinas quoniam forte uellet prodesse /fol. 58r/ et nocebit et cetera. Concordat Constantinus in *Theorica* libro primo ubi dicit: De hac intencione ideo tractauimus ut hanc viam ingredientibus lumen prebeamus. Est enim quasi secus [cecus: Sloan] qui viam ingreditur quam ignorat. Similiter contra tales loquitur compilator *Compendii Sal⟨erni⟩* ubi sic ait: Cognitis causis propria curacio poterit adhiberi. Nam qui causam ignorant quando [quomodo: Sloan] curat, quomodo scit utrum sanat an occidat? Si fortet [*sic*; forte: Sloan] curet non est illius sed fortune. Remota autem causa, remouetur effectus aut statim aut in breui': BL MS Royal 12B XXV, fols. 57v–58r. Cf. Haly Abbas, *Pantegni, Practica* iii.2: 'De dietis omnium egritudinum', in *Opera omnia Ysaac* (Lyons, 1515), fol. 86va; Galen, *Comment. I in Hippocratis Liber Epidemiarum I*, in *K* 17/1, p. 16; Haly Abbas, *Pantegni, Theorica* i.2 'Que sciri conveniat ab introducendis', fol. 1rb.

12 'Rursus ut dicit Constantinus in *Speculatiua* [= *Theorica*]: "Sex sunt que oportet medicum scire antequan curare incipiat id est: Libri intencionem, eiusdem utilitatem, titulum, ad quam partem doctrine tendat [intendat – Sloan], nomen autoris, libri diuisionem." [. . .] Quid enim melius est medicina cum sibi homines subiectos faciat. Similiter ingenium naturale medici multum adiuuat artem ut dicit Jo.[hannes] Da.[mascenus]: "Et habundanter libros veterum [veterorum: Sloan] peritorum relegere et secreta eorum diligenter excutere hominem sapientem iuuat" [. . .]. Contra dicit Hermes in *Libro de 15 stellis et 15 lapidibus*: "Beatus est qui probat quoniam probacio est mater scienciarum et quilibet sapiens appetit scienciam procus autem non." Unde dicit Constantinus in *Practica* libro primo

Palpable throughout this text is the sheer entangledness of medicine and religion. One can study the history of medieval medicine by examining the medical writings or the legal documents which specifically deal with physicians. But this is not enough. Not only does a plurality of non-medical texts – synodal canons, theological disputations, inquisition records, sermons, preachers' manuals and chronicles – contain much that is hidden or unexplored, but they also do what the narrowly medical sources cannot do. They make the theme three-dimensional and, in particular, they illuminate the intertwined roles of science and faith in matters of health. This feature is common to all the articles in this book. They all deal with key topics in the history of medieval medicine by examining sources which one would not normally use when writing about medieval medicine or the medical milieu. In so doing they widen the scope of the study of medieval medicine and correct deep-rooted misconceptions. Like our contemporary culture medieval culture was permeated by medical themes at all levels. It is for the historian to integrate these themes into the larger historical narrative, and the purpose of collecting articles in this book is to show just how useful this approach is, and to encourage further exploration of the *terra* still largely *incognita*, Religion and Medicine in the Middle Ages. Our own chart is not only provisional but also – accidentally rather than deliberately – selective. Important areas not represented in it include monastic medicine, magic and astrology, medicine in hagiography, and the encounter of different religions in the medical setting.

Published at the beginning of this collection of articles is the annual York Quodlibet lecture by Vivian Nutton, who provides a general account of the

capitulo 7°: Oportet medicum si aliquod probatum inuenerit ad curandum egros sufficiens, non laborare in aliis probandis molestum enim est. Ideo medicaminum pauca sunt /58v/ tenenda nisi quorum iuuamentum sepius expertus confidere possit. Tocius enim multitudo noticia incomprehensibilis est. Neque enim si volueris per singula inquirendo discurrere [percurrere: Sloan] multiplici diuersitate sensus distractus in nullo fidem poteris adhibere. "Propterea non oportet in humanis corporibus medicinam probare sed que probata sunt ab antiquis sufficiant." Unde Jo.[hannes] Da.[mascenus] dicit: Non ergo sis temerarius in dando medicinam et maxime fortem antequam sciueris dosim omnium medicinarum usualium et que fortibus et que debilibus et delicatis sunt exhibende [adhibende: Sloan]. Alioquin pacientem complexionem corrumpendo in deteriorem deduces consistenciam. Unde Ypocras: "Vita breuis, ars vero longa", et cetera': BL MS Royal 12B XXV, fols. 58r–v. Cf. Haly Abbas, *Pantegni, Theorica* i.2 'Que sciri conveniat ab introducendis', fol. 1rb; Yuhanna ibn Masawayh (Jean Mesue), *Le Livre des axiomes médicaux (Aphorismi)*, ed. and trans. D. Jacquart and G. Troupeau (Geneva, 1980), nos. 3 and 15, pp. 113 and 123; *De quindecim stellis, quidecim lapidibus, quindecim herbis et quindecim imaginibus*, in L. Delatte, *Textes latins et vieux français relatifs aux cyranides* (Liège and Paris, 1942), pp. 242–3. On *De quindecim stellis* attributed to Hermes see L. Thorndike, 'Traditional Medieval Tracts Concerning Engraved Astrological Images', in *Mélanges Auguste Pelzer* (Louvain, 1947), pp. 217–74 (224–7); Haly's discussion of medical proof in *Pantegni, Practica* ii.8 'De cognoscenda medicina per calorem', fol. 66rb–va.

assimilation and absorption of the Galenic medical corpus into Christian medieval culture. The medicine of Classical pagan Antiquity became acceptable to Christians, Muslims, and Jews not only because it was thought to work but also because its underlying theories were well adapted to those of a religious universe. Nutton shows that the essential Christian distrust of leading practitioners of Classical medicine in late Antiquity did not prevent its predominance in the Byzantine Empire and later on in the Muslim Orient and Latin Occident. Galen's world was dominated by purpose, order and organization, providing a strong argument in favour of the existence of God. Galen's view of the moral, godfearing physician operating within a divinely created universe strongly appealed to Christians. The basic canon of Galen's medical writings was theologically neutral or compatible with basic monotheistic theology while other texts (mainly philosophical) were more difficult to assimilate. Nutton examines the strategies chosen to overcome these obstacles, by straightforward adaptation to Christian purposes, or by the replacement of offending words and concepts by more neutral equivalents. He ends his broad survey of the depaganization of Galenic medicine with an account of the Renaissance legend according to which later in life Galen acquired the Christian faith.

There was the problem of medical knowledge which is incompatible with religious beliefs or practices, which had to be tackled by all those who became exposed to such knowledge. They had various options. They could censure the problematic section or even ban an entire book. They could simply ignore the problematic section and refrain from reading it. They could discuss the harmful medical opinion and either refute it, or by means of scholastic hermeneutics render it acceptable. To our knowledge it was only in Counter-Reformation Europe that there was an orchestrated effort on the part of ecclesiastical authorities to ban sections from medical books or entire books, by putting them on the indices of prohibited books. Before that period it was more a kind of self-censorship that reigned, and users of medical books merely avoided the problematic sections, or did whatever adaptation of the medical view was neccessary to make it acceptable to religious orthodoxy.

This is Danielle Jacquart's area. She looks at three *loci* in Jacques Despars' commentary on Avicenna's *Canon*, where the physician seems to be struggling with an apparent dissonance between religious dogma and medical theory, and thereby draws our attention to the range of forbidden opinions that physicians had to conceal, avoid, or explicitly reject. The first topic is how one could reconcile, on the one hand, belief in God's absolute power and, on the other hand, the medical notion that nothing, not even infinite power to renew daily the loss of life-sustaining moisture, can prevent the desiccation which leads inevitably to death. Secondly, in his *On the Usefulness of the Parts of the Body* xi.14 Galen had written about bodily hair (and in particular the enigma of the eyebrows and eyelashes which, unlike other facial hair, have a fixed length), and Despars incorporated Galen's statements into his commentary on Avicenna's discussion of the complexions of different parts of the body. The problem was that Galen had sided with Plato and other Greek philosophers in their opposition to the notion (attributed to Jewish philosophy) that God could do everything, even counter-natural things. The third theme is Despars' commentary on Avicenna's treatment of male homosexual practices and the way his analysis employed the naturalistic explanations of the phenomenon in Aristotle's (attributed) *Problems*. Self-censorship characterized Despars' writing, and Jacquart sets this against the broader background of medical themes in the propositions which were condemned in Paris in 1277. These had included in particular medical views on sexuality, on astral determinism and on the entangled relationship between physical and psychological states, and their proscription had set the limits to the free use of medical theory.

Another source of potential tension between Galenic physicians and Christian theologians was Galen's discourse about the soul. Vivian Nutton shows in his article how Galen's agnostic views on the soul were ignored by his Greek commentators, who interpreted them as applying only to the soul once it has entered the human body, not to its physical origins nor to its condition after the body's death. Michael McVaugh adds the medieval dimension to the long but successful process of depaganizing Galen and his texts. McVaugh looks closely at the particular case of Arnau de Vilanova's double career as a scholastic physician and a visionary mystic. This is a very fruitful area of research, examing the relationship between the medical and non-medical writings of physicians who were thereby engaged in 'interdisciplinary' intellectual activity. For by contextualizing medicine, it highlights the broader cultural role of medicine and medical practice and leads to further insights into medicine's extra-medical significance. Stimulated by recent research into Arnau's enigmatic behaviour, McVaugh looks at Arnau's treatment (in *Tractatus de intentione medicorum* ii.4) of Galen's alleged views that the complexion *is* the soul, tracing Arnau's sources and carefully analysing Arnau's explanation. Arnau who may have drawn some of his knowledge concerning Galen's views about the soul from Dominican theologians in Barcelona, argues that Galen cannot really have meant what he is supposed to have said. McVaugh reaches the conclusion that it is wrong to connect this defence of the Galenic notion of the soul with Arnau's therapeutic spirituality in the 1290s. The result of this reading of Arnau's medical text is a refinement of recent descriptions of the fusion between Arnau's medical and spiritual thinking. In the beginning there were two independent careers, which gradually grew towards one another in the 1290s and really fused only around 1300.

How far can one generalize about the ambiguous boundaries between medicine and theology or spiritual contemplation from the specific example of Arnau de Vilanova? Arnau has so far remained an anomalous case, and few other learned physicians played as major a religious role as he did. If it proves fruitful to look more carefully at the writings of other physicians who trod a similar path, from medicine to theology, then William Courtenay's article will have helped to signpost the route. Courtenay has compiled an updated list and a study of medical doctors (mostly from Paris in the period 1337–46) who had also studied or held degree in theology. The fact that the sequence – the logic and function of which still awaits exploration – was from medicine to theology is yet another indication of the permeable disciplinary boundaries between medicine and theology.

A meticulous analysis of north French synodal legislation is used by Kathryn Taglia to correct those historians who have stressed the oppressive nature of the regulations of midwives from the fourteenth century onwards. These regulations should be read in the context of the concern of the ecclesiastical legislators for the proper celebration of baptism and their conviction that it was their role to teach the laity in general how to baptize correctly. The ecclesiastical authorities recognized the essential role the midwives had in assisting in births according to the medical norms of the time. But at the same time they increasingly recognized that midwives played an important role in pastoral care, which had to be regulated. There is no sign in this legislation that the ecclesiastical legislators were overtly concerned about midwives as sources of witchcraft. At the same time Taglia's evidence bears incidentally but very significantly upon the very definition of the midwife. A 1311 Paris synod laid down that there should be 'skilled midwives' in all vills, while the provision (in a Meaux synodal collection of 1365) for sworn midwives in each parish, specifically 'one or two *according to the parish's population*' (our emphasis), goes even further in suggesting midwifery as something specialized.[13] More broadly Taglia's paper suggests that the study of medicine in canon law and its glosses, is a highly pertinent field of research. Themes such as abstinence and fasting,[14] clerical continence, and sexual practices in general were all controlled by ecclesiastical regulations and demanded the use of medical knowledge.

The involvement of ecclesiastical authorities in securing and providing services of public health is a well known phenomenon already in late Antiquity. Peregrine Horden has recently shown how in urban communities throughout the early Middle Ages the religious approach to public health (via rituals of prayer, penitence, processions, and invocations of saints) was blended with the material approach (via the management of drainage, water supply, sewage, overseeing of food supplies, and the provision of nursing services). In both cases the primary responsibility for regulating such

[13] These two synodal texts are given in nn. 22–3 of Taglia's paper.

[14] On medical thinking in discussions of abstinence and fasting see Arnau de Vilanova, *De esu carnium*, ed. D. M. Bazell, AVOMO XI (Barcelona, 1999) (on Carthusian vegetarianism). A starting point for the study of medical thinking and abstinence in late Antiquity can be T. M. Shaw, *The Burden of the Flesh: Fasting and Sexuality in Early Christianity* (Minneapolis, 1998), especially ch. 3, and V. E. Grimm, *From Feasting to Fasting: The Evolution of a Sin: Attitudes to Food in Late Antiquity* (London, 1996), pp. 165–6.

measures lay with bishops.[15] This 'medical pluralism' of public health surely persisted beyond the year 1000 and its full history still needs to be told. But at least one of its aspects, the history of hospitals, has benefited in recent years from the growing interest of scholars in the topic.

Carole Rawcliffe has reiterated that the cure of the souls was accorded absolute priority in medieval English hospitals and should be perceived as their *raison d'être*.[16] Three chapters in this collection add further insights to the spiritual dimension of hospitals' activity and role in the medieval Latin West. Jessalynn Bird's contributions to the history of medieval hospitals add a comparative dimension to Rawcliffe's account. By looking at Jacques de Vitry's sermons to the personnel and patients of hospitals and *leprosaria*, and at his description of hospitals in his *Historia occidentalis*, she highlights the institution of the hospital and hospitallers in the late twelfth and early thirteenth centuries as agents for the supply of charity where lay and religious interests mingled. She provides the cultural and ecclesiastical contextualization of the hospitals in northern France and the Low Countries and maps the social role of hospitals and *leprosaria*, their patients and personnel. In another chapter, and in line with this series' established tradition of producing editions and translations of key texts, Bird provides an annotated translation of the most important thirteenth-century description of hospitals, chapter 29 of Jacques de Vitry's *Historia occidentalis* ('On the hospitals of the poor and leper houses'), and she also provides an edition of his sermons to those who worked in hospitals.

In both chapters the tight relationship of spiritual and temporal, body and soul, is apparent. In thirteenth-century continental hospitals the first line of treatment for bodily illness was reconciliation with God and spiritual healing. But, Bird points out, these hospitals did not shun recourse to physical or material medicine, glimpses of which can be seen through Jacques' sermons. Hospital personnel go round clearing away dirt and keeping the beds clean. 'In some places', where this is not done, 'more die through stench and the corruption of the air than through their bodies' illness.' While going around the beds, hospital personnel ask the ill what they want to eat and drink, thereby allowing some who 'labour with an acute fever or some hot illness to ask for meat and wine'. Bad practice is being criticized – 'more die from contrary foods than from their illness' – and according to Jacques this is as bad as enabling suicide by giving a sword to a frenetic.[17]

Peregrine Horden ventures into an extraordinary, exciting, and hitherto

[15] P. Horden, 'Ritual and Public Health in the Early Medieval City', in *Body and City: Histories of Urban Public Health*, ed. S. Power and H. Sheard (London, 2000), pp. 17–40; P. Squatriti, *Water and Society in Early Medieval Italy, AD 400–1000* (Cambridge, 1998), pp. 12–17 and 46–7.

[16] Rawcliffe, 'Medicine for the Soul', and *Medicine for the Soul*, esp. pp. 102–3, 131. Some important case histories of medieval therapeutics which highlight the religious context of medieval hospitals are in Risse, *Mending Bodies*, pp. 69–229.

[17] Chs. 7–8 below, pp. 91–134.

unstudied domain, namely the use of religious chant as part of the therapeutic process in the medieval hospital. Once again there is the ambiguity mentioned above: religion can be perceived as medicinal. This study opens up a new domain of research, the intertwining of medicine and liturgy. For example, monastic liturgical texts include information about both the proper days for phlebotomy and also the actual carrying out of the treatment. Although systematic enquiry will be needed into all monastic liturgical manuscripts, it is already clear that blood-letting was tightly connected with the liturgical activity of a monastery.

Lack of religious orthodoxy and medicine have been often depicted as sisters. Vivian Nutton mentions the medieval view that atheism and medicine go hand in hand, while Danielle Jacquart parades for view a variety of medical opinions which could be branded heretical if not adapted. Did the materialism and often the determinism involved in medical theory make physicians more sceptical than others about the Christian interpretation of life and death or, in other words, did the story of Christ incline them to indifference? Or were physicians really prone to heresy, in other words to an unorthodox but enthusiastic Christianity? These questions, insofar as they relate to the realm of learned, academic heresy, await their separate answers. Here, however, we include a study which makes a step towards the reconstruction of the medical world of not-so-learned heretics, the thirteenth-century Cathars and Waldensians of southern France. Peter Biller presents new data extracted from inquisitors' records which show, first of all, the dense provision of medical care in the rural communities of Languedoc. The strong presence of female medical practitioners substantiates Monica Green's hypothesis that female medical practitioners were more numerous than shown in the conventional biographical dictionaries, which use sources that tend to conceal women and emphasize elite practitioners. Both Cathar and Waldensian preachers supplied medical aid, and its character seems conventional, but thereafter there were significant differences. For the Waldensians this task was intrinsic to their original ideal, literal obedience to evangelical counsels which were taken as precepts and included the injunction 'Heal the sick', whereas with the Cathars it was incidental, brought about by the accident of Cathar recruitment among people who were trained and included lawyers and medics. A notable area of medical practice among the Cathars was phlebotomy, which acquired a ceremonial role and may have been used to curb and avoid sexual desire and sin. This suggests comparison with phlebotomy in the Church's monasteries. Depositions in front of inquisitors come tantalizingly close to affording windows into the souls of a few practising medieval physicians and barbers. Cathar dualist theology suggests areas of tension with medical practice, one of which is gendered. Bearing in mind that Waldensian clients came fairly near to an even sex ratio, the smaller proportion of female clients among Cathars may be related to a reluctance among Cathar practitioners to touch female patients: the body was abhorrent, created by an evil principle, and female bodies bore the brunt of this abhorrence. Radical abhorrence of the material world and a desire to accelerate escape from it may have led to an even darker area, tension with the medical aspiration to preserve life.

The last section of this book presents two essays which explore the intricate question of the mutual relationship between physicians and theologians when writing about the same topics or discussing matters of common interest. Maaike van der Lugt traces in her article the debate about the *incubus* from late Antiquity to the Renaissance. She uncovers two separate traditions of explanation to the phenomenon: the physiological explanation that was expounded by physicians and dream theorists (a bad dream which creates the sensation of nocturnal suffocation), and the alternative explanation that was upheld by the laity and the clerical authorities (the nocturnal suffocation is caused by a demon or another evil being which attacks people during sleep). Both traditions were aware of each other's existence. They were neither static nor monolithic and each developed a variety of nuances, however they never fused into a single explanation. Van der Lugt shows how belief in sexual demons infiltrated learned physicians' accounts of *incubus* in the fifteenth century, but she stresses that despite some concessions to theologians and popular beliefs, they continued to privilege their own naturalistic explanations.

Joseph Ziegler explores theological explanations of Adam's immortality in the State of Innocence. Mainly on the basis of commentaries on Peter the Lombard's *Sentences,* he shows how medical concepts and theories infiltrated theological debate from the twelfth century onwards. This intensified in the mid-thirteenth century. Theologians were aware of current medical ideas, terms and books, and did not hesitate to use them. Their discussions became dominated by the themes and vocabulary of the radical and nutrimental moistures and the *complexio equalis*. Sometimes, in order to incorporate the medical concept into their explanation, they had to alter the definition of the medical concept or openly to argue with the medical explanation. The theological explanation of Adam's immortality was not overturned, but its style and shape underwent a sea-change as the miraculous receded and gave a large place to absolutely up-to-date medical theory. The book begins with the depaganization of Galen and Classical medicine, and it concludes here, with the most dramatic demonstration of its theme, in this marriage of Theology and Medicine in the terrestrial paradise.

The 1999 York Quodlibet Lecture

God, Galen and the Depaganization of Ancient Medicine

Vivian Nutton

In the middle years of the fourth century, around 350, a young man from a wealthy Christian family travelled to Alexandria to study medicine at what his brother called the 'factory of universal learning both in reputation and in reality'.[1] Caesarius proved to be a brilliant student, and a faithful Christian. He picked out what was valuable in geometry and astronomy, a branch of learning dangerous to others: from the order and harmony of the heavens he came to admire the Creator's handiwork. In the marvellous art of medicine his understanding of natures, temperaments and the first principles of diseases by which to exterminate illness, root and branch, was second to none. Above all, he avoided the dangers that had entrapped others. He did not consort with the wicked (i.e. pagans), and he refused to attribute to the motion of the stars all being and becoming, thereby setting up creation in opposition to its Creator.[2] His own moderation proved that he had no need to take the Hippocratic Oath in order to act properly, and his career flourished at court and within the imperial administration.[3] Caesarius is held up by his brother as the very model of a Christian in a profession that was largely pagan, and in which the speculative philosophy of Galen, Hippocrates, and their opponents carried dangers for those less committed to Christianity.[4] Nine hundred years later, a former professor of medicine was elected Pope. Peter of Spain, whose medical lectures at the University of Siena had indeed touched on the philosophy of Galen and Hippocrates, became Pope John

[1] Gregory of Nazianzus, *On the death of his brother Caesarius, Orations* vii.6–7; *PG* 35, 761–2.

[2] Doctors needed a knowledge of astronomy for their practice, but a Christian doctor would reject the firm predictions of the astrologers in favour of a stochastic prediction of the uncertain future: Gregory of Nyssa, *Contra Fatum*, ed. J. A. McDonough (Leiden, 1987), pp. 49–50; *PG* 45, 164.

[3] For the Oath, Gregory, *Orations* vii.10 (*PG* 35, 767), a comment made *en passant* when describing Caesarius's career in Constantinople and hence not necessarily related solely to that period. Some pagan medical students may well have taken the Oath at Alexandria, and Gregory clearly sees it as a mark of the medical profession, but the casual way in which he refers to it here shows that it was not compulsory.

[4] Cf. Gregory, *Orations* vii.20 (*PG* 35, 783). 'Philosophizing' is an ambiguous term, and Gregory sees the creation of a truly Christian philosophy as very difficult.

XXI.[5] The same transition can be neatly illustrated by juxtaposing two monuments. The first is the tombstone of Fadianus Bubbal of the third or fourth century. Fadianus, a local doctor from Cherchel in modern-day Morocco, is depicted with his book and his surgical knife beneath the pagan symbol of the moon.[6] The second is a fresco in the crypt of the cathedral of Anagni in southern Italy, painted around 1250–5.[7] It shows the two most famous doctors of Antiquity, Hippocrates on the right and Galen on the left, conversing together. Their presence here is explained by the proofs they offer of God's creation, of the Christian universe made up of elements.[8] They are virtuous pagans, and, indeed, as we shall see, Galen on some accounts even becomes a Christian. A pagan medicine becomes depaganized.

How this transformation takes place is the theme of this paper. In particular, I want to look at the ways in which the medicine of Classical pagan Antiquity was made acceptable to Christians, Muslims, and Jews to become the formal medicine of the later Middle Ages, and even beyond. For although the discoveries of the sixteenth and seventeenth centuries effectively supplanted ancient ideas on anatomy and physiology, clinical medical teaching in Europe continued to make use of ancient Greek medical texts well into the nineteenth century.[9] In the Muslim world, and among immigrant communities in this country and France, for example, the system of *yunani*, that is Greek, medicine still flourishes in the form given it by the great medieval Muslim physician Ibn Sina (Avicenna).

This is not a simple story of a struggle between science and religion,

[5] Basic details in J. N. D. Kelly, *The Oxford Dictionary of Popes* (Oxford, 1988), pp. 200–1, to which add F. Salmón, *Medical Classroom Practice: Petrus Hispanus' Questions on* Isagoge, Tegni, Regimen Acutorum *and* Prognostica *(c. 1245–50)*, Articella Studies 4 (Cambridge, 1998).

[6] A. Hillert, *Antike Ärztedarstellungen*, Marburger Schriften zur Medizingeschichte 25 (Frankfurt, 1990), pp. 151–2, and pl. 32.

[7] A good photograph in *Les textes médicaux grecs: Tradition et ecdotique*, ed. A. Garzya and J. Jouanna (Naples, 1999), frontispiece. The dating and the whole series of frescos are discussed by M. Q. Smith, 'Anagni: An Example of Medieval Typological Decoration', *Papers of the British School at Rome* 33 (1965), 1–47, and L. Pressouyre, 'Le cosmos platonicien de la Cathédrale d'Anagni', *Mélanges d'Archéologie et d'Histoire* 78 (1966), 551–93.

[8] Galen's open book reads: 'Mundi presentis series manet ex elementis'; that of Hippocrates: 'Ex his formantur quae sunt quaecumque chreantur'. The source, if there is one, is a medieval cosmological poem in hexameters. A link with contemporary science and philosophy in southern Italy is clear. Less so is any connection with Byzantine frescos showing Galen and Hippocrates among the heralds of Christianity like Homer and Plato, see G. Nandris, *Christian Humanism in the Neo-Byzantine Mural Painting of Eastern Europe* (Wiesbaden, 1970), pp. 24–44; M. D. Taylor, 'A Historiated Tree of Jesse', *Dumbarton Oaks Papers* 34–5 (1980–1), 125–76; I. Duichev, *Antike heidnische Dichter und Denker in der alten bulgarischen Malerei* (Sofia, 1978), pp. 90–1, 118–19.

[9] Temkin, *Galenism*. Valuable information on nineteenth-century Hippocratism is given by *Médecins érudits de Coray à Sigerist*, Actes du colloque de Saint-Jullien en Beaujolais (Juin 1994), ed. D. Gourevitch (Paris, 1995).

between pagan believers in rational medicine, and Christians who preferred to leave it all in the hands of God, for there were pagans too who believed that the healing power of a deity was a safer, more effective, and certainly less expensive remedy than the intervention of a doctor.[10] Besides, those who trusted only in a medicine of faith, as laid down by the Epistle of St James 5. 14–16, were always a minority. Most Christians recognized the difficulty of a medicine whose success depended on one's being in love and charity with one's neighbours. That, wrote Bishop Diadochus, might be all well and good for a hermit in the middle of the desert; it was well nigh impossible in a monastic cloister.[11]

Nor is the story of the take-over by the later Middle Ages of Galenic-Hippocratic medicine a story of the triumph of scientific truth over religious obscurantism. Hippocrates was no Copernicus, Galen no Galileo. The effectiveness of Galenic-Hippocratic therapeutics compared with that of its rivals was hotly disputed in the Classical world. Galen himself lamented on more than one occasion that the writings of Hippocrates were studied by only a handful of Greek doctors, and he felt himself to be very much in the minority.[12] Until the eleventh century, the learned doctors of latin Europe knew little or nothing of Galenic or Hippocratic medicine; the most popular works among the Carolingians represented a much more practical, non-theoretical type of medicine, that derived from a different, and arguably more effective tradition, that of the so-called Methodical physicians.[13] Galenic medicine was far from being the obvious choice it might seem to us, and its eventual triumph owed not a little to its compatibility with Christian, Muslim, and Jewish theology. It succeeded, not only because its remedies were thought to work, but also because its underlying theories could be adapted better to those of a religious universe. The process of depaganization brought benefits to both Galenists and Christians.

There is an irony in this, for Galen himself was scathing about the intellectual failings of the Christians. He was familiar with some Christians of his own day and he was interested in Judaism and Christianity as types of saintly Stoicism. He approved of their highly moral conduct, but derided their views on miracle as logically deficient.[14] Christian writers of the early Middle Ages held similarly robust views about medicine. The average

[10] *Inscriptiones Graecae* (Berlin, 1873–), V.1.1119, p. 206. Cf. O. Weinreich, *Antike Heilungswunder: Untersuchungen zum Wunderglauben der Griechen und Römer* (Giessen, 1909).

[11] Diadochus, *Oeuvres spirituelles*, ed. and trans. E. des Places, Sources Chrétiennes 5 (Paris, 1955), p. 115.

[12] Galen, *De optimo medico cognoscendo. On Examinations by which the Best Physicians are Recognized*, ed. A. Z. Iskandar, Corpus Medicorum Graecorum, Supplementum Orientale 4 (Berlin, 1988), p. 69.

[13] A. Beccaria, *I codici di medicina del periodo presalernitano*, Storia e Letteratura 53 (Rome, 1956).

[14] Walzer, *Galen on Jews and Christians*; S. Gero, 'Galen on the Christians: A Reappraisal of the Arabic Evidence', *Orientalia Christiana* 56 (1990), 371–411.

doctor and all that he stands for is a stock opponent in a variety of lives of the saints. Medical forecasts are shown up as frivolous, human endeavours as fruitless, the pain and torture of an operation as unnecessary if one believes sufficiently strongly in God and his saints. Whether we look at hagiography from a Latin, Byzantine, or Near Eastern perspective, the pattern is the same; the doctor is at best an ambiguous figure, capable of bringing help and succour to the sick, but, at the same time, over-confident, over-charging, and reluctant to accept Christian truth unless it was forced on him.[15] Anecdotes from historians describe doctors slipping away to pay sacrifice to Asclepius, and ever determined to pursue the old ways.[16] No wonder that at the Syrian town of Nisibis in the late sixth century, students of theology at the famous school were forbidden to associate with doctors, for fear that the Children of Light would be contaminated by contact with the children of this world – and, one might suspect, give up theology for the more lucrative practice of medicine, a concern that resurfaces regularly in Church canons of both East and West.[17]

Besides, no one could deny that pagan medicine had been visibly successful, and continued to be so well into the fifth century. The magnificent buildings of the great shrine of Asclepius at Pergamum, erected around 140 with imperial support, or the great temples of Sarapis at Alexandria and Memphis in Egypt, gave proof of that success, and archaeologists have shown that in many instances this prosperity continued well down into the fourth or fifth century. The little shrine of Nodens near Lydney in Gloucestershire enjoyed its best days and was refurbished in the mid fourth century, although evidence for its continuation into the next century is much slimmer than was once thought.[18]

A Christian assault on pagan healing took a variety of forms, not least violence. A pitched battle was fought at Alexandria before the temple of Sarapis was destroyed,[19] and the remarkable lack of cult objects found among the excavations of the Asclepieia at Pergamum and Epidaurus suggests that destruction here was carefully targeted and extremely thorough. Elsewhere,

[15] P. Horden, *Saints and Doctors in the Early Byzantine Empire: The Case of Theodore of Sykeon*, SCH 19 (1982), pp. 1–13, gives a more sober view than H. J. Magoulias, 'The Lives of the Saints as Sources of Data for the History of Byzantine Medicine in the Sixth and Seventh Centuries', *Byzantinische Zeitschrift* 57 (1954), 127–50, who is unreliable but adds further details. A comparative study of hagiographical views of medicine along the lines pioneered by C. Stancliffe, *St Martin and his Hagiographer: History and Miracle in Sulpicius Severus* (Oxford, 1983), is a desideratum.

[16] A. Moffatt, 'Science Teachers in the Early Byzantine Empire: Some Statistics', *Byzantinoslavica* 24 (1973), 15–18.

[17] A. Vööbus, *The Statutes of the School of Nisibis*, Eesti Usuteadlaste Selts Paguleses 12 (Stockholm, 1963), Statutes of Henana 19–20, pp. 100–1. For later Western canons, Amundsen, *Medicine, Society and Faith*, pp. 227–35.

[18] P. J. Casey and B. Hoffmann, 'Excavations at the Roman Temple in Lydney Park, Gloucestershire, in 1980 and 1981', *The Antiquaries Journal* 79 (1999), 81–144.

[19] Sozomen, *Historia ecclesiastica* vii.15; pp. 319–20.

there was direct competition: St Cyrus and St John, two healing saints who gave their services for free, set up their surgery deliberately across the road from the healing shrine of Isis at Menuthis (Aboukir in Egypt) in order to attract away those who might be tempted to seek healing from pagan gods.[20] There were also takeovers of sites, although whether a Christian church arose immediately on top of a destroyed pagan healing shrine or only some time later is a matter for some controversy. There is certainly an early church built in the remains of the Asclepieion of Epidaurus perhaps in the fourth or early fifth century.[21] Nor can it be simple coincidence that one of a complex of legends about the holy healers Cosmas and Damian locates them at Aegae in southern Turkey, site of one of the most famous shrines of Asclepius.[22] The healing spring of the Asclepieion of Rome became in time the font for the church of St Bartolommeo, while a hospital has occupied the rest of the Tiber island since the eleventh century, if not before.[23] Besides, if the pagan healing gods were displaced, many of the rituals and beliefs of pagan healing continued almost unchanged. As Ramsey Macmullen has noted, incubation rites are transferred to Christian saints, and many of the practices associated with pagan healings are still recorded in substantial numbers well into the Middle Ages, if not until today – binding of threads around candles, eating of dust from around the altar or tomb, placing of a sacred book or object on the affected part, chants, charms, phylacteries, and so on.[24] But these practices, while part of medicine and healing, occupy an ambiguous position both in medical and in religious terms. For every Bishop Victricius of Rouen, rejoicing in the healing powers of relics, we can call on a St Augustine, disquieted at his flock's adherence to their old ways even in a Christian context.[25] Likewise in medicine, Galen and Caelius Aurelianus generally frown on doctors who use such practices, whereas a leading Greek physician of the sixth century, Alexander of Tralles, is quite prepared to record chants and charms, alongside his more orthodox remedies.[26] Alexander, brother of

20 R. Herzog, 'Der Kampf um der Kult von Menuthis', in *Pisciculi. Studien zur Religion und Kultur des Altertums: Franz Joseph Dölger zum sechzigsten Geburtstage dargeboten von Freunden, Vererhren und Schülern*, ed. T. Klauser and A. Rücker, Antike und Christentum: kultur- und religionsgeschichtliche Studien, Ergänzungsband 1 (Münster, 1939), pp. 117–24.

21 F. Robert, *Epidaure* (Paris, 1935), p. 41.

22 L. Robert, 'De Cilicie à Messine et à Plymouth, avec deux inscriptions grecques errantes', *Journal des Savants* (1973), 161–211; M. Van Esbroeck, 'La Diffusion orientale de la légende orientale des saints Cosme et Damien', in *Hagiographie, cultures et sociétés, IVe–XIIe siècles*, ed. E. Patlagean and P. Riché, Etudes Augustiniennes (Paris, 1981), 61–77; R. Ziegler, 'Aigeai, der Asklepioskult, das Kaiserhaus der Decier und das Christentum', *Tyche* 9 (1994), 187–212.

23 M. Besnier, *L'Île Tibérine dans l'Antiquité* (Paris, 1902), pp. 184–246.

24 R. MacMullen, *Christianizing the Roman Empire (A.D. 100–400)* (New Haven, 1985); *Christianity and Paganism in the Fourth to Eighth Centuries* (New Haven, 1997) .

25 Victricius of Rouen, *De laude sanctorum*, ed. R. Demeulenaere, CCSL 64 (1985); MacMullen, *Christianity and Paganism, passim*.

26 V. Nutton, 'From Medical Certainty to Medical Amulets: Three Aspects of Ancient

the architect of Santa Sophia, and of Justinian's favourite lawyer, also claims that he would have liked to have mentioned many more, had not circumstances been against him – a polite reference to Christianity.

An ambiguity towards pagan medicine at a popular level contributes to a certain suspicion of doctors at a higher level. As Valerie Flint has put it, they occupy a position in healing midway between the saint and the sorcerer, never clearly demarcated from either.[27] Her evidence comes largely from the early Latin West, from Gregory of Tours for example, but it can be extended both in space and in time. Arnobius of Sicca at the end of the third century might boast that even doctors were now turning to Christianity, but in the East, doctors in local elites, professors at Alexandria, and even court physicians are frequently and overtly pagan in sympathy well into the sixth century.[28] Asclepiodotus of Aphrodisias around 480 had visited the country of the magi and practised astrology and theurgy to go with his knowledge of plants and herbs.[29] His contemporary, the doctor, Eusebius of Emesa, had travelled to find the remains of a fallen star, a meteorite, which he affixed to the wall of a temple: the stone spoke, and Eusebius began a second career as its interpreter.[30] Most striking is the story of the Alexandrian professor Gesius, an honoured friend of Byzantine emperors in the early sixth century. He was baptized a Christian, but his sympathies were with the old gods – both his friends and his enemies agree in this. He protected Heraiscus the philosopher from the wrath of the emperor Zeno when he opposed a Christian takeover of the shrine at Menuthis, and gave him an appropriate burial. A little later, Gesius himself fell ill, punished, it was alleged, for his impiety in explaining Christian miracle cures at the shrine in purely secular terms: this was the treatment of Hippocrates, this of Galen, and so on. Only when Gesius had made a contrite confession to St Cyrus and St John did he recover his health, proof of the superiority of the saints over human healers.[31]

In the face of such Christian distrust of leading practitioners of Galenic medicine, one might wonder how this medicine ever came to predominate in the Byzantine Empire and, afterwards, in the Muslim world and that of the later Western Middle Ages.

The key lies in the career and influence of Galen of Pergamum, who lived

Therapeutics', in *Essays in the History of Therapeutics*, ed. W. F. Bynum and V. Nutton, Clio Medica 22 (Amsterdam, 1991), pp. 3–12.

27 V. J. Flint, 'The Early Medieval "Medicus", the Saint – and the Enchanter', *SHM* 2 (1989), 127–45; *The Rise of Magic in Early Medieval Europe* (Oxford, 1991).

28 Arnobius, *Adversus Gentes* ii.5; *PL* 5, 816–18.

29 Suidas, *Lexikon*, s.v. *Asclepiodotos*, ed. A. Adler, 5 vols., Teubner edn (Leipzig, 1928–38), I, 383–4, no. 4174; Photius, *Bibliotheca*, 344b, ed. R. Henry, 8 vols., Association Guillaume Budé, Collection Byzantine (Paris, 1959–77), VI, 33–5.

30 Photius, *Bibliotheca*, 348b, ed. Henry, VI, 43–5.

31 Suidas, *Lexikon*, s.v. *Gesios*, ed. Adler, I, 520–2, no. 207; Sophronius, *Miracula sanctorum Cyri et Johannis* 30, *PG* 87.3, 3513–20.

from 129 to 216 or 217. He was a prolific polymath, writing on subjects as varied as cancer and the anatomy of the brain, or logic and lexicography. For almost seventy years, he wrote on average two-three pages at least every day, in addition to a busy and varied clinical practice. The range of his learning is truly amazing, even if we allow for the fact that, as the son of a millionaire, he had an enormous private library. But his learning was also allied to a considerable range of empirical skills: he was highly dextrous with his hands, witness his complex anatomical experiments on the brains of sheep, pigs, goats, and monkeys; he experimented with a variety of pharmaceutical preparations; he was an expert on diagnosis, not least of stress diseases. One could go on, but five points are directly relevant to his later success.[32]

First, in later Antiquity, in an age when facilities were beoming fewer, when books were scarcer, and when intellectual institutions of quality, especially in medicine, shrank to a mere handful, Galen's achievement appeared miraculous and unsurpassable. He had both preached and practised a unified medicine that, so a sixth century commentator lamented, could no longer be achieved in a poorer world.[33]

Secondly, he was a brilliant speaker and advocate; where his logic failed to point out the weakness in an opponent's case, and that was rare, his urgent rhetoric could convince his readers that his was the only true explanation.

Thirdly, he emphasized again and again the need for the doctor to understand and use philosophy. One of his treatises bears the title 'The best doctor is also a philosopher', arguing that a successful medical career can be achieved only by a man who puts into practice the philosophical virtues of temperance, courage, wisdom, and the like; whether he knows that that is what he is doing is immaterial. Philosophy, and especially moral philosophy, was always of interest to Galen, and he wrote on such topics as the avoidance of grief or good and bad habits. Mental health, in his view, contributed to physical health, and vice-versa.[34]

Fourthly, the universe in which he placed his medicine was that of Plato and Aristotle. If his human anatomy and physiology depended largely on Plato and, for its activation, on Plato's tripartite soul, his physical world was that of Aristotle, the world of the four elements, the four qualities, and the whole schema of Aristotelian physics. It was a world dominated by purpose, by teleology; nature, or the divine creator, had created nothing in vain, and

[32] Useful short summaries of Galen's life and career are in Temkin, *Galenism*, chs. 1 and 2; V. Nutton, in *The Western Medical Tradition, 800 BC to AD 1800*, ed. L. I. Conrad, M. Neve, V. Nutton, R. Porter, A. Wear (Cambridge, 1995), pp. 58–70; P. N. Singer, *Galen: Selected Works* (Oxford, 1997), pp. vii–xlii.

[33] Palladius, *In Hippocratis Epidemiarum librum VI commentarius*, in *Scholia in Hippocratem et Galenum*, ed. F. R. Dietz, 2 vols. (Königsberg, 1834), II, 157.

[34] In addition to the works cited above, n. 32, see M. Zonta, *Un interprete ebreo della filosofia di Galeno: gli scritti filosofici di Galeno nell'opera di Shem Tob ibn Falaquera*, Eurasiatica (Turin, 1995).

the very order and organisation of the universe was a strong argument in favour of the existence of God.[35]

Finally, and most convincing of all, Galen's own theology, his strong belief in the existence of God or gods, made for at least a qualified acceptance. Of the existence of God or gods, whatever they might be, Galen was certain on two grounds. The first, already mentioned, is the purposefulness he saw within the human body and throughout the universe: macrocosm and microcosm matched perfectly to show a divine foresight, a divine care, a divine *pronoia*. The notion of the Epicureans or the methodical physicians that the world was a mere chance assemblage of atoms he rejected as vigorously as any theologian in Reformation and Counter-Reformation Europe, where this bogey surfaced again.[36] The final book of his great interpretative tract on anatomy, *On the usefulness of the parts of the body*, is a hymn, an epode he called it, to the wisdom and forethought of the Creator or Nature. The leg of a flea or the trunk of an elephant, perfectly adapted to their purposes, display the wisdom and power of the Creator: 'Who could be so stupid or so hostile and antagonistic to the works of Nature, as not to recognise at once, from the skin of one's hands first of all, the skillful handiwork of the Creator?'[37]

Allied to this was the conviction that divine intervention in this world was possible, indeed certain. God or the gods are not remote beings, always out there beyond the firmament. Asclepius had protected Galen and others from illness and shipwreck; the god had even sent advice to Galen in a dream on how to cure his own medical problems, and those of others.[38] This divine intervention differs, however, from Christian and Jewish miracle in one important, and for Galen crucial, way: the god works within his own creation, he obeys his own rules, and his cures, we might say, are scientifically explicable.[39]

All this helps to explain why Galen's medical ideas triumphed, and along with them those of Hippocrates, for Galen claimed always to be the most faithful and scrupulous interpreter of Hippocrates, and the Middle Ages did not disagree.[40] One can see also how his view of the moral, godfearing physician operating within a divinely created universe would appeal to Christians, Jews, and Muslims alike. No wonder that the Byzantine author of the life of the St Procopius, writing around 890, could include Galen among the 'philosophers of the cosmos' whose arguments proved the truth of

35 R. J. Hankinson, 'Galen and the Best of All Possible Worlds', *Classical Quarterly* 39 (1989), 206–27.

36 V. Nutton, 'Wittenberg Anatomy', in *Medicine and the Reformation*, ed. O. P. Grell and A. Cunningham, The Wellcome Institute Series in the History of Medicine (London, 1993), pp. 11–32 (pp. 20 and 25).

37 Galen, *Usefulness of the Parts of the Body*, II, 724–33; translation adapted from p. 729.

38 Galen, *De propriis placitis. On my Own Opinions* ii.1–3, ed. and trans. V. Nutton, Corpus medicorum Graecorum V.3.2 (Berlin, 1999), with the commentary ad loc., pp. 134–40.

39 Walzer, *Galen on Jews and Christians*, pp. 23–37.

40 Temkin, *Hippocrates*, pp. 47–50.

Christianity.[41] Their message, claims the hagiographer, was one and unequivocal. By contrast with the God who made the heavens, all other gods had been created by men, or had been simply called gods; they were thus inevitably doomed to destruction and decay.

Leaving aside the strange company in which Galen here finds himself, next to Plato, Aristotle, Socrates, Homer, Hermes Trismegistus and the mysterious Scamander, the hagiographer's exposition runs up against one major obstacle. Galen was a pagan, an active worshipper of Asclepius (the Greek word for worshipper, *therapeutes*, indicates, in the context in which Galen uses it, that he was more than merely a passive spectator, more than just the man in the pew), and Asclepius was one of the most celebrated examples of a human, or half-human, turned god.[42] Pagan phrases are found throughout the Galenic Corpus. Most difficult of all for the would-be Christianizer of Galen, Galen specifically attacked Christianity in several places, and his detailed views on God and creation, and his agnosticism about the nature and immortality of the soul, were at variance with Christian teaching.[43]

How best to reconcile Galen with monotheism, to smooth over the divergencies, was not easy.

The first attempt, made even in Galen's own lifetime, was a notorious failure. According to the church historian Eusebius, a group of Christians, led by an immigrant to Rome called Theodotus the shoemaker, tried to correct their Christianity in accordance with Galen's criticisms.[44] Whether it was their logic or their understanding of the words of the Bible that required correction is not clear, but they were swiftly denounced, and their heresy seems to have disappeared quickly. Their adoration of Galen (I use Eusebius's word) was misplaced.

The process of reconciliation was, however, favoured by Galen's own logorrhea, his unsurpassed productivity, which enforced on his followers the necessity to select, to precis, or to abridge his writings in order to bring them into a manageable, and affordable, compass. By 500, at the very latest, a selection of his writings, the so-called 'Twenty Books', had formed a medical canon that was being studied widely, at Alexandria, and, by the mid-sixth century, in Latin at Ravenna in Italy and in Syriac in the Christian Near East.[45]

41 H. Delehaye, *Les légendes grecques des saints militaires* (Paris, 1909), p. 219.

42 F. Kudlien, 'Galen's Religious Beliefs', in *Galen: Problems*, pp. 117–27, but with a less precise interpretation of 'therapeutes' as simply meaning 'worshipper'.

43 For his attack on Christianity, see Walzer, *Galen on Jews and Christians*, and for his agnosticism, Galen, *On my Own Opinions, passim.*

44 Eusebius, *Historia ecclesiastica* V.xxviii.14, ed. E. Schwartz (Leipzig, 1908), p. 217. Walzer, *Galen on Jews and Christians*, pp. 76–7, argues for a philosophical reworking of Christianity; H. Schöne, 'Ein Einbruch der antiken Logik und Textkritik in die altchristliche Theologie', in *Pisciculi*, ed. Klauser and Rücker, pp. 252–66, less plausibly raises the possibility that Theodotus adopted Galen's methods of textual exegesis. See also Gero, 'Galen on Christians'.

45 The oriental canon is conveniently listed by Lieber, 'Galen in Hebrew', p. 173. The Latin commentaries are discussed by I. Mazzini and N. Palmieri. 'L'École médicale

The books that formed this syllabus were, on the whole, brief, terse, and severely practical; philosophical and moral musings were largely absent from them, individual incidents and elegant stories were infrequent. This was Galen the basic doctor, and as such, this syllabus formed the groundwork of all subsequent learned medicine in Byzantium, and in the Near East. Theologically, it was uncontroversial, and one can imagine that when a biographer of St Cosmas and St Damian referred to them as having learned thoroughly the works of Hippocrates and Galen he saw no problem in this, any more than Cassiodorus in the Latin West had in recommending for his monastery at Vivarium a different, but still more basic, series of medical writings associated with the names of earlier doctors.[46]

But Galen is a seductive author; he encourages you always to investigate further, to move from the purely practical and descriptive to an understanding of why and how things work, to theory and to philosophy. He repeats, again and again, that some of his texts are merely for beginners, and that for detailed understanding one must seek elsewhere in his writings. If the basic canon of his writings was theologically neutral, other texts by him and by his master Hippocrates were more difficult to assimilate.

Two strategies were followed. The first, and least common, was a straightforward adaptation to Christian purposes. Here the best example is the fate of the Hippocratic Oath, which begins with an invocation to 'Apollo, Asclepius, Hygieia, Panacea, and all the other gods and goddesses my witnesses', hardly the oath of a pious Christian. One solution, particularly in the early medieval West, was to combine sentences of the Oath with a variety of more specifically Christian obligations, emphasizing love and charity.[47] But in the Greek and Muslim worlds the offensively pagan opening was simply replaced by another suitable formula. To emphasize the religious element still further, in three manuscripts of the Oath, the words are written out in the form of the cross.[48]

de Ravenne', in *Les Écoles médicales à Rome*, ed. P. Mudry and J. Pigeaud (Geneva, 1991), pp. 285–310. For Greek summaries, B. Gundert, 'Die Tabulae Vindobonenses als Zeugnis alexandrinischer Lehrtätigkeit um 600 n. Chr.', in *Text and Tradition*, pp. 91–144. For the Syriac, H. Hugonnard-Roche, 'Note sur Sergius de Res'aina, traducteur du grec en syriaque et commentateur d'Aristote', in *The Ancient Tradition in Christian and Islamic Hellenism: Studies on the Transmission of Greek Philosophy and Sciences Dedicated to H.J. Drossaert Lulofs*, ed. G. Endress and R. Kruk, CNWS Publications 50 (Leiden, 1997), pp. 121–43.

[46] 'Vita sanctorum Cosmae et Damiani', *Analecta Bollandiana* 1 (1882), 589–90; cf. G. Rupprecht, *Cosmae et Damiani Vita et Miracula* (Berlin, 1935); Cassiodorus, *Institutes* I.xxxi.2; ed. R. A. B. Mynors (Oxford, 1937), pp. 78–9.

[47] L. C. MacKinney, 'Medical Ethics and Etiquette in the Early Middle Ages: The Persistence of Hippocratic Ideals', *BHM* 26 (1952), 1–31; L. Firpo, *Medicina medievale* (Turin, 1972), pp. 36–48.

[48] W. H. S. Jones, *The Doctor's Oath* (Cambridge, 1924); T. Rütten, 'Retextuirungen des Hippokratischen Eides im Vorfeld seiner Editio Princeps unter dem Einfluss seiner Christianisierungs-geschichte', in *Les textes médicaux grecs*, ed. Garzya and Jouanna, pp. 509–33 (p. 517).

Such adaptation was, however, rare. A second solution, favoured especially by the translators into Syriac and Arabic, was the replacement of offending words by more neutral equivalents. While the Creator can remain, lesser gods are transformed into spirits or angels, and Galen's devotion to Asclepius becomes piety towards God or adherence to a leader or exemplar. This strategy, however, fails when faced with the task of translating Galen's commentary on the Hippocratic Oath, which contains a major discussion on the role of pagan gods as founders and inspirers of medicine. Here the Christian Arabic translator of the ninth century, Hunayn ibn Ishaq (Johannitius), not only modifies Galen's phrasing: sacrifices are offered to God *in the name of* Asclepius; medical cures are attributed *to God through* Sarapis and Asclepius, but he also provides his own commentary, explaining the deification of Asclepius in terms of the assimilation of Asclepius's rational soul to the divine, which adorned it with all the virtues.[49] In so doing, and in part by treating Galen's gods as historical personages, Hunayn makes Galen's comment acceptable to Christians and Muslims. The commentary on the Hippocratic Oath thus becomes a piece of antiquarian scholarship, rather than the personal testament that Galen had envisaged.

But one difficulty still remains; translation can reduce the overt signs of Galen's paganism, but it cannot abolish his theological doubts and criticisms entirely. His often repeated agnostic views on the creation and on the eternity of the world, and still more, his agnosticism about the nature of god and the soul, could not entirely be avoided by those who concerned themselves deeply with Galen. In the Greek tradition, it is his comments on the eternity of the world that attract attention, if only briefly, and they are rejected as based on incorrect logic.[50] His agnostic views on the soul are not mentioned, and his claim, made in some writings at the end of his long life, that the soul's habits depend on the mixture of the body, are not debated as such. Instead, they are interpreted to apply only to the situation of the soul once it has entered the human body, not to the physical origins and make-up of the soul. Medicine is thus confined to the understanding of the body, at which Galen was supreme. Hence George of Pisidia, writing his *Hexaemeron* in the first half of the seventh century, could within two hundred lines warn his readers against trusting Galen as a physician of the soul and call God 'the Galen of our souls'.[51]

Medieval Arabic and Jewish philosopher-physicians, however, were more subtle in the understanding of Galen and, in all likelihood, had access in translation to more of Galen's philosophical writings than survived in

[49] F. Rosenthal, *Science and Medicine in Islam*, CS330 (Aldershot, 1990), article no. III, pp. 52–87; G. Strohmaier, 'Asklepios und das Ei', in *Beiträge zur alten Geschichte und deren Nachleben: Festschrift für Franz Altheim zum 6.10.1968*, ed. R. Stiehl and H. E. Stier, 2 vols. (Berlin, 1969–70), II, 143–53.

[50] Temkin, *Galenism*, pp. 74–5.

[51] George of Pisidia, *Hexaemeron*, lines 1388–9 and 1544, in Claudius Aelianus, *Varia historia*, ed. R. Hircher, 2 vols., Teubner edn (Leipzig, 1864–6), II, 646 and 651.

eleventh- or twelfth-century Byzantium, let alone in the medieval West. A distinguished line of scholars, including Rhazes, Averroes, al-Biruni, al-Ghazali, and Maimonides, all took issue with Galen's theological views.[52] They pointed to his apparent changes of opinion over the years, and they criticized what, in justice, might seem to be Galen's wish to have his theological cake and eat it. They rightly noted that at the end of his life, Galen came very, very close to accepting that the soul was something physically determined, if not something physical, and that this argument would, if rightly developed, lead to a belief in the mortality of the soul. Maimonides, more charitably, noted how Galen's exposition of his views on the soul followed logic as far as his logic could take him; Galen was prepared to acknowledge the existence of God; but any exposition of God's attributes he felt was beyond him.[53] What was needed for that was faith, and a greater understanding of logic. A Spanish follower of Maimonides, the Hebrew philosopher Shem Tov ibn Falaquera in the latter half of the thirteenth century, quotes Galen often in his own theological and moral treatises, and appears to have had access, directly or indirectly, to some of the less familiar philosophical treatises circulating in Arabic – whether they were also available in Hebrew is a more difficult question.[54] Certainly he seems to have had a much greater knowledge of and respect for Galen's moral treatises than any of his Latin contemporaries, and he brings the rehabilitation of Galen almost to completion.

How much of these debates in Arabic or Hebrew did Christian Europe or Byzantium know? As far as Byzantium is concerned, the answer is very little indeed; for many of the relevant primary texts had long disappeared in Greek. The treatise *On scientific demonstration*, where Galen treated many of these problems at length, and which had been used in the fifth century by Bishop Nemesius of Emesa, had been lost in Greek by the eleventh century.[55] So too had most of Galen's philosophical autobiography, *On my own beliefs*, and what remained circulating largely under an entirely different and misleading title derived from its last few sentences.[56] More was available in Latin; although not all of the relevant Galenic treatises were turned into Latin, traces of the Muslim debate might be found in Latin versions of Averroes. But if translations were available and being copied, were they being read or, if they were read, were they understood?

[52] Temkin, *Galenism*, pp. 76–80; J. C. Bürgel, 'Averroes "contra Galenum"', *Nachrichten der Akademie der Wissenschaften in Göttingen*, Philologisch-historische Klasse 9 (1967), pp. 265–340 (pp. 276–90); G. Strohmaier, 'Bekannte und unbekannte Zitate in den Zweifel an Galen des Rhazes', in *Text and Tradition*, pp. 263–88.

[53] M. Meyerhof, *Studies in Medieval Arabic Medicine: Theory and Practice*, ed. P. Johnstone, CS204 (London, 1984), article no. IX, pp. 53–76.

[54] Zonta, *Un interprete ebreo*.

[55] Müller (von), 'Galens Werk'.

[56] Galen, *On my Own Opinions*, ed. Nutton, pp. 14–22. The misleading title is *On the substance of the natural faculties*.

Here the answer must be almost entirely negative. Charles Burnett has recently pointed to a Spanish Dominican, Ramon Martí, who seems to know of this debate around 1280,[57] and the list of Galenic treatises assembled around 1320 and often ascribed to Walter Burley includes a reference to Niccolò da Reggio's very recent translation of *On the substance of the natural faculties*.[58] But these are exceptions. When some of Galen's philosophical writings were translated from Greek, between 1300 and 1350, they did not circulate widely – and were read even less. A copy in southern Germany was distinguished by the smell of its rotting leaves, high up on an inaccessible shelf of a monastic library.[59] Even when a translation was available, few bothered to read it. Galen's *On my own beliefs* was translated into Latin as *De sententiis*, and was included in several large collections of his works. At Paris, it was found in the 'big book' on which the Dean of the Medical Faculty took his oath of office, but I have evidence for only one actual reader, Pierre de Saint-Flour in the 1350s. Not surprisingly, this large manuscript volume over the centuries disintegrated entirely; a few leaves still remained at the end of the eighteenth century, and had disappeared by the middle of the next.[60] Why such philosophically and medically interesting writings should, even when available, have remained unstudied is a question for the psychologist, rather than the historian, but one might point to the development of a university teaching syllabus that excluded Galen's more speculative or theoretically challenging treatises. In the early fourteenth century, when these new translations became available, they were difficult to fit into an already existing syllabus. They lacked an obvious practical purpose, or intellectual champions such as had promoted the new Galenism only a generation or so earlier.[61]

What filled their place was legend and confusion. An easy misunderstanding of Galenic quotations from a treatise on cosmetics ascribed to the most famous beauty of antiquity, the so-called *Cleopatra's guide to beauty care*, led to the conclusion that Galen had learned all about women and women's medicine from her.[62] He must thus have been alive in her lifetime. Another

57 C. Burnett, 'Encounters with Razi the Philosopher: Constantine the African, Petrus Alfonsi and Ramon Martí', in *Pensamiento medieval hispano: Homenaje a Horacio Santiago-Otero*, ed. José María Soto Rábanos (Madrid, 1998), pp. 973–92 (pp. 981–91).

58 When I suggested (Galen, *On my Own Opinions*, ed. Nutton, pp. 41–2), that this text contained a reference to *On my Own Opinions* under the heading *De fide*, I did not know of the extremely complex textual and authorial problems outlined by M. Grignaschi, 'Lo pseudo Walter Burley e il "Liber de vita e moribus philosophorum"', and 'Il catalogo delle opere di Ippocrate e Galeno nel "De vita et moribus philosophorum"', *Medioevo* 16 (1990), 131–90 and 357–95.

59 R. Stauber, *Die Schedelsche Bibliothek* (repr. Nieuwkoop, 1969), p. 249.

60 Galen, *On my Own Opinions*, ed. Nutton, pp. 25–7.

61 N. G. Siraisi, *Taddeo Alderotti and his Pupils: Two Generations of Italian Medical Learning* (Princeton, 1981), pp. 27–42; L. García-Ballester, 'The New Galen: A Challenge to Latin Galenism in Thirteenth-century Montpellier', in *Text and Tradition*, pp. 55–83.

62 Quotations in K, XII, 403; 432; 492, cf. K, XII, 446. His source was probably the

legend, this time circulating in Greek, reported a conversation between Galen and none other than Mary Magdalene; when she told him that Christ had cured the man blind from birth (John 9. 1–12), Galen explained to her that Christ must have had a substantial knowledge of minerals, for otherwise he could not have performed such a cure.[63] The apparent praise of Galen here in a twelfth-century story contrasts with the condemnation of Professor Gesius for doing the same thing seven hundred years earlier. How the link with Mary Magdalene came about is not clear, but I suspect that we may be dealing with a reminiscence of yet another famous, if pseudonymous, writer on alchemy and mineral drugs, Mary the Egyptian, sometimes identified with the Virgin Mary or with Mary Magdalene.[64] The objection that an author who lived in the time of Christ could not have been alive 150 years later under Marcus Aurelius was met with the reply that if as good a doctor and expert on gerontology as Galen could not live so long, who could?[65]

The Cleopatra story, with its dating to the time of Christ, may also explain yet another conflation, this time in Hebrew; where Galen becomes conflated with the famous rabbi Gamaliel, and medicine becomes 'the art of Gamaliel'.[66] A similarity of letters in Hebrew and Arabic will have helped to merge the two individuals.

Of even greater consequence was a story widely circulating throughout Europe and the Middle East that goes back at least to the tenth century and is reported at length by an Arabic biographer of Galen, al-Mubassir ibn Fatik, who lived in the eleventh century. It is this biography that formed the basis for the celebrated medieval collection known in various vernaculars as the *Dicts and Sayings of the Philosophers*, the *Bocados d'oro*, and so on. al-Mubassir's biography is a neat mixture of fact and fiction, based in part on Galen's own words, supplemented by pleasant invention. Al-Mubassir describes how Galen had learned all he knew about women from Cleopatra,

cosmetic writings of Statilius Criton (fl. 110), rather than direct acquaintance. For the later stories, M. Ullmann, 'Kleopatra in einer arabischen alchemistischen Disputation', *Wiener Zeitschrift für das Kunde des Morgenlandes* 63/64 (1972), 158–75 (pp. 159–61). The much reorganized Arabic version of *On theriac for Piso*, which contains a detailed discussion of Cleopatra's death (K, XIV, 235–7) gives the impression to the unwary that it was written by Galen in the time of Nero.

[63] Michael Glycas, *Annales* iii.231; *PG* 158, 436–7.

[64] Ullmann, 'Kleopatra', citing Greek as well as Arabic alchemical texts.

[65] The story was known to John Tzetzes, *Historiae* xi.397 (ed. P. A. M. Leone, Università di Napoli, Istituto di filologia classica, Pubblicazioni 1 (Naples, 1968), lines 1010–29, pp. 468–9), who described it as nonsense, quoting Galen's *De Antidotis* to show that he must have lived after Andromachus the Elder, and under Marcus Aurelius. Cf. also John Tzetzes, *Epistulae*, ed. P. A. M. Leone, Teubner edition (Leipzig, 1972), p. 121. The (non-medieval) response is that of L. Caelius Rhodiginus, *Lectiones antiquae* xvi.39 (Venice, 1516), p. 842; in later enlarged edns, e.g. Basle, 1550, the passage occurs at xxx.12.

[66] G. Vajda, 'Galien-Gamaliel', *Annuaire de l'Institute de Philologie et d'Histoire orientales et slaves* 13 (1953) [1955], 641–54.

and talks of his death in Egypt at the age of eighty-seven. He was buried at Perama, on the borders of Egypt and Syria; in fact ancient Pelusium, at the easternmost mouth of the Nile.[67] That this story was circulating well before al-Mubassir is clear from the Arabic geographer al-Istakhri, writing two or three generations earlier, who reports that in his day visitors were being shown the tomb of Galen at Perama.[68] What was Galen doing there? The answer from al-Mubassir is that he had gone to the Levant in search of drugs, but had died on his way from Egypt to Syria, an explanation based on a much earlier journey by Galen in that region.[69] But there was a much more attractive explanation, found particularly in Christian sources; Galen had died while on a voyage to Jerusalem to see the actual location of Christ's miracles.[70] Where he died, and both Pergamum and Sicily as well as Pelusium were mentioned as possible sites, was less important than the fact that Galen had died while on a pilgrimage, for this is the version that came down to Western Europe in the fourteenth century.[71] Travellers to Sicily were shown the tomb of Galen 'on the left, going from Qasr al-Amiri [Misilmeri] towards the capital [Palermo]', where he had stopped off on his journey to Syria to find the friends and acquaintances of Jesus.[72] That this story was a nice invention did not stop it from being repeated in works of scholarship well into the seventeenth century or from being taken as proof that, at the very end of his life, Galen had acquired the Christian faith that had eluded him for so long.[73] A man of consummate virtue – and Renaissance scholars, both Protestant and Catholic, spent pages showing how Galen's virtues matched those of the ideal Christian – he could now be

[67] English translation by F. Rosenthal, *The Classical Heritage in Islam* (London, 1975), pp. 33–6.

[68] Al-Istakhri, *Geography*, ed. M. J. de Goeje, *Bibliotheca Geographorum Arabicorum*, 8 vols. (Leiden, 1870–94), I, 53.

[69] V. Nutton, 'The Chronology of Galen's Early Career', *Classical Quarterly* n.s. 23 (1973), 158–71 (especially pp. 169–70).

[70] Vajda, 'Galien-Gamaliel', 649–50; W. Hertz, *Gesammelte Abhandlungen* (Stuttgart and Berlin, 1905) pp. 403–4. The story would appear to go back at least to the eleventh century.

[71] M. Amari, *Biblioteca arabo-sicula: ossia raccolta di testi arabici che toccano la geografia, la storia, le biografia e la bibliografia della Sicilia*, 3 vols. (Turin and Rome, 1880–9), I, 346 (Ibn Sabbat); II, 503 (Ibn Abi Usaybi'a).

[72] Amari, *Biblioteca arabo-sicula*, 'Appendice', III, 3, citing al-Harawi, *Kitab al-Istarat*, of *c.* 1185, who took his information ultimately from al-Bakri (*c.* 1100). M. Amari, 'Sul sopposto sepolcro di Galeno alla Cannita', *Archivio storico siciliano* n.s. 11 (1887), 427–39, notes that there was a Classical (and earlier Punic) burial ground at this site, about five miles from Palermo. Hertz, *Gesammelte Abhandlungen*, p. 403, identifies the tomb of Galen with one said to be that of Socrates or Aristotle high up in the cathedral of Palermo, but no source specifies Palermo as the location of Galen's tomb and al-Harawi's description is very precise.

[73] Both Perama and Palermo could be derived from phonetic or orthographic renderings of Pergamum in Arabic, while the story of a Sicilian visit could be a misunderstanding of the story of Galen's hurried escape there from Rome in 166.

fully accepted as a Christian, for why else should he go to Jerusalem, if he was not prepared to believe in Christ's miracles?[74]

None of these Renaissance scholars, however, knew of the elaboration of this story, which located Galen firmly within the family of the early church: his sister was the mother of St Paul.[75]

With these legends, the depaganization of Galenic medicine is complete. Galen ascends to heaven, and his medicine is passed fit for a Christian to use. To reach this point we have travelled a long and complicated route, across political, religious, and linguistic boundaries, and we have touched on lives of the saints as well as on academic medicine and philosophy. By 1400, the fount of academic medicine, Galen of Pergamum, is now purged of all taint of heresy. Gone are the doubts and the criticisms of the Asclepius-worshipper, replaced by the image of Galen the sage, the seeker after Christian miracle, and the epitome of moral rectitude. That modern scholars find difficulty in believing that the egotistical, boastful, and unscrupulous Galen could ever be held up as a model of peaceful and charitable virtue is by the way. For the later western Middle Ages, Galen had become fully assimilated: he had known Christians, and had, according to some, eventually, believed. His view of the universe, created, fostered, and watched over by the providence of the divine creator, was entirely compatible with a Christian medieval world view. Indeed, Galen's observations and his almost infallible logic only added to its strength. His conclusions brought along with them also those of Hippocrates, for again and again Galen had stressed that he had derived his ideas from Hippocrates. Hence their presence together in the Anagni fresco, offering solid explanations for the universe. Although there were those in the later Middle Ages who continued to repeat the old jibe *ubi tres medici, ibi duo athei* – 'where there are three doctors, there are two atheists'; although there were those who described how the face of the gentle doctor who approached the bedside swiftly turned into that of the devil when he submitted his bill; and although there were those who still feared the presence of an unbeliever at the bedside of the dying or the pregnant, and sought the presence of a priest as much as that of a doctor, their fears could be easily assuaged.[76] Those who followed closely the learned Galenic and Hippocratic medicine were now firmly on the side of the angels.

[74] V. Nutton, 'Biographical Accounts of Galen, 1340–1660', in *Geschichte der Medizingeschichtsschreibung*, ed. T. Rütten (Wolfenbüttel, forthcoming).

[75] Vajda, 'Galien-Gamaliel', p. 649, from Ibn Abi Usaybi'a's biography of Galen.

[76] For some of these concerns, see Amundsen, *Medicine, Society, and Faith*, pp. 260–8.

Religion and Medicine in the Middle Ages

Moses, Galen and Jacques Despars: Religious Orthodoxy as a Path to Unorthodox Medical Views

Danielle Jacquart

A few lines in Jacques Despars' commentary on Avicenna's *Canon* deserve particular attention for the strange manner in which the author appeals to religious doctrine. Written in Tournai, Cambrai and Paris, between 1432 and 1453, by a former professor at the Paris faculty of medicine, this huge commentary on Book 1, Book 3 and Book 4 fen 1 was printed at Lyons in 1498, forty years after Despars' death. It forms three or four dense folio volumes – depending on the binding – which contain over two thousand pages. The prolific author of this commentary was a very erudite physician and the owner of a very rich private library, which he had built up in part through commissioning his own copies of a lot of long medical works. Their production took up ten years preceding the writing of the commentary, and during their copying Despars was at pains to secure philological accuracy, comparing different translations of the same Greek work and different manuscripts of the same translation. Many reports of cases and consultations in his commentary show that Despars was also heavily involved in medical practice. He held several ecclesiastical benefices, like most Paris medical masters in the first half of the fifteenth century, in his case in Cambrai, Tournai and – at the end of his life – in Paris. His clerical position and transparent piety did not prevent him from teaching and practising an utterly lay medicine. He was even more careful than some of his contemporaries not to introduce any piety into medical practice. For example, he did not include prayer among the ways of protecting oneself from plague, and he reacted with some violence against the practice both of processions including the sick and of resort to the saints. In addition he was vituperative about the theologians of his day for being too absorbed in demonology.[1] Despars, therefore, can be regarded as the very model of a medieval physician able to

[1] On this fifteenth-century commentator on Avicenna's *Canon* see Jacquart: *Médecine médiévale, passim*; 'Theory, Everyday Practice and Three Fifteenth-Century Physicians', *Osiris* 2nd ser. 6 (1990), 140–60; 'Le regard d'un médecin sur son temps: Jacques Despars (1380?–1458)', *Bibliothèque de l'Ecole des Chartes* 138 (1980), 35–86. The last two articles are reprinted in D. Jacquart, *La science médicale occidentale entre deux renaissances (XIIe s. – XVe s.)*, CS567 (Aldershot, 1997), articles XIV and XIII.

distinguish clearly between medical art and religious belief. Given this, any allusion he makes to religious dogma imposing limits on medical theory or practice is going to be of particular interest for the light it casts upon the range of opinions which were forbidden and which a physician did not feel free to uphold.

1. God's Absolute Power and the Significance of a Variant Reading

When dealing with temperaments or complexions according to ages in Book I of the *Canon* (fen 1, doct. 3, c. 3), Avicenna presented an absurd proposition. At stake was the progressive and inescapable loss of innate heat which was supposed to occur after the age of youth and which led human beings towards death. This loss of innate heat was connected with the gradual drying up of radical moisture (*humidum radicale*).[2] Avicenna put forward one of the major causes of this, that the natural virtue or force is unable to resist 'for ever' (*semper*), since all bodily forces are finite. Further, as Avicenna said, even if one imagines that this force could be infinite and that the daily restoration of the body could equal its daily dissolution, the dissolution would increase from day to day, and so it would finally consume the moisture, and in the end the body's matter would be destroyed and its heat extinguished.[3] While commenting on these complicated issues, Despars feels it necessary to clarify the notion of 'infinite', enumerating the three kinds: the first, infinite according to magnitude or number; the second, infinite according to time or duration; the third, infinite according to what was called 'active power or vigour' (*potentia activa seu vigor*).

On the first kind Despars reports the distinction, made by Aristotle in *Physics* III, between an actual and a potential infinite. There can be no *actually* infinite number or magnitude, but the infinite does exist *potentially*, through the infinite division of continuous magnitudes or through the addition of units to a number. In fact, there was no point in saying this, since the commentator had to admit that this kind of infinite was not at issue. What was more at issue was the infinite according to duration, where

2 On the notion of radical moisture, see McVaugh, 'Humidum radicale'. Note that Arnau de Vilanova, in *De humido radicali*, states that the physician can only regulate the restoration process and that only God knows exactly its possible duration; cf. Ziegler, *Medicine and Religion*, pp. 242–3.

3 'Amplius si hec virtus infinita foret et semper permutationem in corpore faceret eius quod dissolvitur equaliter et uno modo, disssolutio tamen uno modo non esset, immo semper quotidie augeretur et corpus dissolutionem tolerare non posset et dissolutio humiditatem finiret, quanto magis cum due res se iuvent ad minorationem faciendam et retrocedendum. Et postquam sic est, oportet necessario ut materia destruatur et calor extinguatur': Avicenna, *Canon* I.i.3.3, fol. 4rb.

Despars agrees with Avicenna. If there could be a restoration which was infinite in time, it would bring a moisture that was actually impure. This impure moisture would not only be unable to restore the innate moisture, but it would, on the contrary, contribute to the destruction of this innate moisture.

Left to deal with was the infinite according to active power. Here Despars concludes, contrarily to Avicenna, that if the natural force of restoration had an infinite active power and could perpetuate the radical moisture in all its purity, this force would be able to resist the gradual process of desiccation and dissolution. Despars goes immediately to a comparison between this *potentia activa* and God's absolute power, and then goes straight to a quotation from Galen's *On the usefulness of the parts of the body*, which mentions Moses.

> Talis namque est virtus omnipotentis dei qui omnia quecumque voluit fecit in celo et in terra, in mari et in omnibus abyssis, licet in hoc Galenus reprehendat Moysen .11. *de utilitate particularum* capitulo .⟨1⟩4. dicens : *Illi enim (scilicet Moysi) sufficit quod velit deus ornare materiam et illa mox ornabitur. Omnia enim esse possibilia deo existimat etiam si cinerem equum vel bovem voluerit facere, nos autem non ita cognoscimus, sed esse quedam dicimus* ***vere*** *impossibilia et hec omnino non attentare deum.* Que si de impossibilibus contradictionem implicantibus intelligeret verus esset sermo eius, sed hanc materiam theologis relinquamus.[4]

> (Of the same kind ⟨as the so-called infinite power which would preserve the radical moisture⟩ is God's absolute power; indeed God made all he wanted in the heavens, on the earth, on the sea and in all abysses, although Galen reprehends Moses in this matter, stating in the eleventh book of *De utilitate particularum*, chapter fourteen: *For him (i.e. Moses) it suffices for God to have willed material to be arranged and straightway it was arranged, because Moses believed everything to be possible to God, even if he should wish to make a horse or beef out of ashes. We, however, do not hold this view, saying rather that some things are* ***truly*** *impossible and that God does not attempt these at all.* If Galen understood impossible things as things implicating any ⟨logical⟩ contradiction, his statement might be true, but let us leave this matter for theologians'.)

Such was the fidelity of Niccolò da Reggio's translation of Galen's work from Greek into Latin that we could use here May's modern translation from Greek into English, at any rate for most of Despars' quotation.[5] But at the end of the passage there is an important discrepancy. Where the Greek text gives 'saying rather that some things are naturally impossible', Despars' quotation runs 'saying rather that some things are truly impossible'. The discrepancy, then, is of one word only: *vere* instead of *nature.* Niccolò da Reggio had

[4] Despars, ad I.i.3.3.

[5] Galen, *Usefulness of the Parts of the Body*, II, 532–3 (*De usu partium* xii.14).

translated accurately, using *nature*.[6] It is easy to explain this confusion paleographically by pointing to the abbreviation normally used in medieval manuscripts and the difficulty of differentiation between the letters 'n' and the letter 'v' written as 'u'. This confusion is not to be attributed to the Renaissance printer, since Despars' comment clearly alludes to a logical contradiction – implying something impossible according to truth – and not to a natural impossibility. Despars' concern with philological accuracy makes this misreading all the more puzzling. Right at the end of his commentary he stated that, before beginning to write, he had collated the manuscripts of Galen's works, as well as those of other Greek and Arab authors, and that he had had them carefully copied for his own use. We know that in 1417 he borrowed the manuscript of Galen's *On the usefulness of the parts of the body* which belonged to the faculty of medicine. It is no longer extant.[7] Did this copy offer the variant reading *vere* rather than *nature*? If this was the case, was it a deliberate correction, one intended to provide an 'authorized' version?

There was an important significance for theological orthodoxy in this replacement of the idea of a natural impossibility with the idea of a logical impossibility. Galen's words about Moses put into question God's power, denying him the power of infringing the laws of nature and, in particular, the material principle. This kind of statement had been clearly condemned in Paris in 1277: 'That the absolutely impossible cannot be done by God or another agent. An error, if impossible is understood according to nature.'[8] So, reading *vere impossibilia* into the quotation from *On the usefulness of the parts of the body* saved the religious orthodoxy of Galen's medieval followers. During the fourteenth and fifteenth centuries the statement, that logical contradiction was the only conceivable limitation on God's power, had become a commonplace. What remained was defining precisely what could be understood by the expression 'logical contradiction', and this became a favourite topic among logicians. In the fields of physics and cosmology the trend was for analysis of the possible to prevail over attention to the understanding of real phenomena.[9] It is in this context that Despars's comment on his quotation from Galen and his allusion to theologians have to be placed.

6 The reading *nature* is clearly provided in Vatican, Biblioteca Apostolica Vaticana, MS Vat. lat. 2380. I thank Dr Marilyn Nicoud for her checking of this manuscript.

7 E. Wickersheimer, *Commentaires de la Faculté de médecine de l'Université de Paris (1395–1516)*, Collection des documents inédits sur l'histoire de France (Paris, 1915), p. 32.

8 'Quod impossibile simpliciter non potest fieri a Deo, vel ab agente alio. Error si de impossibili secundum naturam intelligatur': Piché, *Condamnation parisienne*, p. 124 (art. 147). I have used E. Grant's translation in *Source Book of Medieval Science*, p. 49.

9 Among the numerous works dealing with this topic, see E. Grant, 'The Condemnation of 1277, God's Absolute Power, and Physical Thought in the Late Middle Ages', *Viator* 10 (1979), 211–44; L. Bianchi, *Il vescovo e i filosofi: la condanna parigina del 1277 e l'evoluzione dell'aristotelismo scolastico* (Bergamo, 1990), pp. 122–33; L. Bianchi and E. Randi, *Vérités dissonantes, Aristote à la fin du Moyen Age* (Freiburg-im-Breisgau, 1993), pp. 57–99; J. Sarnowsky, 'God's Absolute Power, Thought Experiments, and

2. Medical Themes in the Condemnation of 1277

Although much has been written about the condemnation of 1277, there has been almost nothing on its medical content or implications for medicine. Among the condemned articles, only a few could affect physicians in their thought and practice. We can take as examples two which were at the border between medicine and natural philosophy:

> Quod raptus and visiones non fiunt nisi per naturam. (That rapture and visions occur only through a natural process.)[10]

> Quod homo per nutritionem potest fieri alius numeraliter et individualiter. (That by nutrition a man can become another numerically and individually.)[11]

In principle the condemnation of both these articles could limit physicians' intervention in mental disorders and medical explanations of the impact of diet on complexions.

More significant were the articles dealing with sexual behaviour and astrology. Translations of medical works from Arabic had played a part in the development of naturalistic views on sexuality, which were potentially in conflict with the principles of Christian ethics.[12] There were possible echoes of these views in three condemned articles:

> Quod delectatio in actibus venereis non impedit actum seu usum intellectus. (That pleasure during sexual acts does not impede the action and use of intellect.)

> Quod perfecta abstinentia ab actu carnis corrumpit virtutem et speciem. (That perfect carnal abstinence corrupts the virtue and the species.)

> Quod peccatum contra naturam, utpote abusus in coitu, licet sit contra naturam speciei, non tamen est contra naturam individui. (That sin against nature, as an abuse during sexual intercourse, is not against the nature of the individual, although it is against the nature of the species.)[13]

the Concept of Nature in the "New Physics" of XIVth Century Paris', and H. Hugonnard-Roche, 'L'Hypothétique et la nature dans la physique parisienne du XIVe siècle', in *La Nouvelle physique du XIVe siècle*, ed. S. Caroti and P. Souffrin (Florence, 1997), pp. 179–201 and 161–77.

10 Piché, *Condamnation parisienne*, p. 88 (art. 33). The English translation is mine. One can find in Piché's book an up-to-date bibliography on the condemnation, its background and implications.

11 Piché, *Condamnation parisienne*, p. 125 (art. 145). The English translation is taken from *Source Book of Medieval Science*, p. 49.

12 On this topic, see Jacquart and Thomasset; J. A. Brundage, *Law, Sex, and Christian Society in Medieval Europe* (Chicago, 1987).

13 Piché, *Condamnation parisienne*, pp. 128 and 130 (art. 172, 169, 166). The English translations are mine.

When dealing with sexual behaviour physicians sometimes felt free to recommend practices which were supposed to facilitate procreation or to ensure the balance of body and mind, even if these actions were in some way beyond Christian rules. Physicians also stressed the dangers of excessively strict abstinence, according to the physical disposition of the individual. While expressing relative tolerance in these matters, physicians did not put forward any natural explanation for homosexual behaviour, in particular when it concerned men. When they had to confront this, they usually confined themselves to the moral level, and expressed strong condemnation. More often than not they avoided the topic, restricting themselves to a repetition of Avicenna's statement, that in some cases, such practices between women could be a remedy for female sterility.[14] The natural explanation of male homosexual practices that they could read in Pseudo-Aristotle's *Problems* iv.26 found almost no echo among them. Whether through conviction or self-censorship, medieval physicians did not contradict Christian moral teaching on male homosexuality. A lone exception is Pietro d'Abano, who took into account the Aristotelian naturalistic explanation in his commentary on the *Problems*, which he had begun in Paris and which he finished in Padua in 1310.[15]

Medical recourse to astrology also encountered some limitation in the condemnation of 1277:

> Quod orbis est causa voluntatis medici, ut sanet. (That celestial sphere is the cause of the physician's will to treat patients.)
>
> Quod sanitatem, infirmitatem, vitam et mortem attribuit positioni siderum et aspectui fortune, dicens si eum aspexerit fortuna, vivet; si non aspexerit, morietur. (That health, disease, life and death are attributed to the positions of the stars and the aspect of [the point called] fortune, stating that if fortune regards someone, he will live ; if it does not regard him, he will die.)
>
> Quod, in hora generationis hominis, in corpore suo et per consequens in anima, que sequitur corpus, ex ordine causarum superiorum et inferiorum, inest homini dispositio inclinans ad tales actiones et eventus. Error, nisi intelligatur de eventibus naturalibus, et per viam dispositionis. (That, at the time of conception, in his body, and consequently in the soul, which follows the body, man receives from the order of superior and inferior causes a

[14] Avicenna, *Canon* III.xx.1.38; cf. Jacquart and Thomasset, pp. 159 and 227 n. 60.

[15] On Pietro d'Abano's endeavour to include practices between men within the framework of what is natural by birth or by habit, see J. Cadden, 'Sciences/Silences: The Natures and Languages of "Sodomy" in Peter of Abano's *Problemata* Commentary', in *Constructing Medieval Sexuality*, ed. K. Lochrie, P. McCracken and J. A. Schultz, Medieval Cultures 11 (Minneapolis and London, 1997), pp. 40–57. On the afterlife of Pietro d'Abano's commentary, see J. Cadden, 'Nothing Natural is Shameful: Vestiges of a Debate about Sex and Science in a Group of Late Medieval Manuscripts', *Speculum*, 76 (2001), 66–89.

tendency which inclines him to such and such actions or events. Error, except if this means only natural events and merely a tendency.)[16]

While the first two of these articles dealt with the influence of the stars on human will and on the determination of death, the third one supposed a natural determinism of both soul and body. This natural determinism could be supported not only by astrology and physiognomy but also by the medical theory of complexions. Although it is difficult to gauge precisely the impact these condemnations had, the three articles in question certainly marked out the boundaries of acceptable views. Once again, Pietro d'Abano seems to have been less cautious on these topics than most university masters. In his *Compendium phisionomie*, which he wrote in Paris in 1295 and therefore within twenty years of the famous condemnation, he combined astrology, physiognomy and theory of complexions in order to describe psychological predispositions. Despite his claims and endeavour to expound an orthodox theory of the soul, he was not completely safe from the suspicion that he was upholding a kind of psychological determinism.[17] The combination of his position on this and his naturalistic views on homosexuality are perhaps sufficient to explain his suffering inquisition proceedings three times in his life, first in Paris and then, later on, in Padua.[18]

It is clear that physicians had to be cautious in their views on sexuality, astral determinism and the interweaving of physical and psychological states. These were the issues most likely to stir up conflict between medical explanation or advice and religious demands or theological doctrine. As for

[16] Piché, *Condamnation parisienne*, pp. 119 and 143 (art. 132, 206, 207). The English translations are mine. Note that in art. 207, the expression 'in corpore suo et per consequens in anima, que sequitur corpus' echoes the beginning of Pseudo-Aristotle's *Physiognomy*: 'Quoniam et anime sequuntur corpora . . .', in *Scriptores physiognomici graeci et latini*, ed. R. Foerster, 2 vols. (Leipzig, 1893), I, 5. The question of the link between physiognomic and astrological explanations had therefore to be tackled with some caution by medieval writers. On the reception of this Pseudo-Aristotelian work in Paris, see J. Agrimi, 'La ricezione della *Fisiognomica* pseudoaristotelica nella Facoltà delle arti', *AHDLMA* 64 (1997), 126–88. On the relationship between body and soul according to physicians around 1300, see Ziegler, *Medicine and Religion*, pp. 152–7.

[17] G. Federici-Vescovini, 'Peter of Abano and Astrology', in *Astrology, Science and Society: Historical Essays*, ed. P. Curry (Woodbridge, 1987), pp. 31–9, and 'Pietro d'Abano e la medicina astrologica dello *Speculum physionomiae* di Michele Savonarola', in *Musagetes: Festschrift für Wolfram Prinz zu seinem 60 Geburtstag am 5 Februar 1989*, Frankfurter Forschungen zur Kunst 17 (Berlin, 1992), pp. 167–77; D. Jacquart, 'L'influence des astres sur le corps humain chez Pietro d'Abano', in *Le corps et ses énigmes au Moyen Âge: Actes du Colloque, Orléans, 15–16 mai 1992*, ed. B. Ribémont (Caen, 1993), pp. 73–86.

[18] Much has been written, from late medieval writers to modern scholars, on the substance of these prosecutions. It remains, nevertheless, unclear. See P. Marangon, 'Per una revisione dell'interpretazione di Pietro d'Abano', in *Pensiero ereticale*, pp. 66–104. One can find a general survey of Pietro d'Abano's life and works in E. Paschetto, *Pietro d'Abano medico e filosofo* (Florence, 1984).

the problem of God's absolute power, this does not seem to have been a major concern for physicians: had it been, it would have called into question the very foundations of Galenic medicine. Given this, it was better not to mention it.

There was a further consideration. One superficial interpretation of God's absolute power could have led to the reintroduction of the problem of the miraculous. Despars himself took care to employ the perfect tense of verbs in use when describing God's achievement in the realm of nature (*omnia quecumque voluit fecit*). In this way Despars managed to refer only to the time of the Creation, allowing no room for the problem of later miraculous intervention, which would have embarrassed him. He was a constant defender of an entirely secular medicine and he usually favoured strict limitation of religious intrusion into medicine. It comes as a surprise, then, to find him raising the miraculous on another occasion. Why did he tread on this dangerous ground?

3. A Quotation out of Context

Galen himself alluded to Moses and God's omnipotence, when dealing with the length of eyelashes and eyebrows. Since it was better for these bodily hairs always to stay at the same length, the Creator had to provide a suitable material for their implantation.

> Has, then, our Creator commanded only those hairs to preserve always the same length, and do the hairs preserve it as they have been ordered either because they fear the injunction of their Lord, or reverence the God who commands it, or themselves believe it better to do so? Is this the way in which Moses reasons about Nature (and it is a better way than Epicurus')? Yet it is best for us to adopt neither, but continuing to derive the principle of generation from the Creator in all things generable, as Moses does, to add to this the material principle. For our Creator has made these hairs feel the necessity of preserving always an even length for the reason that this was the better thing. And since he had decided that it was necessary to make them so, he spread beneath some of them [the eyelashes] a hard body like cartilage [the tarsus] and under the others [the eyebrows] a hard skin united to cartilage by means of the brows. Now it was not enough merely to will that they should be so; for even if he wished to make a rock into a man all of a sudden, it would be impossible. And this is the point at which my teaching and that of Plato and the other Greeks who have treated correctly of natural principles differ from that of Moses. For him it suffices for God . . .[19]

When commenting on the chapter in Avicenna's *Canon* that is devoted to the complexions of the diverse parts of the body, Despars had not quoted verbatim Galen's statement about bodily hair, contenting himself with a

[19] *De usu partium* xi.14, in Galen, *On the Usefulness of the Parts of the Body*, II, 532.

summary. After reminding his readers that hair, eyelashes and eyebrows were intended, according to the Creator's design, for the protection of the head and the eyes, he pointed out that these hairs did not grow casually, but 'naturally, through a prime intention' (*ex natura secundum primam intentionem*).[20] There was no allusion to Moses, or to God's absolute power. One century earlier, Gentile da Foligno (d. 1348) had alluded to Moses, but in an oblique way.

> Que sit diversitas in pilis faciei, barbe et capitis et aliorum partium lege Gal. prolixe et rhetorice loquente in libro *de utilitate partium* XI capitulo XIV° contra Moysem prophetam, de quo fortiter increpat eum Raby Moyses .25. particula *afforismorum* .54. capitulo.
>
> (On the question of what the diversity is between the hairs of the face, the beard and other parts, read Galen, who in his book *On the usefulness of the parts of the body*, [Book] XI, Chapter 14, speaks lengthily and rhetorically against the prophet Moses, for which Rabbi Moses [Maimonides] strongly criticizes him [Galen], in Particle 25 of [his] *Aphorisms*, Chapter 54.)[21]

In this way Gentile da Foligno avoided quoting the exact passage in Galen's work, but took care to mention – without detailing it – Maimonides' criticism. In his medical *Aphorisms*, in fact, the Jewish philosopher stated that since God was almighty he was even capable of contravening the laws of nature as they happened to be known later by men, but that all what he did was dictated by wisdom and goodness. Galen's error was to think that God came with the world, whereas he created everything *ex nihilo*.[22] The obliqueness of Gentile's reference to Galen, Moses and Maimonides shows that he was reluctant to explore thoroughly the theme of God's absolute power. It should be pointed out that, when Gentile came to comment on the chapter in Avicenna's *Canon* dealing with male homosexual practices, he referred to Pseudo-Aristotle's *Problem* iv.26, but avoided quoting its content and its naturalistic explanation.[23] Recognizable in both these cases are the traces of self-censorship.

As for Despars, the problem is probably more complicated. First of all, he did not give the Galenic quotation in its proper context. Secondly, he favoured a reading which was consonant with religious orthodoxy, whereas there is no doubt that Gentile da Foligno had the genuine version in mind. Was Despars' intention just to provide an 'authorized' version of this

[20] Despars, ad I.i.3.2.

[21] Gentile da Foligno, comm. *Canon*, I.i.3.2 (Venice 1494).

[22] Cf. *Aphorismi Rabi Moysis medici antiquissimi ac celeberrimi*, *Sectio* 24, *De quibusdam locis sibi contrariis apud Galenum*, c. 41 (Basel, 1579), pp. 517–27 (520–7). On Maimonides' criticism, see Walzer, *Galen on Jews and Christians*, pp. 33–4, who relied on J. Schacht and M. Meyerhof, 'Maimonides against Galen, on Philosophy and Cosmogony', *Bulletin of the Faculty of Arts of the University of Cairo* V.1 (1939), 54–88.

[23] Gentile da Foligno, comm. *Canon* III.xx.1.6. On Gentile's allusion to *Problem* iv.26, see Jacquart and Thomasset, pp. 156–9.

quotation? It is not clear. He used the notion of a divine power capable of acting against the laws of nature as an example, in order to suggest that these laws, as established by medical doctrine, were not inviolable. He did this in the way that natural philosophers did, when they happened to contradict some principles of Aristotelian physics. By comparing the infinite active power, that could stop the extinction of radical moisture, with God's absolute power, Despars was suggesting that it could be possible – at least, hypothetically – to impede the natural process which leads to this extinction. It is necessary here to point out that Despars seems to have been very interested in alchemy, and that the radical moisture was at issue in alchemical discussions of prolongation of life.[24] If Despars had been less cautious and more willing to state his intent clearly, he could have alluded to another article condemned in 1277: *Quod Deus non potest dare perpetuitatem rei transmutabili vel corruptibili* (That God is not able to give perpetuity to a transmutable or perishable thing).[25] The condemnation of this article was clearly intended to preserve the doctrine of the resurrection of the body, but it was not immune to other and imprudent interpretation. Doubtless Despars was not prepared to put forward the possibility of perpetuating life for ever, but he thought its prolongation by artificial means possible. A few pages before alluding to God's absolute power, Despars had raised the question: 'What is the limit of old age?' (*Quis est naturalis terminus senii?*). After summarizing the various views of medical authorities, he gave his own opinion that the natural term seemed to be a hundred years. But he pointed out that the prolongation of life beyond one hundred years was not impossible, whether through divine miraculous intervention, in accordance with propitious celestial conditions, or by means of some medicine.[26] Although Despars was constantly promoting in his commentary an entirely secular medicine and despite his strong reserve about astrology,[27] here he was prepared to allude both to miracle and (more vaguely) to celestial influences, so that he could postulate the possibility of prolonging life, in particular through regenerating radical moisture. Returning in the same chapter to the topic of prolonging life, he mentioned *myrobolans* and an

[24] On Jacques Despars and alchemy, see Jacquart, *Médecine médiévale*, pp. 488–501. On alchemy and the theme of *prolongatio vitae*, see M. Pereira, 'Un tesoro inestimabile: elixir e *prolongatio vitae* nell' alchimia del '300', *Micrologus* 1 (1993), 161–87 and 'Teorie dell'elixir nell' alchimia latina medievale', *Micrologus* 3 (1995), 103–48; A. Paravicini Bagliani, 'Il mito della *Prolongatio vitae* e la corte pontificia del duecento, Il *De retardatione accidentium senectutis*', in his *Medicina e scienze della natura alla corte dei papi nel duecento* (Spoleto, 1991), pp. 283–326.

[25] Piché, *Condamnation parisienne*, p. 86 (art. 25). The English translation is mine.

[26] Despars, ad I.i.3.3: 'Teneo tamen quod terminus naturalis senii hominis sani semper quem describit Galenus primo *Tegni* non est procul ab anno centesimo . . . Teneo 2° quod nichil prohibet aut divino miraculo aut influentiis celi vehementer faventibus et propiciis aut medicine beneficio terminum senii longe ultra .100. annum protendi.'

[27] On Despars' reserve about astrology, see the works cited in n. 1.

indian drug called *trifera* among the substances that could reinforce radical moisture. He concluded thus: 'it is possible to delay death, which, without the help of art, will come at a fixed time according to the laws of nature' (*possibile est retardare mortem certo tempore venturam secundum principia nature non adiuta ab arte*).[28] After this reference to the possibilities of art, he referred once again to propitious celestial influences and divine favour. With all these tortuous suggestions, Jacques Despars gives us an illuminating example of the use of religious orthodoxy in the defence of unorthodox medical views.

[28] Despars, ad I.i.3.3.

Moments of Inflection: The Careers of Arnau de Vilanova

Michael R. McVaugh

It was about the year 1290, we know, that Arnau de Vilanova began to assume a new identity – or, more accurately, what would become two new entangled identities. Until that time he had been merely a medical practitioner, though one of some distinction. Unusually for the age, he had received formal education in medicine at Montpellier in the 1260s and had risen to become physician to King Pere II of Aragon, but when Pere died in 1285 Arnau had returned to his own home in Valencia; documents dated as late as March 1289 show him busy with his affairs there. Yet something must have propelled him into his new identities almost immediately thereafter. Already by 1291 he had moved to Montpellier, and from that moment on two different careers engaged him simultaneously and would continue to do so for the twenty years he had left to live: one, that of an academic physician pursuing medical learning (though he can have taught relatively little, if at all, after 1301), and the other, that of a lay theologian and prophet. And the new careers expressed themselves in an abrupt burst of literary productivity: in the 1290s Arnau composed at least five monographs on medical theory[1] and five works on theological matters.[2] He would continue to write on both subjects during the following decade.

A variety of accounts of how Arnau combined these two subjects in his own mind, of how one influenced the other over the twenty years he pursued these two careers, have already been offered by several scholars – most recently by Joseph Ziegler, who has used Arnau to exemplify the potential for a kind of fusion between medical and spiritual concerns in Latin Christendom in the years around 1300.[3] Ziegler shows that while Arnau did not

[1] See the argument in Arnau de Vilanova, *Aphorismi de gradibus*, ed. M. R. McVaugh, *AVOMO* II (Granada-Barcelona, 1975; repr. Barcelona, 1992), pp. 80–1; since that was published, it has been established that the *Repetitio super 'Vita brevis'*, cited there, was finished in 1301. I take *De intentione medicorum, De considerationibus operis medicine, De dosibus tyriacalibus, Aphorismi de gradibus* and probably *De humido radicali* to be works composed by Arnau in the 1290s.

[2] *Introductio in de semine scripturarum* [1292?], *Allocutio super tetragrammaton* [July 1292], *Alphabetum catholicorum* [1295–7], *De prudentia catholicorum scholarium* [before 1297] and *De adventu antichristi* [1290?, 1297–1300]. I follow the list given in F. Santi, *Arnau de Vilanova: L'obra espiritual* (Valencia, 1987), pp. 250–3.

[3] Ziegler, *Medicine and Religion*.

incorporate specific details of medical theory into his spiritual writings (or vice versa), his figurative world depended heavily on a medical imagery that he extended to spiritual pathologies; and he argues that Arnau's conviction that medicine had a spiritual dimension and that medical certainty could come from God allowed him to believe that he was qualified to move between one sphere and the other. I have no intention of trying to improve on this as an overall portrayal of Arnau's views, for it seems entirely convincing to me.

Instead, I want to try to do something that scholars have not yet done: to look at the interaction of religious and medical themes in Arnau's mind at one particular moment – a moment of inflection, or redirection, within those twenty years. It is not really surprising that this has not yet been done, because it is often difficult to assign a specific date to Arnau's individual writings, but it has meant that accounts of his thought tend to have a kind of flatness; they inevitably make it appear static and unchanging, fully matured, from the moment his new identities began, and they imply that medical and spiritual concerns were fused there from the start.[4] I mean to take advantage of the fact that we can identify with some confidence the works that – simultaneously – *launched* those two identities. I want to look closely at those works to see if we can understand them and their relationship not only as they were emerging at that moment within Arnau's mind, as it were, but also as they were emerging out of his earlier biography. The other contributors to this conference have addressed our theme as it played out in medieval society; let me offer some thoughts about its application to a single exemplary individual.

I

I want to begin by discussing the earliest of Arnau's scholastic medical works, the treatise he called *De intentione medicorum* – 'On the priorities of physicians'. We know that it was the earliest of his academic productions because it is quoted in almost every other one (while it quotes none of the others), and this suggests that we would not be far wrong if we dated it to the beginning of his Montpellier period – that is, to about 1291. The fact that he referred to it over and over again in those other medical works indicates how important it was and how central to his thought. As the title suggests, it dealt not with some specific point of pathology or therapeutics, but far more

[4] Cf. Santi, *Arnau de Vilanova*, p. 85: 'Hi ha una relació constant entre els escrits religiosos i els escrits mèdics.' Even Ziegler, who asks 'was Arnau of 1300–11 a different person from Arnau of the 1280s and 1290s?', in the end goes no further than to say that 'the fact that in both periods he concomitantly produced spiritual and medical texts suggests that he never clearly separated his spiritual from his medical interests' (*Medicine and Religion*, p. 33), without exploring the possibility of a development in Arnau's thought.

generally with what it was that should characterize a physician's practice. Arnau believed that medical knowledge involved a particular kind of truth: not absolute, abstract, ineluctable, logical philosophical truth, but a practical or heuristic truth, an instrumental truth. It is this that he argues in *De intentione*, that the physician does not need to worry about truth as certified by the natural philosopher; all he needs to do is to adopt a model or theory that does what he wants it to do – namely, allows him to treat patients so as to bring them back to health.

Arnau illustrates what he means by discussing, in turn, three areas where natural philosophers and physicians disagree about nature, explaining the same thing differently; in each case he shows that, while the philosophers are indeed giving a true account of affairs, the physicians' account, though not strictly true, is one that will allow them to treat their patients most effectively. The first of these, for example, is the well-known disagreement between Aristotle and Galen, and so between philosophers and physicians, over whether there is one principal member or four. Aristotle has said that the heart is prior to all the other members; Galen has declared that heart, liver, brain and testes are all equally fundamental. Arnau argues that while in principle no doubt Aristotle is correct, in practice the physician is concerned immediately with the proper functioning of the parts of the body, and therefore 'he will necessarily judge those members to be principal in which is directly manifest the function of powers disposing other members'.[5] There are four such proximate directors of functional activity, directing life, growth, activity and generation, and so the physician is right to think of *them* as the principal members, for if he insisted that, philosophically speaking, the heart was the only principal member, he would do damage to his patients:

> For if a flaw should occur merely in the act of sensing, and the physician called the heart rather than the brain the principle of sensing, he would then suppose that a passion or preternatural disposition existed in the heart, not the brain, which is evidently false, in that it is impossible that the heart should suffer illness without some power other than the sensitive one experiencing a flaw in its functioning, like the power moving the breath and pulse, which is called *vital* by the physician; and if an error should befall his judgement or understanding, a physician will inevitably fall into error in practising, for he would apply to the parts of the heart the healing remedy that he ought to apply to the region of the brain.[6]

[5] '[E]a membra necessario iudicabit principalia in quibus immediate manifestabitur operatio virtutum ceteris disponentium membris': Arnau de Vilanova, *De intentione* ii.1, p. 105 lines 5–7.

[6] 'Si namque vitium cadat in opere sentiendi solum, et medicus cor dicat esse sentiendi principium et non cerebrum, iudicabit tunc in corde passionem seu dispositionem preter naturam existere, non in cerebro – quod tamen falsum relinquitur evidenter, eo quod est impossibile quod cor patiatur absque eo quod alia virtus preter sensitivam vitium in opere non incurrat, utpote virtus hanelitum et

In the same way Arnau deals with two other disagreements between natural philosophers and physicians: the question of whether a middle or neutral state exists between sickness and health (philosophers say no, physicians say yes), and of whether medicines can change the body without themselves being changed (again, philosophers say no, physicians say yes). In each case, he argues that the physician's answer, though not indeed strictly true, is true in an instrumental sense in that it shows the kind of treatment that is required in order to return the patient to health. Arnau insisted for the rest of his life on the fundamental importance of this instrumentalism for the physician, who must value his patient's well-being above philosophical 'truth'.

Simultaneously with *De intentione* Arnau somehow found time to produce a series of prophetic treatises on a subject that for some reason had suddenly become of overwhelming interest to him: the end of history and the second coming of Christ, which he found foretold in scriptural and other sources as scheduled for the following century. His earliest work along this line was finished about 1290 but was shown to no one for many years; subsequently it was revised several times, and it no longer survives in its original form.[7] His next two works, however, both completed by 1292, *were* made public. The first of these, the *Introductio in librum Ioachim de semine scripturarum*, was a commentary on an apocalyptic work that Arnau believed had been written by Joachim da Fiore, a work that assigned letters of the alphabet to past centuries in order to reveal the pattern of history. By applying this technique to the book of Daniel, Arnau could predict the transformations that would begin in the fourteenth century when Antichrist would appear, and would end in the fifteenth when history would come to a close. That the letters can have such significance is for Arnau the consequence of a more general principle, that *all*

pulsum exercens, que vitalis a medico nuncupatur; et si error in iudicio seu cognitione ceciderit, necessario medicus operando incidet in errorem, nam causam sanitatis quam deberet applicare cerebri regioni cordis partibus applicabit': Arnau de Vilanova, *De intentione* ii.1, p. 105 lines 18–28.

7 This work is the so-called *De adventu antichristi*, beginning 'Constitui vos', which in its surviving form has one portion carrying the internal date 1297 and another dated 1300; it was the latter version that earned Arnau a brief imprisonment late that year at the hands of the Parisian faculty of theology. Elsewhere he referred to the earlier history of this work, 'quam scripturam non divulgavi, nec etiam comunicavi, nisi quibusdam cartuscientibus in eorum monesterio longe post, bene per .vii. annos. Deinde post, fere per quadrienium, missus per regem Aragonum ad regem Francie, causaliter divulgavi Parisius': M. Batllori, 'Dos nous escrits espirituals d'Arnau de Vilanova', *AST* 23 (1955), 45–70 (p. 61). It is on this basis that I date the original draft to 1290. Batllori (p. 52) argued that this passage meant that the original had been written in 1288, subtracting the total of eleven years from 1299, when he thought Arnau had been imprisoned. But we now know that the king's embassy to Paris took place in the latter half of 1300 rather than the previous year (see M. R. McVaugh, 'Further Documents for the Biography of Arnau de Vilanova', *Dynamis* 2 (1988), 363–72 [pp. 367–8]), and Arnau's phrase 'fere per quadrienium' could certainly mean three-plus years, from early 1297 to late 1300. Lee, '*Scrutamini Scripturas*', p. 33 n. 2, also suggests the year 1290, though on somewhat different grounds.

human knowledge contains within itself the elements for prophecy – which means that as human knowledge grows, our prophetic understanding too will grow. Here Arnau reminded his readers of I Corinthians 13. 9–10: 'For we know in part and we prophesy in part. But when that which is perfect is come, that which is in part shall be done away.'[8] In effect, Arnau has had to develop an account of the nature and power of human knowledge, in order to justify his procedure. He concludes the *Introductio* with a remarkable enumeration of the spheres of human knowledge, each with its achievements leading on *misterialiter* to higher things and more perfect truth: grammar, arithmetic, music, astrology, natural philosophy, metaphysics and so forth. Of the geometer's knowledge, for example, he exults:

> here is that geometrical circle with which every angle and multilateral figure is described suitably by the logic of mystery, and where all multigonal figures, resolved ultimately in a triangle, terminate in its occurrence, that mystery of the beginning of all things which we surely know to be the indivisible Trinity.[9]

It comes as a kind of break in this itemization of intellectual potential, therefore, to find Arnau treating medical knowledge less exaltedly, less confidently, very differently from these other forms:

> He who loves well-being – that is, the physician – pursues it so that he may confer health; [but] studying the variety of natural, non-natural and contranatural things, he applies his understanding to them only so far as is necessary *misterialiter* to bring about well-being, following the Apostle's command, 'Know only what you need to know.'[10]

Medical knowledge is different from these other kinds of knowledge, Arnau seems to be saying; it does not claim to look forward to eternal truths, indeed *it* conforms to a very different injunction from St Paul: 'Know only what you need to know' (Romans 12. 3, my translation).[11] And when we remember that

[8] 'Ex parte enim cognoscimus, et ex parte prophetamus. Cum autem venerit quod perfectum est, evacuabitur quod ex parte est': Manselli, 'Religiosità', p. 48. Lee, '*Scrutamini Scripturas*', pp. 42–8, provides a fuller summary of the work.

[9] 'Hic est etiam ille geometricus circulus infra quem omnis angularis et multilatera figura describitur convenienter ad misterii rationem, ubi etiam omnes figure multigone, finaliter in triangulum resolute, ipsius passionibus initunter, haud dubium non sine misterio principii rerum omnium quod firmiter esse scimus individuam Trinitatem': Manselli, 'Religiosità', pp. 57–8. The translation is that of Lee, '*Scrutamini Scripturas*', pp. 46–7.

[10] 'Hic salutis amator accedit ut conferat sanitatem, videlicet, medicus, qui, rerum naturalium, non naturalium, et contra naturam diversitatem enumerans, tantum in ipsis profundat indaginem intellectus quantum adquisitioni salutis misterialiter est necesse – iuxta illud Apostoli, "Non plus sapere quam oportet"': Manselli, 'Religiosità', p. 58.

[11] The interpretation that I am suggesting Arnau placed on this passage would seem to agree with that of the *Glossa ordinaria*, 'Quod iusticie terminos non egrediatur quod nobis solum utile fit': *Biblia Latina cum glossa ordinaria*, IV, 299b.

Arnau was simultaneously working out the thesis of *De intentione medicorum*, the break in his argument here in the *Introductio* becomes understandable. He was developing a theory of knowledge in the early 1290s from two different perspectives at the same time, that of medicine and that of theology, and he is trying to reconcile them here: medical instrumentalism, he knew, had to be sharply distinguished from philosophical knowledge, yet it was philosophical knowledge that was related *misterialiter* to prophecy. The consequence would seem inevitably to be that the *misterium* of medicine can apply only to the acquisition of health, not to the prophetic understanding. We might remember that the passage that he quoted from Romans goes on to remind readers that 'in one body we have many members, but all the members have not the same office (*in uno corpore multa membra habemus, omnia autem membra non eumdem actum habent*)'.

This interpretation seems to find some support in the work Arnau composed immediately after the *Introductio*, the *Allocutio super Tetragrammaton*. He completed the *Allocutio* in the summer of 1292, while at the castle of Meuillon in Provence, fifty kilometres north of Avignon.[12] It was an outgrowth of the study of Hebrew that he had undertaken in the early 1280s, and in it he applied the exegetical techniques he had laid out in the *Introductio* to an analysis of the symbolic meaning of the Hebrew symbols *yod, he, vav, he,* standing for the Name of God (IHVH). He argued that in fact the Hebrew characters, properly understood, revealed the nature of the Christian Trinity: *yod,* the simplest character and the origin of all the others, has the nature of 'a beginning without a beginning (*principium sine principio*)' and represents God the Father; *vav,* formed from two *yods* and, like *yod,* a source of all the other letters, 'has the nature of a beginning from a beginning (*habet rationem principii ex principio*)' and represents the Son; while the aspirate *he,* following both the Father and the Son, reveals the Holy Spirit.[13]

> It follows manifestly that [the Tetragrammaton] signifies that there are three persons in God, of which one has the nature of a true and perfect father, the second of a perfect son, and the third of their mutual love.[14]

To back up his argument, Arnau points to the realm of biological generation, where a *principium ex principio* is properly called 'son (*filius*)' and a *principium*

[12] The text is published by J. Carreras Artau, 'La *Allocutio super Tetragrammaton* de Arnaldo de Vilanova', *Sefarad* 9 (1949), 75–105.

[13] Carreras Artau, 'La *Allocutio*', pp. 93–4. Lee, '*Scrutamini Scripturas*', pp. 48–53, gives a more systematic explication of the work. See also E. Colomer, 'La interpretación del Tetragrama bíblico en Ramón Martí y Arnau de Vilanova', *Sprache und Erkenntnis im Mittelalter*, ed. J. P. Beckmann and W. Kluxen, 2 vols., Miscellanea Mediaevalia 13/2 (Berlin, 1981), II, 937–45.

[14] 'Manifeste relinquetur quod propriissime significat in Deo esse tres personas, quarum una rationem habet veri Patris et perfecti. Alia vero perfecti Filii. Tertia vero rationem mutui amoris': Carreras Artau, 'La *Allocutio*', p. 94.

sine principio is properly called either a 'father' or a 'mother'; but only 'father', he says, is appropriate to a perfect God, since paternal generation is perfect and maternal generation imperfect. A mother, he explains, generates not actively but passively, *non ex se sed ab alio,* whereas a father generates *active et ex se.*[15]

Joseph Ziegler has already recognized that in this passage Arnau was accepting the Aristotelian interpretation of conception, according to which the mother contributes only matter, menstrual blood, to the fetus, while the father's seed carries the activating soul, and he has pointed out perceptively that Arnau had chosen here to say nothing about the very different Galenic understanding of the process, where both male and female seed are viewed as formal contributors to the fetus.[16] I would go on to propose that Arnau's silence on this point is particularly significant in the light of the theory of knowledge that we know he had just developed in *De intentione* and the *Introductio.* The position he had worked out in the former treatise would have allowed him to argue in the *Allocutio* that the medical and philosophical interpretations were both true, each in its own way, if he had wanted to remind the reader of the autonomy and value of the medical perspective that he as a physician possessed, because the difference between the Aristotelian and Galenic theories is exactly the sort of controversy he had already repeatedly resolved instrumentally in *De intentione medicorum.* However, the ideas he developed in the *Introductio* had led him to the conviction that where exegesis and prophetic understanding are concerned, a specifically medical, instrumental, truth has no value, and it would have been irrelevant here even to point out that such heuristic 'truths' might exist and be of use in providing for physical health. Rather than representing a way of being 'theologically medical', it seems to me, his discussion here might be better understood as being deliberately *'non-*medical'.[17] If I am right, his two careers, his two identities, were at this stage still quite distinct.

II

Yet at this early stage in their development one could still inform the other, as the contents of *De intentione* also reveal. That work begins, as we saw, by addressing and smoothing over three medical disagreements with natural philosophers, all widely discussed in medical faculties. But Arnau concluded his treatise by addressing a fourth question that seems not to have worried earlier medical masters, one concerning the nature of

[15] Carreras Artau, 'La *Allocutio*', p. 94.

[16] Ziegler, *Medicine and Religion*, pp. 62–3.

[17] Ziegler, *Medicine and Religion*, p. 250.

the soul:[18] is the essence of the soul the complexion, as Galen said, or is the Philosopher correct to deny that soul is such a 'harmony of miscibles'? Arnau says no more than this about Aristotle's views, perhaps because the details would have been familiar to any arts graduate, who would have known that the notion that the soul was a harmonious blend of the elements had been criticized by Aristotle in *De anima* i.4, five hundred years before Galen:

> [They] say that the soul is a kind of harmony, for (*a*) harmony is a blend or composition of contraries, and (*b*) the body is compounded out of contraries. Harmony, however, is a certain proportion or composition of the constituents blended, and soul can be neither the one nor the other of these.[19]

As in the other three disputes, Arnau is ready to concede the basic truth of the Aristotelian position; this time, however, he is not so much trying to defend an alternative medical viewpoint instrumentally as he is concerned to show that Galen cannot really have meant what he is supposed to have said. It is, in fact, an instance of what Vivian Nutton describes in this volume as 'the depaganization of Galen'.

But what exactly had Galen said, and where had Arnau come upon his remarks? Curiously, while Galen commented many times in his works on the problem of the soul, it was invariably to insist on its intractability, to declare that we know nothing at all about the essence of the soul.[20] Only towards the end of his life, in the work *Quod animi mores corporis tempora sequantur*, did he outline an argument that the soul must be a mixture or *krasis* of the four qualities, and then only hypothetically; he himself vouched for nothing more than that evidence demonstrated some sort of dependence of soul on body. In this sense, the title of the work (which is Galen's own) is somewhat misleading.[21] And in any case *Quod animi mores* could not have been available

[18] The complete text of Arnau's discussion of this subject is in Arnau de Vilanova, *De intentione* ii.1, pp. 124–6.

[19] 'Dicunt enim quod [anima] est aliquod armonicum. Armonia enim est admixtio et compositio contrariorum, et corpus est compositum ex contrariis. Licet armonia sit proportio inter res admixtas aut compositio; anima autem non est alterum duorum': Aristotle, *De anima* i.4, 407b27 et seq.; Averroes, *Commentarium Magnum in Aristotelis de Anima libros*, ed. F. S. Crawford, Corpus Commentariorum Averrois in Aristotelem, Versionum Latinorum 6,1, Medieval Academy of America 59 (Cambridge, MA, 1953), p. 75. The translation is that of *The Works of Aristotle*, ed. J. A. Smith and W. D. Ross, 12 vols. (Oxford, 1910–52), III, 407b.

[20] Cf. A.-E. Chaignet, *Histoire de la psychologie des grecs*, 5 vols. (Paris, 1890; repr. Brussels, 1966), III, 357–8; Temkin, *Galenism*, pp. 81–4; P. Moraux, 'Galien comme philosophe', in *Galen: Problems*, pp. 87–116 (pp. 91–3).

[21] L. García-Ballester, 'Alma y cuerpo, enfermedad del alma y enfermedad del cuerpo en el pensamiento médico de Galeno', *Revista de la Asociación Española de Neuropsiquiatría* 16 (1996), 710–20, and 'Soul and Body, Disease of the Soul and Disease of the Body in Galen's Medical Thought', in *Le opere psicologiche di Galeno*, ed. P. Manuli and M. Vegetti (Naples, 1988), pp. 117–52 (pp. 124–37). These works emend and

to Arnau in a Latin translation in the 1290s, for it was first translated by Niccolò da Reggio in the early fourteenth century.[22] Indeed, a few years before, when Pietro d'Abano had reported in his *Conciliator* that 'some moderns say Galen believed the soul to be a crasis', he added that he could find no such statement in Galen's writings.[23] So what is the source of Arnau's firm assertion?

Arnau himself here says only that 'Galen declares in many of his books, especially in *De demonstrationibus*, that the essence of soul is the complexion, or rather a harmony of miscibles, writing on this too in connection with *virtus* in *De rebus contra naturam*'; a little later he again singles out '*De demonstrationibus*' as a principal source for this doctrine.[24] *De demonstratione* was a long and important Galenic book that is lost today, though an overall reconstruction of its contents has been attempted on the basis of the references to it and quotations from it that can be found in Greek and Arabic sources. Much of it was translated into Arabic by Hunayn and his successors in the ninth century and quoted extensively by Rhazes in his *Hawi* in the tenth, but by that time it was already becoming difficult to find the complete text. Its later history in the Arabic-speaking world is uncertain; Averroes may still have been able to consult the text in the twelfth century, but today the Arabic translation as well as the Greek original has disappeared.[25]

The Latin West, therefore, knew of *De demonstratione* simply from scattered references by Rhazes and by some Greek authors translated into Latin, and one of the latter – the fourth-century bishop Nemesius of Emesa – provides in his *De natura hominis* a reason for believing that Galen did indeed discuss the nature of the soul as *krasis* in *De demonstratione*:

> Galen [Nemesius wrote] says nothing about the soul, and further in *De demonstratione* declares that he has said nothing about it. Yet it may be presumed, from what he does say, that he inclines to identify the soul with

revise García-Ballester's earlier discussion in *Alma y enfermedad en la obra de Galeno* (Valencia–Granada, 1972), esp. pp. 181–200.

Galen refers to this work by this title in *De libris propriis* (K 19, p. 46: *Galeni scripta minora*, ed. I. Mueller, 3 vols. (Leipzig, 1891), II, 122); however, *De libris propriis* was not known in the Middle Ages either, and thus not even the misleading title could have been the origin of Arnau's statement.

[22] Lynn Thorndike, 'Translations of Works of Galen from the Greek by Niccolò da Reggio (*c.* 1308–1345)', *Byzantina Metabyzantina* 1 (1946), 213–35 (p. 229); the medieval translation begins 'Quoniam corporis complexionem sequuntur . . . '.

[23] 'Quidam . . . modernorum imposuerunt Galenum velle ipsum animam fore crasim': Pietro d'Abano, *Conciliator*, diff. 17, fol. 27ra.

[24] 'Dicit enim magnus Galienus in multis librorum suorum, specialiter tamen in libro de demonstrationibus, essentiam anime fore complexionem, aut magis proprie miscibilium armoniam, illud idem scribens etiam de virtute in libro de rebus contra naturam': Arnau de Vilanova, *De intentione* ii.4, p. 124 lines 16–20; see also p. 125 lines 20–4.

[25] Only fragments of this work survive; they have been reconstructed by von Müller, 'Galens Werk'. See also G. Strohmaier, 'Galen in Arabic: Prospects and Projects', in *Galen: Problems*, pp. 187–96 (p. 191).

temperament. For he says that differences of behavior are consequent upon temperament, constructing his argument with the help of Hippocrates.[26]

Nemesius's work was twice translated into Latin in the Middle Ages, by Alphanus of Salerno in the eleventh century and by Burgundio of Pisa in 1165, this latter version subsequently mined for quotations by Albertus Magnus and Thomas Aquinas.[27] Although Arnau does not mention Nemesius's book, there is some reason to suspect that it was his source, at least indirectly, and that he had learned about it by chance in the early 1280s, in the course of his study of Hebrew.

At about the time that Pere II brought Arnau to Barcelona as physician to the court, in 1281, the Dominican order appointed Ramon Martí as lector in the school of oriental languages it had established in the same city twenty years before, and Martí taught there until his death sometime after 1284;[28] in this school, Arnau tells us in the *Allocutio super tetragrammaton*, he had studied Hebrew with Ramon Martí himself. Arnau also tells us there of his admiration for Martí's great *Pugio fidei*, completed in 1278, today recognized as 'the magnum opus of medieval missionizing among the Jews'.[29] Arnau describes it enthusiastically as 'a glorious book that I firmly believe he wrote under divine inspiration';[30] it had provided him with the starting point for his interpretation of the meaning of the Tetragrammaton, and he seems still to have had a copy of the work in his library at the time of his death.[31]

[26] This translation is that made from the Greek in *Cyril of Jerusalem and Nemesius of Emesa*, ed. W. Telfer, Library of Christian Classics 4 (Philadelphia, 1955), pp. 271–2; the Greek is available in von Müller, 'Galens Werk', p. 463. Alphanus's version of this passage is 'Galenus autem testari videtur in demonstrativis sermonibus, tamquam nihil de anima appareat loquens; sed videre ex his, quae dicit, ut magis velit crasin id est temperantiam esse animam (hanc enim consequuntur morum differentiae), ex dictis Hippocratis confirmas rationem': *Nemesii episcopi Premnon Physicon . . . a N. Alfano . . . translatus*, ed. C. Burkhard (Leipzig, 1917), p. 33. In Burgundio's version, it reads: 'Galenus autem enuntiat quidem nihil, sed et contestatur in Demonstrativis suis sermonibus quod nihil erat de anima enuntiaturus; videtur autem ex quibus dicit existimare magis complexionem esse animam, hanc enim sequi morum differentiam, ex his quae Hippocratis sunt construens hunc sermonem'; *Nemesius d'Emèse* De natura hominis, ed. G. Verbeke and J. R. Moncho, Corpus Latinum commentariorum in Aristotelem Graecorum, Suppl. 1 (Leiden, 1975), p. 32.

[27] M. Morani, *La tradizione manoscritta del* De natura hominis *di Nemesio* (Milan, 1981).

[28] A. Berthier, 'Un maître orientaliste du XIIIe siècle: Raymond Martin, O.P.', *AFP* 6 (1936), 267–311 (p. 277); on Martí's date of death, see *Raimundi Martini capistrum judaeorum*, ed. A. Robles Sierra (Würzburg, 1990), p. 9.

[29] R. Chazan, *Daggers of Faith: Thirteenth-Century Christian Missionizing and Jewish Response* (Berkeley, 1989), p. 115.

[30] 'Illud gloriosum opus quod credo firmiter editum divino spiramine per ministerium et laborem predicti viri': Arnau de Vilanova, *Allocutio*, in Carreras Artau, 'La *Allocutio*', p. 80.

[31] Colomer, 'La interpretación', pp. 937–9. Inventoried among Arnau's books after his death was 'una summa in pergameno et in ebraico scripta et glosata in latino contra judeos' (R. d'Alòs, 'De la marmessoria d'Arnau de Vilanova', *Miscel.lània Prat de la*

The *Pugio* is not all anti-Judaic apologetics, as a matter of fact; the first book is in part a critique of Greek and Muslim philosophical errors corrected in the light of the Christian faith, and one of Martí's targets here is *Galenus falsiloquus*.[32] Arnau the physician would certainly have been taken aback by this denunciation, would surely have read closely the particular Galenic doctrine that Martí singled out for attack – which was, as it happens, the idea that the soul is to be identified with the complexion. Martí summarizes this view as follows:

> [Galen] asserted that the complexion was the soul, influenced by the fact that he recognized that the various passions that we attribute to the soul are caused by different complexions: those who have a sanguine complexion rejoice for no reason, melancholics easily become sad, the choleric grow angry for no reason, phlegmatics react slowly.[33]

He does not identify the work from which his reference is taken, however, so that the *Pugio*-text cannot be the *only* source of Arnau's allusion to Galen's teaching.

There remains, nevertheless, a further possibility. Historians have long been aware that the first book of the *Pugio fidei* draws frequently on Thomas Aquinas's *Summa contra gentiles* (written 1259–64) for its arguments – it is one of the earliest texts to do so – and Martí's criticism of Galen on the soul proves to be based on Thomas's work.[34] The *Summa*'s discussion of the problem is a fuller one, which refutes it in two chapters: to begin with, 'Quod anima non sit complexio, ut posuit Galenus'.[35] Thomas follows by proving 'quod anima non sit harmonia', a view he says is really similar to the first one because its adherents 'are not saying that the soul is a harmony of sounds but of the contraries out of which they recognize that animated bodies are formed'; among those adherents he identifies Empedocles, cited by Aristotle in *De*

Riba (Barcelona, 1923), I, 289–306 (p. 305); the identification with the *Pugio* was proposed by J. Carreras Artau, 'La llibreria d'Arnau de Vilanova', *AST* 11 (1935), 63–84 (p. 69).

32 'Galenus cum maxima naturalium et physicorum turba apparebit falsiloquus': Ramon Martí, *Pugio fidei adversus Mauros et Judaeos* I.i.7 (Leipzig, 1687), p. 194.

33 '[Galenus] animam posuit esse complexionem, motus ex hoc, quod vidit ex diversis complexionibus diversas passiones causari, quae attribuuntur animae: sanguineam namque habentes complexionem pro nihilo gaudent, melancholici vero tristantur de facili, colerici irascuntur pro modico, tarde moventur phlegmatici': Martí, *Pugio* I.iv.10, p. 206.

34 Berthier, 'Un maître', pp. 299–301; M. D. Jordan, 'Medicine and Natural Philosophy in Aquinas', in *Thomas von Aquin: Werk und Wirkung im Licht neuerer Forschungen*, ed. A. Zimmermann, Miscellanea Mediaevalia 19 (Berlin, 1988), 233–46 (p. 236), and 'The Disappearance of Galen in Thirteenth-Century Philosophy and Theology', in *Mensch und Natur im Mittelalter*, ed. A. Zimmermann and A. Speer, 2 vols., Miscellanea Mediaevalia 21/2 (Berlin, 1992), II, 703–13 (pp. 703–4).

35 Thomas Aquinas, *Summa contra gentiles* ii.63 in *Liber de Veritate Catholicae Fidei contra errores Infidelium seu 'Summa contra Gentiles'*, ed. C. Pera with P. Marc and P. Caramello, 3 vols. (Rome and Turin, 1961–7), II, 199.

anima, and 'Dinarchus', cited, Thomas says, by Gregory of Nyssa.[36] In this latter reference lies a clue to the source of Thomas's information about Galen: here and elsewhere Thomas makes frequent use of a work by 'Gregory of Nyssa' which we now know to have been in fact the *De natura hominis* of Alphanus, and it turns out to be demonstrably that work from which Thomas is drawing in these two chapters.

It does not seem too far-fetched, therefore, to speculate that Arnau first became sensitized to the issue of the soul as complexion through his acquaintance with Martí and the *Pugio fidei*, and that he was led to Alphanus's account of the Galenic position by his Dominican teacher, who knew of it from the *Summa*. Certainly there is no reason to think that Arnau was directly acquainted with Thomas's work and drew on it rather than on Martí's, though a copy of the *Summa* would have been available to him at the Dominican *studium* in Barcelona. Although the *Pugio* repeats the language of the *Summa contra gentiles* almost verbatim in posing the problem, the two refute the view attributed to Galen in quite different ways. Arnau's *De intentione* seems to be rephrasing an argument found in the *Pugio*; it has nothing in common with those of the *Summa*. Arnau concedes that Galen may have said that soul and complexion are identical, but he denies that Galen can actually have meant this; he does so by positing that variability cannot inhere in the soul and asserting that since the activities of which it is ultimately the author *do* vary, there must be an intermediate variable agent between *anima* and *operatio*, which 'can only be a *complexio* or, more properly, a harmony of miscibles'.[37] This strongly suggests a recasting of Ramon Martí's argument that

> the complexion is always changing and undergoing a constant transformation, because of transforming causes like the natural heat and external heat; so if the aforesaid essence of man were the complexion, it could never be the same as it had been years before, yet it is a fundamental axiom that that essence is now what it was then. So this kind of essence cannot be the complexion, which has changed over a thousand times during that period.[38]

[36] Thomas Aquinas, *Summa contra gentiles* ii.64, pp. 199–200.

[37] 'solum reperiatur complexio (vel magis proprie miscibilium armonia) . . .': Arnau de Vilanova, *De intentione* ii.4, p. 125 lines 7–8.

[38] 'Complexio propter causas dissolventes, ut est calor naturalis et calores exteriores . . . semper est in dissolutione & permutatione continua; si ergo essentia hominis supradicta esset complexio, nullo modo poterit invenire seipsum esse illum qui fuit ante permultos annos: sed ipsum esse illum quoque nunc, qui fuit tunc, est firmissima mentis ejus conceptio. Hujusmodi ergo essentia ejus non potest esse complexio, quae ab illo tempore forsitan est plusquam millesies permutata': Martí, *Pugio*, p. 206. Thomas makes a related point in passing when he reasons that 'complexio, cum sit quiddam constitutum ex contrariis qualitatibus quasi medium inter eas, impossibile est quod sit forma substantialis; nam substantiae nihil est contrarium, *nec suscipit magis et minus* [my emphasis]. Anima autem est forma substantialis et non accidentalis . . .; anima igitur non est complexio': Aquinas, *Summa contra gentiles* ii.64, p. 199. But certainly this brief phrase (which Aquinas is quoting from Aristotle, *Categories* 5) is far less likely than the passage just given from

This reconstruction of Arnau's intellectual development in the early 1280s would make it more understandable why, a few years later, this relatively obscure theological issue should have been on his mind and should have been included in *De intentione*, attached to three others of far greater importance to current medical debate within the schools.[39]

To be sure, this neat story has its difficulties. First, Nemesius's report of Galen's views is far less positive than is Arnau's presentation of them. Nor does the specific phrase given three times by Arnau (twice directly attributed to Galen), that 'animam esse miscibilium armoniam', appear in either of the translations of Nemesius. And the title Arnau gives to Galen's work, *De demonstrationibus*, is not that which it has in both of those translations.[40]

Hence it remains conceivable that Arnau learned of *De demonstratione*, not from Ramon Martí (or not simply from him), but from a further source still unknown. There are other references to this work in his writings, and they seem to reflect themes that are mentioned by no one else. Towards the end of *De intentione* ii.4, for example, Arnau seems to be going a little further in his account of Galen's book:

> In his book *De demonstrationibus* Galen teaches that the physician calls the soul a harmony of miscibles, and calls the complexion or power resulting from it a *virtus*; but he postpones a more thorough treatment lest he be distracted from his purpose.[41]

the *Pugio* to have given rise to Arnau's emphasis on stablity/variability as the feature distinguishing *anima* from *complexio*.

39 The Parisian condemnations of 1277 were promulgated just a year before Martí's *Pugio fidei* was finished, and some of the positions condemned there by Etienne Tempier could perhaps be taken, by extension, to include the supposed Galenic teaching that because the powers of the soul depend on the complexion, the soul must be equivalent to the complexion: for example, 'Quod in hora generationis hominis in corpore suo et per consequens in anima, quae sequitur corpus, ex ordine causarum superiorum et inferiorum inest homini dispositio inclinans ad tales actiones vel eventus'; or again, even more directly, 'Quod anima est inseparabilis a corpore; et quod ad corruptionem harmoniae corporis corrumpitur anima': P. Mandonnet, *Siger de Brabant et l'averroïsme latin au XIIIme siècle* (Louvain, 1908), part 2, pp. 184 and 185; nos. 105 and 133. But I think the parallel can only be a coincidence; after all, Bishop Tempier and his advisors were not the only authorities disturbed by the growing naturalism of their age. I see no reason to believe that Martí was aware of the Parisian condemnations when he set down his critique of 'Galen', and no reason either to think that they played a part in Arnau's own intellectual development.

Yet another, different, critique of the soul=complexion doctrine that Martí (and Arnau) could have cited but did not is provided in Avicenna's *Liber de anima* i.2, ed. S. van Riet, 2 vols., Avicenna Latinus (Louvain, 1968–72), I, 43 and 47.

40 Above, n. 26.

41 'Secundum hanc ergo considerationem proprie loquendo docuit Galienus in libro de demonstrationibus medicum dicere animam esse miscibilium armoniam, complexionem vero ab ea resultantem tanquam potentiam eius vocare virtutem; postponit autem altiorem considerationem ne ab opere retardetur': Arnau de Vilanova, *De intentione* ii.4, p. 125 lines 20–4.

Again, in the *Repetitio super canone 'Vita brevis'* (1301) Arnau cited the treatise 'de demonstrationibus medicinalibus' as one of the works in which Galen explained the distinction 'inter dyalecticam et medicinalem scientiam vel investigationem'.[42] These references to thematic material may merely be creations of Arnau's imagination, but they may also be valid indications of the lost contents of *De demonstratione*. It is possible that they are drawn from allusions to *De demonstratione* made by other authors who have not yet been identified – Rhazes, for example. In his *Hawi* (the Latin *Continens*) Rhazes quotes widely and extensively from many Galenic works, including *De demonstratione*, and the *Continens* is so large a book that no full index of his authorities has yet been made.[43] Arnau is unlikely to have known the *Hawi* in its Latin translation, since that was completed only in 1279, but he might well have come upon a part or all of it in Arabic.[44] It is not even impossible that he

42 'Ad primum autem cognoscendum dat Galienus in pluribus locis doctrinam et specialiter in primo de interioribus ubi docet distinguere inter dyalecticam et medicinalem scientiam vel investigationem in tractatu diffinitionis medicine et de demonstrationibus medicinalibus': Arnau de Vilanova, *Repetitio super canone Vita brevis*, in *Opera Arnaldi* (Lyons, 1504), fol. 337ra. Here, to be sure, Arnau may be developing Galen's own reference to *De demonstratione*, at the end of the *Tegni* ('Oportet . . . ut exerceantur in libro meo quem edidi in demonstratione qui vult uti hac arte per viam ratiocinationis et exerceri in ea'), in the light of Haly Ridwan's commentary on this passage: 'Docuit per hunc sermonem modum necessitatis que est de arte dialectice in arte medicine. Manifestum est enim quod non scitur rectum et certum nec rectificatur ab errore nisi per artem dialecticam solam' (text and commentary both in *Articella* (Venice, 1523), [II] fol. 155rb).

43 Likewise Rhazes' *al-Shukuk 'ala Jalinus* – 'Objections to Galen' – is now known to quote widely from *De demonstratione* and to provide more passages from it than were known to von Müller, though apparently the Arnaldian citation is not one of them: see G. Strohmaier, 'Bekannte und unbekannte Zitate in den *Zweifeln an Galen* des Rhazes', in *Text and Tradition*, pp. 263–87. Rhazes considered *De demonstratione* as 'le plus sublime et le plus utile des livres après les divines écritures, objet de la révélation'; S. Pines, 'Razi critique de Galien', *Actes du VIIIe Congrès International d'Histoire des Sciences* (Paris, 1953) pp. 480–7 (also in *Studies in Arabic Versions of Greek Texts and in Mediaeval Science*, The Collected Works of Shlomo Pines (Jerusalem and Leiden, 1986), II, 256–63).

44 In his medical writings, Arnau expresses particular admiration for Rhazes, as J. A. Paniagua pointed out long ago ('L'Arabisme à Montpellier dans l'oeuvre d'Arnau de Vilanova', *Le Scalpel* 117 (1964), 631–7 (p. 631); reprinted in *Studia Arnaldiana* (Barcelona, 1995), p. 319). Indeed, Arnau praises Rhazes much more warmly than he does Avicenna, despite his regular use of the *Canon*. It is at least conceivable that his admiration led him to look for works by Rhazes that were not available in Latin, and that he came upon the *Hawi* in this way. It is worth pointing out that two of Rhazes' writings praised by Arnau are today unknown under the Latin titles he gives them: a work 'De comprehensione multorum' is mentioned in *De consideracionibus operis medicine*, ed. L. Demaitre, *AVOMO* IV (Barcelona, 1988), p. 249, for example, while *De intentione* itself acknowledges a particular debt to Rhazes' 'libello . . . de concordia philosophorum et medicorum'. Perhaps in each of these cases Arnau was rendering into Latin a title that he had found attached to an Arabic text. The first could well be an allusion to the *Hawi* – or even to the lost *al-Jami' al-kabir* that is supposedly different from *al-Hawi*: see M. Ullmann, *Die Medizin im Islam* (Leiden,

was acquainted with *De demonstratione* itself – that is, with that part of it which still survived in Arabic translation in the later Middle Ages – and that these references testify directly to its contents. Neither of these suggestions is inconsistent with his having first learned of the work through Ramon Martí, for he could then have tried to obtain more information about it from Arabic sources; it is worth remembering that Arnau was not only studying Hebrew in the early 1280s, he was also seeking out Arabic-language medical works and rendering them into Latin, as his Arabic–Latin translation of Galen's *De rigore* (completed in Barcelona in 1282) reveals.[45]

The second work that Arnau cited as a source for Galen's views on the soul, the 'liber de rebus contra naturam', is nearly as intriguing as *De demonstratione*. No Galenic work is known by this title in either Greek or Arabic, and it would be tempting to dismiss the reference as mistaken or imaginary if it were not for three very specific further allusions to the title in Arnau's *De considerationibus operis medicine*. These three references identify the work in question, for they correspond to passages in Books 2, 3 and 4 of the work known to the Middle Ages as *De accidenti et morbo*. This 'book' was in reality a compilation by the Alexandrian commentators of late antiquity of four originally independent Galenic works: *De morborum causis* (Book 1 of *De accidenti*); *De morborum differentiis* (Book 2); *De symptomatum differentiis* (Book 3); and *De symptomatum causis* (Books 4–6). The collection was translated into Arabic by Hunayn under the title *Kitâb al-ʿilal wa'l-aʿrâd* ('Book of illnesses and symptoms'); its Latin translator is still unidentified, but the translation seems to have been completed by the thirteenth century.[46]

Here again it is not impossible that Arnau's references to the 'liber de rebus contra naturam' reflect a knowledge of an Arabic text. His citations to

1970), p. 131, and the forthcoming article by E. Savage-Smith, 'The Working Files of Rhazes: Are the *Jamiʿ* and the *Hawi* Identical?', which argues that the two titles actually refer to the same work. Arnau's second reference, however, does not seem to correspond to any of Rhazes' known writings (see the lists in Ullmann, *Medizin*, pp. 128–36; and F. Sezgin, *Geschichte des arabischen Schrifttums*, 9 vols. (Leiden, 1970), III, 274–94).

45 Arnau de Vilanova, *Translatio libri Galieni de rigore*, ed. M. R. McVaugh, *AVOMO* XVI (Barcelona, 1981).

Vivian Nutton has pointed out to me that a knowledge of *De demonstratione*'s views on the soul could also have been acquired by Arnau (perhaps via Martí) from contemporary Hispano-Jewish philosophers such as Shem Tov ibn Falaquera of Tudela (d. 1295), who often made extensive use of Greek texts in Arabic translation. Indeed, in his *Sefer ha-nefesh* ibn Falaquera referred to the idea that the soul is complexion (though he did not ascribe it to Galen; his language suggests that he was reporting it from Avicenna's *De anima* [above, n. 39]), declaring that it had been shown to be absurd – see R. Jospe, *Torah and Sophia: The Life and Thought of Shem Tov Ibn Falaquera* (Cincinnati, 1988), p. 348.

46 On *De accidenti* and its history in Arabic, see Ullmann, *Medizin*, p. 42; Sezgin, *Geschichte*, III, 89–90; Lieber, 'Galen in Hebrew', pp. 172–3 and n. 27. R. J. Durling, 'Corrigenda and Addenda to Diels's Galenica', *Traditio* 37 (1981), 373–81 (p. 377), gives references to two thirteenth-century manuscripts of the Latin version.

Books 2, 3 and 4 correspond accurately to the Latin, but his specific language is not obviously based on the corresponding passages in the Arabic–Latin translation.[47] His title for the work, distinct from both the Latin and the Arabic title, is an accurate reflection of *De accidenti*'s contents – the 'contra-naturals' were, in scholastic medical theory, those things invariably opposed to health, namely *morbus et causa morbi et accidens morbi*[48] – and it may be Arnau's own coinage or the translation of a chance title in an Arabic manuscript. In any case, in the 1290s it was not yet widely known even in Latin.[49] Arnau probably came upon it, in whatever form, in searching for passages in Galen's other works that could illuminate the perplexing assertion in *De demonstratione* that soul was to be identified with complexion.

As it turns out, Galen *does* briefly allude to the nature of the soul in Book 5 of *De accidenti*, but his point there is not what we would expect, given Arnau's citation: rather than define *anima*, he explicitly refuses to do so, just

[47] Arnau's references to the work, and the passage to which he is apparently referring as it appears in the Arabic–Latin translation, are as follows:

(a) 'De preteritis non curet medicus nisi ut per ea veniat in notitiam presencium, quemadmodum G. docuit in secundo de rebus contra naturam' (*De consideracionibus*, ed. Demaitre; *AVOMO* IV, 182). Cf. 'Sed cum intentio mea sit in hoc loco dicere preteritas et presentes causas morborum simplicium quatenus ad presentia venire possumus . . .': *De accidenti et morbo* ii.2, in *Galieni Opera* (Venice, 1490), II, fol. 141rb.

(b) 'Sunt autem prime differencie accidencium sicut ostensum est in tercio de rebus contra naturam, lesio operationis, immutacio exeuntis a corpore, et immutacio qualitatis corporis' (*AVOMO* IV, 179). Here Arnau seems to have in mind the discussion in *De accidenti et morbo* iii.2, which explains that *accidentia* are divided into three: 'alia enim qualia corporis vocantur, alia repugnantia actioni et alia subsequentia, quorum alia sunt corpus minuentia nimis vel ultime, alia sonitus qui fiunt intra corpus et cetera que corpore sentiuntur'. These topics are covered in succeeding chapters: iii.3 and iii.4 deal specifically with *nocumentum actionis;* iii.5 with *accidentibus que fiunt in qualitate corporis;* and iii.6 with *exiens a corpore. Galieni Opera* II, fols. 142vb–143vb.

(c) 'Scit autem medicus sicut ostensum est in quarto de rebus contra naturam quod vehemens dolor sicut et vehemens delectacio non fiunt nisi in sensu tactus' (*AVOMO* IV, 223). Cf. 'Delitia vero et contrarium eius in omnibus sensibus fiunt, non tamen in omnibus equaliter, quia in visu minus quam in aliis efficiuntur, in tactu vero et gustu magis ceteris': *De accidenti et morbo* iv.6, in *Galieni Opera* II, fol. 145vb.

None of these seems to me to supply convincing evidence either that Arnau was or that he was not summarizing the Arabic–Latin translation in these passages.

[48] So Arnau himself explains the term in his *Speculum medicine*, c. 88: 'De rebus contra naturam' (*Opera Arnaldi*, fols. 32vb–33ra).

[49] In 1309 it was introduced as a study option in the curriculum of the medical faculty at Montpellier (*Cartulaire de l'université de Montpellier*, 2 vols. (Montpellier, 1890), I, 220). On its place in university medicine see L. García-Ballester, 'Arnau de Vilanova (*c.* 1240–1311) y la reforma de los estudios médicos en Montpellier (1309): El Hipócrates latino y la introducción del nuevo Galeno', *Dynamis* 2 (1982), 97–158 (pp. 131–4), although the genuineness of the commentary on *De accidenti* there tentatively ascribed to Arnau remains questionable.

as he so often does elsewhere.[50] In the midst of a discussion of *rigor*, explaining that, while this condition is caused by heat, nevertheless in it the extremities become cold, he digresses into an explanation that leads him to consider the physiological consequences of the passions, the *accidentia anime*:

> [This happens because] the natural heat is prior and superior to the other motions that are inside and outside the body. The same thing happens with the emotions, which also can move the spirits. Sometimes spirits or heat are drawn inside towards their origin, and sometimes moved outside. It is not appropriate here [*inconveniens est*] to define the nature of soul – if occasion offers we might at some point explore this subject, though it calls for boldness and even rashness. But leaving aside what soul *is*, let us see whether soul uses heat and spirit and blood as its instruments or whether perhaps it does not act through them but they act on their own. You can see and study this clearly in the emotions: for example, fear carries blood, heat and spirit within, namely back to their origin, the heart, so that the external parts of the body are cooled.[51]

Galen goes on to discuss the other emotions, showing that they too are produced in this way, before returning to *rigor* and saying that 'since rigor depends on hot humours, it is not surprising that the body's extremities should be cooled, because the ensouled power [*animata virtus*] rushes to the inner parts of the body along with blood and spirit, so that coldness seizes the extremities'.[52]

If this passage does not bear out Arnau's statement that Galen said *anima* was a harmony of miscibles, it does conform remarkably well to what Arnau claims he *meant* by that statement. Galen's point here seems to be that, whatever *anima* may be, it produces effects in the human body through the *animata virtus*, which, together with blood and spirit, is the vehicle for the

[50] As indeed Pietro d'Abano points out: *Conciliator*, diff. 17, fol. 27ra.

[51] 'Causa autem quare hoc contingit investiganda est; inde dico quod calor naturalis prior et dignior est ceteris motibus qui sunt in corpore interius et exterius quod in anime accidentiis contingit, cum quo etiam spiritus movetur; et aliquando spiritus sive calor moventur interius in suam originem et interdum ad exteriora moventur. Et dico quod diffinitio que essentiam anime ostendit, scilicet quid sit, hec dicere inconveniens est. Si vero oportunum tempus contigerit, forsitan aliquando inde disputabimus, quod quidem temeritati atque audacie pertinet. Et pretermisso hoc, quid sit ipsa anima, dicemus utrum anima exerceat hec scilicet calorem atque spiritum atque sanguinem sicut instrumentum aut nihil operetur in istis sed ipsimet per se exerceant. Hoc palam intelligere et videre poteris in accidentiis anime, verbi gratia timor sanguinem calorem atque spiritum reportat ad interiora, scilicet ad suam originem, id est ad cor, atque exteriora corporis refrigerantur': *De accidenti et morbo* v.5, in *Galieni Opera* II, fol. 149va.

[52] 'Non est mirum cum rigor contingat ex calidis humoribus si corporis extremitates refrigerantur, quia animata virtus ad corporis interiora fugit cum sanguine et spiritu, et propter hoc frigiditudo loca exteriora obtinet et non interiora': *De accidenti et morbo* v.5, in *Galieni Opera* II, fol. 149vb.

natural heat that is the first physical cause of bodily motions; the same general theme is widespread in Galen's other writings, that *virtus anime*, bodily complexion and psychophysiological effect are closely related.[53] And it is essentially this that Arnau now proceeds to argue in the concluding section of *De intentione* (ii.4).

It has been suggested that this section shows Arnau trying to bridge the gap between illnesses of the body and illnesses of the soul, and that it prepared the way for him 'to cure infirmities of the soul which have nothing to do with the well-being of the body'.[54] I am hesitant to believe that the passage warrants this inference, and that it allows us to see Arnau's later spiritual ideas already prefigured here in this medical work. In *De intentione*, after all, he is not trying to defend the literal truth of the supposed Galenic view that soul is to be identified with complexion, but to explain that Galen did not mean what he seems to have said; Arnau is insisting that Galen clearly and sharply – and correctly – distinguished the unchangeable soul from the variable cause of bodily illness and health.

Arnau's argument runs as follows. A physician cannot treat a patient effectively unless he understands the changing causes of the different members' function. These causes derive ultimately from the soul, but the immediate cause of the members' activity is the complexion, and Galen is simply referring to complexion *as though* (Arnau repeatedly uses the word 'tanquam') it were a variable soul or power of the soul that is informing a *virtus* responsible for a member's function. 'Virtus' in this sense cannot be what the philosophers say it is, either, namely a power of the soul, for then we could not speak of *virtutes* as inherent in the different members. Thus the physician is giving both 'anima' and 'virtus' a new instrumental definition that does not correspond to their meaning in philosophy; indeed, Arnau says, for a physician it is actually dangerous to understand *virtus* as the philosopher does, as a *potentia anime*, rather than as a cause of activity dependent on the complexion and identical in a sense with it.[55]

[53] Cf. *De interioribus* iii.7 (*Galieni Opera* II, fol. 125rb; K 8, p. 191; trans. R. E. Siegel, *Galen on the Affected Parts* (Basel, 1976), p. 93): 'Periti medici concordati sunt quia humores et corporis compositio et natura mutant actionem animi; quod monstravi una particula, quia virtus anime complexionem corporis imitatur.' This also appears to have been Pietro d'Abano's conclusion: 'Concessum est ab optimis medicis, et philosophis, et a me per unum monimentum monstratum est, quod per crases corporis sequentes demonstravi animae virtutes': *Conciliator*, diff. 17, fol. 27ra. See also the works of García-Ballester cited above in n. 21, and R. Siegel, *Galen on Psychology, Psychopathology and Function and Diseases of the Nervous System* (Basel, 1973), pp. 117–22.

[54] Ziegler, *Medicine and Religion*, p. 136.

[55] 'Diximus autem quoniam medicorum sermones cognitionem ad opus utilem non transcendunt. Cum igitur corporis dispositiones quas considerat discernat operibus, causas considerat actionum, et solum eas quibus transmutatio fit in organo quo dicta operatio exercetur, ideo videlicet ut illis causis sufficienter cognitis valeat recte movere membrum. Cum autem in anima et virtute consideratis secundum essentiam proprie variatio non contingat, et ea dicat esse operationum principia, et

To identify *virtus* and *complexio* in this way was actually a sharp departure from scholastic medical theory, for the list of seven *res naturales* (the entities on which life depends) hallowed by its presentation at the outset of Johannitius's *Isagoge* included them both, and in commentaries on the *Isagoge* they are routinely discussed separately, with no attempt to link them.[56] Arnau, however, maintained this position firmly for at least the next few years.[57] To those who might protest that *complexio* and *virtus* are distinct *res naturales*, Arnau responds that that is only true *quantum ad rationes*, not *quantum ad rem*; one and the same thing is called a *virtus* insofar as it is a *principium operationis*, but a *complexio* insofar as it informs the body.[58]

As I have said, I find it difficult to find in this conclusion to Arnau's first important medical treatise an anticipation of his eventual conviction that the physician of the body is qualified to treat the soul as well, since his instrumentalist soul is explicitly presented as something different from what we think of as the human soul – it is not really 'soul' at all. But I

intelligat quantum opus exigit ea fore variabilia, et inter remota vel prima operationum principia variabilia solum reperiatur complexio (vel magis proprie miscibilium armonia), hinc est quod eam tanquam primum operationis principium in organo variabile animam esse dicit, essentiam autem virtutis complexionem existere tanquam animam virtutem influentem que principium operationis existit proximum. Si enim per virtutem intelligeret medicus potentiam anime, sicut facit naturalis, non diceret aliqua membra habere virtutem innatam, cum omnia membra a corde recipiant virtutem vite; sed intelligit per virtutem complexionem que manat ab armonia miscibilium, et hoc sufficit medico et non nocet, ut hic ostenditur. Similiter etiam non diceret virtutem vitalem aliam esse ab aliis, cum secundum veritatem virtus vitalis in quantum potentia anime est ab aliis non differat secundum rem, immo est eadem cum eis': Arnau de Vilanova, *De intentione* ii.4, p. 124 line 24–p. 125 line 24.

56 For example, by Cardinalis at Montpellier: in his *Isagoge*-commentary in Kues, St Nikolaus-Hospital, MS 222, the discussion of *commistio/complexio* begins on fol. 4v, and then, after sections on the humours and the members, the discussion of *virtus* follows at fol. 10v.

57 Arnau repeated his conclusion in *De consideracionibus*: 'Cum autem ulterius vult cognoscere causam subtrahentem organo virtutem sentiendi receptam ab origine aliqua, considerat similiter quid est virtus illa que transmittitur ad organum a predicta origine. Per consideracionem autem suam inquantum medicus est non dicit esse virtutem senciendi nisi spiritum animatum transmissum a cerebro ad predictum organum; et ideo dicimus virtutem senciendi quia virtutem naturalem medicus dicit esse complexionem, sicut in de intencione medicorum ostendimus' (*AVOMO* IV, 220–1). However, in the *Speculum medicine* (written apparently by 1308), a work loosely constructed around the plan of the *Isagoge*, Arnau treats *virtus* and *complexio* separately among the *res naturales* (in chs. 6 and 3 respectively) and does not try to equate them.

58 'Si quis autem obiciat quia medicus dicit complexionem et virtutem esse duas res naturales ad invicem differentes et ex opposito condivisas, dicendum quod illud dicit quantum ad rationem et non quantum ad rem, secundum suam considerationem; una enim et eadem res in quantum est informans corpus dicitur complexio, in quantum autem est principium operationis dicitur virtus': Arnau de Vilanova, *De intentione* ii.4, p. 125 line 25–p. 126 line 1.

think we do find there an anticipation of his later *medical* theories, which as time went on looked increasingly to a doctrine of complexions as a fundamental unifying principle to which all physiological and therapeutic phenomena could be reduced.

III

We are all aware, reflecting on our own lives, of how certain choices or actions seem to have determined their direction. But it is rare that we can recognize these moments in the lives of our acquaintances; and it happens only exceptionally that we know enough about someone in the distant past to talk confidently about specific moments of inflection that redirected his life – Charles Darwin is one of these rare exceptions. Sometimes these moments are conscious epiphanies, like the one we know Darwin had after rereading Malthus 'for pleasure' in September 1838; sometimes, on the contrary, they are impulsive choices that *we* can see would turn out to have unforeseen consequences, like Darwin's application to join the *Beagle*'s company seven years before.

I suppose I think that Arnau de Vilanova had a kind of 'Malthusian epiphany' of his own at the beginning of the 1290s, when he began to fashion two new identities at once,[59] and I have been suggesting why I do not think he appreciated where the decision was going to lead him: the tendencies that Ziegler has identified in Arnau's later works do not seem to me to be present yet in the ones I have considered from 1291–92. The connection between the two, the medical and the spiritual, was far from being automatic and instantaneous. They began, I suspect, as independent careers, self-consciously compartmentalized, only to grow towards one another gradually during the 1290s, as Arnau's spiritual thinking and his sense of the physician's professional role each gained depth and subtlety. I am tempted to suggest that they really fused only in 1300, the year of his confrontation with the Paris theologians and of the *Medicationis parabole* that the confrontation inspired, but to develop that suggestion would call for much more study.

But I also think that Arnau had already had an earlier moment of inflection, a kind of *Beagle* voyage of his own – that is, an earlier decision with quite unforeseen consequences for his life: namely, his simple decision to study Hebrew in the Barcelona *studium* with Ramon Martí at the beginning of the 1280s. In that study, as we have seen, he encountered certain specific themes that seem suddenly to have taken on new meaning for him, ten years later, in his Montpellier environment, and to have provided him with a starting point

[59] Lee, '*Scrutamini Scripturas*', identifies the Montpellier period immediately after 1290 as a kind of moment of inflection in Arnau's spiritual development (see his p. 56), but discusses it in isolation from Arnau's medical career.

for *both* his medical *and* his spiritual development in the 1290s. No doubt Arnau – and Darwin too, for that matter – had other moments of inflection that will always remain hidden from us. But to the extent that the historian can plausibly reconstruct *any* such moments, the shape of the lives he studies is bound to take on added meaning and suggestiveness.

Curers of Body and Soul: Medical Doctors as Theologians

William J. Courtenay

Two decades ago Danielle Jacquart noted the phenomenon at Paris of medical doctors pursuing a second higher degree in theology or law.[1] In the case of law, the acquisition of a double degree was obtained in several universities, including Paris and Montpellier, but for those medical doctors who had also studied or held a degree in theology, Paris was overwhelmingly the university where this combination existed. In the cases she noted, the frequency of an additional degree in law was highest in the late fourteenth and early fifteenth century, while the choice of theology peaked in the fourteenth century and declined markedly in the fifteenth.[2]

Surprisingly little attention has been given to either phenomenon. In the case of theological study, one might well understand the desire to acquire a second degree in medicine or law, since those disciplines were thought of as lucrative professions with an opportunity for remunerative private practice that had no parallel for a theological graduate. The reverse pattern – medical doctors seeking a degree in theology – would seem far less likely in light of the differential in potential income of the respective disciplines and because the course of study in theology was twice as long as that in medicine. Yet when the cases of double study in medicine and theology are examined, a remarkable pattern emerges. The sequence was from medicine to theology. Theological study was almost invariably undertaken after having first obtained the licentiate or doctorate in medicine.

What explains such a career shift or, at least, a doubling of career paths and possibilities? At Paris the pattern may already be in evidence with the first known dean of the faculty of medicine, Pierre de Limoges, who may be identical with the master of that name who became a bachelor of theology, was attached to the Collège de la Sorbonne, and gave it a large legacy of books from his library, including works in medicine.[3] Numerous examples

[1] Jacquart, *Milieu médical*, p. 393, tables 33–4.

[2] For double degrees in medicine and theology, she listed (table 34) three instances in the second half of the thirteenth century, nineteen in the first half of the fourteenth, thirty in the second half of the fourteenth, and eleven in the first half of the fifteenth.

[3] Wickersheimer (*Dictionnaire*, p. 645) rejected the identification, but Jacquart (*Supplément*, p. 237) left the question open. On the theologian, see P. Glorieux, *Aux origines de la Sorbonne*, vol. 1: *Robert de Sorbon* (Paris, 1966), p. 323; on the doctor of medicine, see *CUP* I, 468, 488. Pierre was dean at least during the years 1267–70.

followed, and the pattern was particularly in evidence during the pontificates of Benedict XII and Clement VI. Nancy Siraisi has suggested that the very presence of a faculty of theology encouraged such a combination of studies.[4] Faye Getz, in noting a similar pattern at Oxford, suggested that at this early stage of the academic development of the discipline of medicine, its close association with arts and philosophical training allowed it to be viewed as preparatory training for 'the ultimate degree, the doctorate in theology'.[5]

These explanations have merit, but they do not adequately account for the phenomenon under discussion. Medicine had achieved recognition as a higher faculty of study at Paris by the middle of the thirteenth century, and the arts degree was as preparatory for medicine as it was for theology. In the second half of the thirteenth century arts and medicine were no more interrelated disciplines than were arts and theology. Consequently, the pattern of seeking a degree in theology after having achieved the licence or doctorate in medicine – a pattern frequently encountered in the fourteenth century – cannot be explained on the grounds that medicine shared with arts a preparatory function.

Academic proximity of the disciplines of medicine and theology in some northern European universities also does not tell us much. The fact that theological study was an option at Paris and Oxford does not explain why doctors of canon law, a higher discipline also present at Paris and Oxford, almost never availed themselves of the same opportunity.[6] It also does not explain why, for those who sought a second higher degree, the medical degree was obtained before the theological degree. Other factors must surely have come into play to produce such a one-directional flow among higher faculties from medicine to theology, never the reverse, and rarely to or from any other higher faculty. Some possibilities can be ruled out immediately. One of these is the hypothesis that medical doctors sought a degree in theology in order to become eligible for ecclesiastical benefices and prebends. Doctors of medicine were just as eligible for appointment to income-producing positions in the church as were other masters of arts. Moreover, early in the development of the practice of universities submitting rolls of supplications for benefices (*rotuli*), the faculty of medicine was particularly aggressive in seeking access to ecclesiastical income. Where evidence permits

[4] N. Siraisi, 'The Faculty of Medicine', in *A History of the University in Europe*, ed. W. Rüegg, vol. I, *Universities in the Middle Ages*, ed. H. de Ridder-Symoens (Cambridge, 1992), p. 374.

[5] F. Getz, 'The Faculty of Medicine before 1500', in *The History of the University of Oxford*, vol. II, ed. J. I. Catto and T. A. R. Evans (Oxford, 1992), p. 382. Getz states there that the pattern at Oxford is remarkably similar to that at Paris: 'Of the 40 men recorded as having studied medicine at Oxford in the fourteenth century only Henry de la Dale MA BCL BM is known to have held a degree in law, but at least 8 studied theology.'

[6] Except for Philip de Leyden at Paris in 1365 or Henry de la Dale at Oxford in the 1320s, lawyers seem not to have sought a second degree in theology. On Philip, see *CUP* III, 126; on Henry, see Getz, 'Faculty of Medicine', p. 382.

comparison, regent masters in medicine usually outnumbered supplicating regents in theology or canon law at Paris. In the earliest surviving registered results of a university supplication, namely the *rotuli* of 1349, thirty-two members of the faculty of theology and seventeen members of the faculty of decrees were successful in receiving appointment or expectation, while the faculty of medicine had forty-six successful supplicants. The registered letters of expectation resulting from the *rotuli* of 1328 and 1329 reveal the same pattern: three theologians, five canon lawyers, and fifteen doctors of medicine in 1328; three theologians, three canon lawyers, and nine doctors of medicine in 1329. In 1335, the first year of Benedict XII's pontificate, the results of surviving registered letters of expectation are: five theologians, six canon lawyers, and fourteen doctors of medicine.[7]

Doctors of medicine, as regents or non-regents in that faculty, were therefore not shy in successfully pursuing ecclesiastical income. A theological degree did not increase their eligibility, nor did John XXII, Benedict XII, or Clement VI favour medical doctors any less than theologians or canon lawyers. Moreover, the rate of success by which expectative papal graces were transformed into actual appointments to a canonical prebend or a parish church appears to be roughly equivalent for the three higher faculties of theology, canon law, and medicine. Reality and perception of reality are, of course, different matters, and it is possible that some medical doctors assumed a degree in theology might give them an advantage in the quest for ecclesiastical income or higher office in the church. After all, medical doctors who became bishops usually had a second degree in theology. But any astute observer in the fourteenth century would have realized that in every case it was family background, often noble, or an important patronage connection that opened the door to the episcopate. A theological degree, by itself, added little. If improving one's candidacy for high ecclesiastical office were the reason for seeking a second higher degree, there should have been as many medical doctors seeking a degree in canon law as in theology. But such was not the case.

Academic interests should not be ruled out. Medical doctors, unlike their counterparts in law, had been fully trained in the faculty of arts and had 'reigned' in that faculty as masters. They had a philosophical training identical to that of theologians and may have developed an interest in issues of logic and natural philosophy similar to those that reshaped the study of theology in the fourteenth century. And just as continued teaching in the faculty of arts funded their study of medicine, continued teaching in medicine may well have funded subsequent study in theology for those who chose that career path. Religious motivations, although seemingly less likely, should not be excluded. In the thirteenth and fourteenth centuries one encounters the perception that the status of theologian, because of the subject

[7] The information provided here comes from the reconstructed results of the Parisian *rotuli*, which have been edited for publication in the near future.

matter and its non-lucrative reputation, put one in a better preparatory state for the afterlife, similar perhaps to joining a religious order.[8]

The political structure of the university of Paris may have been an important factor. The faculty of theology was the most prestigious faculty within the university, and its masters took the most prominent roles in processions and convocations. College fellowships were primarily for masters of arts and theology, and as colleges gradually came to play a more prominent role for university leaders, college affiliation meant prestige as well as income. The leading college by reputation, if not ultimately by size, was the Sorbonne, which was a college for students and masters in theology. It is probably not simple coincidence that several of the medical doctors who pursued a degree in theology are also known to have been fellows of the Sorbonne.[9] Early and continuing association with their fellow masters of arts who had moved directly into theology may have provided the network or attraction that pulled some medical doctors into the faculty of theology and into the Sorbonne.

The biographical evidence from the second quarter of the fourteenth century provided in the list at the end of this essay shows that the choice of shifting from medicine to theology, or adding a theological degree on top of the medical degree, was not the result of some inability to achieve a successful career in medicine. Persons such as Alfonso of Portugal, Nicolas d'Épernay, Denis Saffray, Nicolas de Cogno of Piacenza, Henri Pistor de Léau, James of Padua, and Geoffroy le Marec were masters of standing in the faculty of medicine and were well connected in the world outside the university. More telling is the fact that in every case where it can be determined, attending lectures in theology (a fourteen-year course of study) began before the completion of the degree in medicine. Rather than a choice made after several years of medical regency, it appears to have been part of a plan developed before or during the years of medical study.

Requirements for the theological degree, which stressed the mature age of the candidate and years of study, posed no additional hardships for medical doctors beyond attending lectures (and eventually giving them), undergoing examinations, and fulfilling the required academic exercises. The years necessary for medical training automatically placed them in an advanced age category. And just as one might begin the study of theology while completing regency in arts, so one might begin attending lectures in theology while completing instructional or regency requirements in medicine. One could not count years of study in one faculty as meeting the requirements in another, but there was no prohibition against double study for the energetic

[8] The question of whether the study of theology made its practitioners more deserving of grace and salvation was discussed by theologians. For example, the opening question of Adam Wodeham's Oxford lectures on the *Sentences* was: 'Utrum studium sacrae theologiae sit meritorium vitae aeternae.'

[9] Of the fifteen examples given at the end of this article, five are known to have been fellows of the Sorbonne.

and career-minded scholar. On the basis of our present knowledge, the phenomenon of medical doctors pursuing a second degree in theology was not a pattern evenly spread across the fourteenth century. The density of examples is highest for the second and third quarters of that century. As other examples of medical doctors turned theologians surface through archival research, we may be in a better position to understand the logic or motivation of this particular career path. For the moment, it would appear to have more to do with the internal structure of universities like Paris and Oxford and with choices made before the completion of medical study. Perhaps the double degree in medicine and theology is somewhat akin to the career path of a double degree in law, the *doctor utriusque juris'*, which placed its holders in a higher category than simple practitioners of civil or canon law.

The following list, arranged in approximate chronological order, contains examples from the second quarter of the fourteenth century, mostly from the period 1337–46. The biographical sketches are provided as illustrations and because several of them contain new information, with source, not found in Wickersheimer's *Dictionnaire biographique* or Jacquart's *Supplément* and *Milieu médical*. For cases before 1330, such as Jean de Basoles, Opicinus de Canistris, Raymond Jarente, and Thomas le Miesier, or cases after 1350, such as Galeran de Pendref, Gérard Mathie de Osterwiic, Guillaume Anglicus, Hugues de Tenolletti de Castro Girardi, Jean Gortenbeke, Jean de Lovanio, Nicolas Fabri, Richard Viard, see their respective entries in Wickersheimer and Jacquart.

Medical Doctors with Degrees in Theology, 1330–49

(? = probable but not certain)

? Petrus de Encra [Pierre d'Ancre (Albert)], clerk from the diocese of Amiens, MA and member of Collège des Chollets by 1329 (W. Courtenay, *Parisian Scholars in the Early Fourteenth Century* [Cambridge, 1999], pp. 198–9, where the identification was doubted); BMed by January 1331; canon of Arras and BTh by February 1335. If same person, he must have been pursuing both courses of study at the same time, having begun medicine earlier. Wickersheimer, *Dictionnaire biographique*, p. 631.

Alfonsus Dionysii de Ulixbona (Lisbon), MA and BMed by March 1330; DMed in 1334; scholar in theology by 1342; BTh by January 1345; DTh and canon at Seville by January 1346 when appointed bishop of Idanna; bishop of Evora in October 1347. Study in theology probably began before completion of medical degree. Wickersheimer, *Dictionnaire biographique*, p. 20; Jacquart, *Supplément*, pp. 16–17.

Bartholomeus Boneti, clerk from the diocese of Clermont; MA, licensed in medicine and a scholar in theology by July 1337, when regent in arts and part of supplication of French nation. DMed by 1342, when provided with a canonry and expectation of prebend at Nevers while still awaiting a benefice in the diocese of Poitiers (Reg. Aven. 70, fol. 85r; Reg. Vat. 156, fol. 179r). Apparently still regent in medicine in May 1349, when no mention is made of his earlier studies in theology. Wickersheimer, *Dictionnaire biographique*, p. 60.

Nicolas [Houduin] de Spernaco (Épernay), clerk from the diocese of Reims; MA and DMed by 1337; cursor in theology by June 1342 and prepared to read Sentences in 1342–3 when he received a canonry with expectation of prebend at Reims (Reg. Aven. 59, fol. 241v; Reg. Vat. 149, fol. 178v). Priest by August 1346 as part of BTh supplication. DTh by May 1349 when he supplicated with faculty of theology. Wickersheimer, *Dictionnaire biographique*, p. 571.

Guillelmus de Escoucheyo, alias de Postigneyo, MA, DMed, priest, and cursor in theology by December 1342, when he received an expectation of a benefice in the diocese of Le Mans in addition to a parish church and an expectation in the diocese of Sées (Reg. Aven. 65, fol. 42v). Wickersheimer, *Dictionnaire biographique*, p. 241.

Dionysius Safredi [Denis Saffray], MA by 1329, DMed before 1331; BTh by June 1342, when he supplicated with other bachelors of theology, not with doctors of medicine, and received provision as a canon at St-Sépulcre at Caen (Reg. Aven. 70, fol. 341v; Reg. Vat. 156, fol. 332v). Wickersheimer, *Dictionnaire biographique*, p. 116.

Nicolas de Cogno de Placentia (Piacenza), MA with expectation in the diocese of Soissons by 1335; DMed and student in theology by 1339; BTh by June 1342, when he supplicated with other bachelors of theology, not with doctors of medicine, and received a canonry with expectation of prebend at Padua (Reg. Aven. 70, fol. 333r; Reg. Vat. 156, fol. 327v). DTh by March 1345 (Reg. Aven. 80, fol. 497r; Reg. Vat. 164, fol. 113v). Took part in supplication of faculty of theology in 1349. Wickersheimer, *Dictionnaire biographique*, p. 568.

Johannes de Daventria, clerk from the diocese of Utrecht; MA, DMed, cursor in theology, and fellow of the Sorbonne by September 1343. Wickersheimer, *Dictionnaire biographique*, p. 390.

Henricus [Pistor] de Lewis (Léau), clerk from the diocese of Liège; MA, BMed, cursor in theology, and fellow of the Sorbonne by September 1343. BTh by 1345 and still in August 1346, when he supplicates with other BThs (Reg. Suppl. 11, fol. 155v). Licensed in medicine by September 1348 and DTh by May 1349 when he supplicates with faculty of theology. Died in 1355. Wickersheimer, *Dictionnaire biographique*, p. 285; *AL: Codices* I, nos. 667, 674, 679, 682, 685, 698, 700.

Johannes de Zantvliete, clerk from the diocese of Utrecht; MA, BMed, cursor in theology, and fellow of the Sorbonne by September 1343. Wickersheimer, *Dictionnaire biographique*, pp. 504–5.

Jacobus de Padua, MA, DMed, fellow of the Sorbonne, and BTh by Oct. 1342; DTh by 1343; still regent in theology in March 1345 (Reg. Aven. 81, fol. 294v; Reg. Aven. 227, fol. 742r; Reg. Vat. 163, fol. 506r) and in May 1349. Still at Paris in 1353 and 1354. Wickersheimer, *Dictionnaire biographique*, p. 334; Jacquart, *Supplément*, p. 137; *AL: Codices* I, nos. 668, 671, 683, 699.

Natalis (Noël) Avenel, priest from the diocese of Le Mans; MA, DMed, and BTh by August 1346. DTh by May 1349, when he supplicates with other masters of theology. Wickersheimer, *Dictionnaire biographique*, p. 582.

Michael de Brachia (de Brèche), clerk from the diocese of Angers; MA and canon at Tours by 1342; DMed, and BTh by August 1346; DTh and canon at Chartres by 1352; bishop of Le Mans in 1355; died 1366. Wickersheimer, *Dictionnaire biographique*, p. 551.

Gaufridus le Marec (Marhec), noble clerk from the diocese of St-Brieuc; MA and DMed by May 1349; at Sorbonne in 1344, and BTh by October 1349 and still in 1351 as familiar of Pierre de Cros, cardinal Autissiodorensis; DTh by January 1353; bishop of Quimper in March 1357; died 1383. Wickersheimer, *Dictionnaire biographique*, p. 179.

Johannes Ogeri de Sancto Medardo supra Montem (St-Médard-sur-le-Mont), clerk from the diocese of Châlons-sur-Marne; MA and licensed in medicine at Paris by 1340; at the Collège de Navarre in 1342 with a bourse in theology; BTh by October 1349 (Reg. Suppl. 21, fol. 43v; Reg. Aven. 107, fol. 453v; Reg. Vat. 194, fol. 251r); DTh by 1353; master of the Collège d'Autun in 1354; canon at Châlons and Reims by 1362; still regent in the faculty of theology at Paris in 1371.

Delivering a Christian Identity: Midwives in Northern French Synodal Legislation, *c.* 1200–1500

Kathryn Taglia

Piecing together a history of midwifery in the Middle Ages is a complicated business – and not just because of the relative scarcity of obvious sources. Historians have offered contradictory claims about the practice of midwifery, sometimes based more on their own prejudices and assumptions than the actual historical record. In one view, medieval midwives and their sisters in the Reformation and early modern eras have been understood as ignorant superstitious women whose care killed more than it saved. Only the imposition of ecclesiastical, civil, and medical regulations and the rise of the male medical obstetrician managed to rescue future generations of mothers and infants from the pathetic fate suffered by so many women and their newborns in the 'dark ages' of medicine.

Other historians have pictured medieval midwives as wise women whose vast empirical knowledge granted other women comfort and healing in times of need. Midwives, in this narrative, were the primary medical caregivers for women. The gradual regulation of their abilities to practice, the professionalization of medicine, and the written libels about their skills were tools used by the male-dominated worlds of the church, state, and doctors to control, marginalize, and almost eliminate this important female profession and to bring reproductive matters and female bodies ever more firmly under masculine supervision.

The majority of support for these two dominant theses is found in evidence from the Reformation and early modern eras; late medieval sources often have ended up playing a secondary role in these two meta-narratives, even when they are ostensibly the primary focus of the historian's interest. Yet the history of midwifery in the later Middle Ages occupies an important interstice between the histories of religion, women, and medicine. Midwives, as is well known, because of their occupation as childbirth helpers, could and were called upon to perform emergency baptisms and possibly caesarean operations. Their history then lies not just in the pages of medical sources, but also in ecclesiastical sources, such as church court records and synodal and conciliar legislation, which were concerned with pastoral care and the maintenance of ecclesiastically sanctioned norms. Situating the practising midwife within the later medieval Church's concerns over pastoral care, Christian identity, and the correct practices of the sacrament of baptism will help us develop a more nuanced, if still incomplete, picture of the midwife and her profession. In this essay I shall look at synodal and conciliar legislation from northern France for what it has to say about how ecclesiastical authorities viewed the midwife's position in the parish and the diocese. The essay starts with a brief discussion of some aspects of previous studies on midwifery, then goes on to examine what the legislation has to say about midwives, and concludes with a short discussion about possible directions for further study.

Histories of Midwifery in Medieval and Early Modern Europe

Medical historians, whose sympathies often have lain with doctors, originally advanced the thesis of (male) medical and regulatory practices triumphing over the (female) irrational, unscientific midwives. This is a story of the victorious progress of technology and medicine, and in this evolutionary history, as in many others, the whole of the Middle Ages is a stagnant, dark, a-historical space between the ancient world and the Renaissance. Midwives are holdovers from those dismal days when 'medieval fatalism' ruled as opposed to 'a more investigative, scientific approach to nature'.[1] Offering no historical evidence, R. Petrelli argues that the unregulated medieval midwife must have been 'uneducated and of low social class . . . feared by those whom she served'. Regulation was thus a blessing that inserted men and their superior knowledge (and class) into the birthing chamber, saving the child and the mother from the 'mercy of the midwife'.[2]

Not surprisingly, many historians of women and feminist historians have reacted strongly to this 'heroic' reading of medical history, seeing it as a too simple picture that effaces the reality of women's lives and skills in order to maintain the centrality of male contributions to medicine. Overcorrecting, some historians have pictured the Middle Ages (or at least the high Middle Ages) as a time of utopian medical freedom for both midwives and their female patients. All too soon this golden age came to an end, when the first attempts to regulate midwives started to appear in the late Middle Ages and early modern era. Dependent, like the pro-doctor historians, on sources written by the regulators and medical authorities, these pro-midwife historians often stress the oppressive nature of the regulations or paint a picture of how male authorities, fearful of the reproductive and medical knowledge of the midwife, attempted to co-opt or demonize her.[3]

[1] T. G. Benedek, 'The Changing Relationship between Midwives and Physicians during the Renaissance', *BHM* 51 (1977), 550–64 (p. 550).

[2] R. L. Petrelli, 'The Regulation of French Midwifery during the Ancien Régime', *Journal of the History of Medicine and Allied Sciences* 26 (1971), 276–92 (p. 276). Other examples include T. R. Forbes, *The Midwife and the Witch* (New Haven and London, 1966) and J. R. Guy, 'The Episcopal Licensing of Physicians, Surgeons, and Midwives', *BHM* 56 (1982), 528–42.

[3] See for example, R. Blumenfeld-Kosinski, *Not of Women Born: Representations of*

While in sympathy with the latter view, indeed admiring of much of the work done on midwifery during the Reformation and early modern period, I think there is a need to be careful when reading medieval sources.[4] Viewing them through the prism of what happens in the early modern era can refract and bend the sources in ways that are not always accurate. It is also important, as M. Green has pointed out in her articles on medieval female medical practitioners, to question our underlying assumptions about how medicine was practised in the Middle Ages. In the debate over midwives and their place in the history of medicine, the unthinking assumption that 'women's health was women's business' has led to the more troubling assumption that childbirth is the only reason that women would need contact with a healer.[5] Even those who would defend midwives and their female patients often became entangled in this reductive thesis that constricts women's health issues solely to the pangs of labour.[6] The best way out of this maze is to turn to a careful historical chronicle of medieval midwifery, paying close attention to what the sources say (and do not say) about midwives. This includes being careful to note the words used by sources to describe the midwife and her duties, and the historical context of the situations in which the midwife was involved.[7] Doing this will, as Green states, '[encourage] us to consider whether "midwife" is really the trans-historical (and hence a-historical) category that it has been assumed to be'.[8]

One interesting source of historical information is found in synodal and conciliar legislation, and in the remainder of this paper I shall examine what

Caesarean Birth in Medieval and Renaissance Culture (Ithaca and London, 1990), p. 110; Greilsammer, 'Midwife', 323; A. L. Barstow, *Witchcraze: A New History of the European Witch Hunts* (San Francisco, 1994), pp. 113–27.

[4] For example, see S. Haney's interesting work on midwives and the construction of the early modern French state ('Engendering the State: Family Formation and State Building in Early Modern France', *French Historical Studies* 16 [1989], 4–27 [esp. pp. 22–3]) or the collection of essays edited by H. Marland, *The Art of Midwifery: Early Modern Midwives in Europe and North America* (London, 1993).

[5] M. Green, 'Women's Medical Practice and Health Care in Medieval Europe', *Signs* 14 (1989), 434–73, reprinted in *Sisters and Workers in the Middle Ages*, ed. J. M. Bennett, E. A. Clark, J. F. O'Barr, B. A. Vilen and S. Westphal-Wihl (Chicago and London, 1989), pp. 39–78 (pp. 39–40). See also Green, 'Documenting'.

[6] For example, after acknowledging Green's point that women's health-care needs go beyond childbirth, Greilsammer continues in her review of the literature on the history of obstetrical practice to equate women's health concerns with the moment of childbirth alone ('Midwife', pp. 289–90).

[7] For example, on Trotula and problems of authorship, see J. F. Benton, 'Trotula, Women's Problems, and the Professionalization of Medicine in the Middle Ages', *BHM* 59 (1985), 30–53; on miracle stories and the information on childbirth and midwives found in them, see P. A. Sigal, 'La grossesse, l'accouchement et l'attitude envers l'enfant mort-né à la fin du moyen âge d'après les récits de miracles', in *Santé, médecine et assistance au Moyen Age*, Actes du 110e congrès national des sociétés savantes, Montpellier, 1985 (Paris, 1987), pp. 23–41.

[8] Green, 'Documenting', p. 340.

the northern French legislation has to say about midwives.[9] The flowering of synodal legislation, starting with the great Paris synod(s) in late twelfth century that predated and influenced Lateran IV, was directly connected to the increasing interest that ecclesiastical authorities showed in pastoral care and the education of clergy and the laity. One of the legislators' primary foci was a correct understanding of the sacraments, including the sacrament of baptism. Personal salvation, a true Christian identity, and communal stability all depended on the correct performance of this rite of initiation. In order to alleviate any anxieties over the Church's claims to be the legitimate and sole source of religious reality, any possibility of ambiguity and anomaly around baptism had to be minimized.[10] Another aspect of concern in the synodal legislation was over moral standards and sinful behaviour. While M. Greilsammer has, for instance, argued that a connection in the minds of the synodal legislators between midwife and witch was clear, I shall show in this essay that the French legislation, at least, reveals no such clear connection.

Midwives and Emergency Baptisms

Medieval Christian thinkers, following Augustine, argued that original sin condemns all those who are not saved to hell (or at best limbo); even the newly born infant is tainted by this fault inherited from Adam.[11] An

[9] The four ecclesiastical provinces of northern France, Rouen, Tours, Sens and Reims, contain the dioceses of Avranches, Bayeux, Coutances, Évreux, Lisieux and Sées (Rouen); Chartres, Meaux, Orléans, Paris and Troyes (Sens); Angers, Le Mans, Nantes, St Brieuc, St Malo and Tréguier (Tours); Amiens, Arras, Cambrai, Châlons-sur-Marne, Soissons, Thérouanne and Tournai (Reims). For this essay, I used mainly published sources – thus, while my investigation into this legislation was extensive, it was not exhaustive. A footnote listing all the printed sources examined (but which yielded nothing for this project) would be quite extensive; instead the reader should consult Mansi and *Répertoire des statuts synodaux des diocèses de l'ancienne France du XIIIe à la fin du XVIIIe siècle*, ed. A. Artonne, L. Guizard and O. Pontal, 2nd edn (Paris, 1969). Although now slightly out of date, the *Répertoire* is still an excellent guide. Printed collections and manuscripts which contained useful material are of course listed in the appropriate notes below.

[10] For a more general overview of the problems of emergency baptism, see K. Taglia, 'The Cultural Construction of Childhood: Baptism, Communion, and Confirmation', in *Women, Marriage, and Family in Medieval Christendom: Essays in Memory of Michael M. Sheehan, C.S.B.*, ed. C. M. Rousseau and J. T. Rosenthal (Kalamazoo, MI, 1998), pp. 255–87.

[11] Augustine saw the need for infant baptism as an apt expression of just how corrupt humanity had become due to original sin. He had no doubt that he, himself, was a sinner from the very day he was born (Augustine, *Confessions*, trans. R.S. Pine-Coffin [Harmondsworth, 1961], p. 27). See also J. Lynch, *Godparents and Kinship in Early Medieval Europe* (Princeton, NJ, 1986), pp. 119–20; J. Pelikan, *The Christian Tradition: A History of the Development of Doctrine*, vol. 1: *The Emergence of the Catholic Tradition (100–600)* (Chicago and London, 1971), pp. 286–93.

As for later medieval thinkers, both Innocent III and Thomas Aquinas assert that

unbaptized, dead infant could have no claim upon the Christian community. This was graphically symbolized in the legislation by the insistence that such a corpse should not be buried in the cemetery.[12] The unbaptized dead infant was in a truly pathetic situation; granted only the briefest span of mortal life, it was denied any identity within the Christian community or any hope of eternal salvation. Baptism was in the Middle Ages not just the announcement of one's private religious beliefs (or of one's family's beliefs), but an initiation rite that marked the baptized with an indelible character and granted him/her membership in Christendom, that is, Christian Western Europe. Failing to deal with the problem of the dying infant and his or her need for immediate baptism would have created serious problems for the universal claims that the medieval Church wished to make about the ordering of the cosmos, the plan of salvation, and the Church's necessary role in the creating and recreating of western Europe's cultural system.

Baptism, thus, was the one sacrament in the Middle Ages that could be performed by anyone – cleric or lay person, man or woman, Christian or not. In the ninth century Pope Nicholas I, in his letter to the Bulgarians, stated that all baptized in the name of the Trinity or in Christ's name (as stated in the Acts of the Apostles) were baptized whether the baptism was performed by a Jew, Christian, or pagan. Important medieval thinkers, such as Peter the Lombard and Pope Alexander III, supported Pope Nicholas I's arguments that the sanctifying aspects of the baptismal ceremony rested on its form, not on the status of the baptizer.[13] Under special and limited circumstances ecclesiastical authorities decided that the need to grant an individual a chance at eternal life outweighed their need to keep baptism totally under their supervision and control. This chance for salvation and membership within the community of Christians (both living and dead) was so important that Gratian allowed in an emergency the setting aside of the spiritual kin relationships created through baptism between the baptizer and the child's parents.[14]

baptism is absolutely necessary for the salvation of infants, as they share in original sin (X 3.42.3; Friedberg II, 644–6; Thomas Aquinas, *Summa theologiae* 3a, qu. 68, art. 9; LVII, 106–11). Peter the Lombard harshly condemns the unbaptized infant to hell, even if s/he died on the way to the baptism (*Sententiae* IV.iv.4; II, 259).

[12] Cambrai synod, n.d. (before 1260), Boeren I, p. 133; Cambrai synod, 1287/8, Boeren II, pp. 131–58 (p. 133); Cambrai synod, *c.* 1300–7, *Veterum scriptorum* VII, 1293; Tournai synod, 1366, Le Groux, p. 4.

[13] This letter was excerpted by Gratian (*Decretum* D. 4 de cons. c. 24, in Friedberg I, 1368 (the complete text of the letter is in Mansi XV, 32). See also Peter the Lombard, *Sententiae* IV.vi.2; II, 268–9; Alexander III, X 3.42.1 (Friedberg II, 644); Lateran IV, canon 1 in *Disciplinary Decrees of the General Councils: Text, Translation, and Commentary*, ed. and trans. H. J. Schroeder (St Louis, MO, 1937), p. 239.

[14] *Decretum*, C. 30 q. 1 c. 7 (Friedberg I, 1098–9). Gratian cites a papal ruling that a father who baptizes his son out of fear that the son is dying should not be separated from his wife because of the spiritual kinship created by baptism. Saving a child from a threat of eternal and everlasting damnation is an act that should be rewarded, not punished. (A possible less meritorious motive for such a baptism is also mentioned,

Although ecclesiastical authorities clearly wanted to keep baptism a priestly ritual publicly enacted within the precincts of the parish church, they also acknowledged that there were times when an emergency baptism was necessary. This meant that there were times when the ecclesiastical desire to control this sacrament of initiation had to be put aside for the important reasons of saving souls and guaranteeing that communal stability was maintained. A canon from the council of Vienne (1311–12), which was taken up in the Clementines decretal collection, forbade private baptisms, except for emergencies or if the candidate was the son of ruler.[15] This canon was quickly taken up by the legislators of various synods in the fourteenth century, perhaps even within five years of the council.[16] A 1421 St-Brieuc statute on private baptisms opens by ruling that such baptisms will be allowed if it is thought that the child would die before being taken to the church font. It is paramount that no one die unbaptized, for, as 'our Saviour asserted, unless anyone was reborn through water and the holy Spirit, s/he cannot enter the kingdom of heaven (John 3. 5)'.[17] Even more importantly than allowing that baptisms could not always be publicly performed, legislators recognized that the office of baptism could not always be performed by a priest. Synodal legislators from Soissons, Tréguier, Chartres and St-Brieuc urge priests not to delay if an infant should need an emergency baptism;[18] however, synodal legislators also instructed priests to teach the laity the correct baptismal formula in their native language.[19] This important

that is, baptizing one's own child in order to create grounds for the dissolution of one's marriage.)

[15] Clem. 3.15.1 (Friedberg II, 1174): 'Praesenti prohibemus edicto, ne quis de cetero in aulis vel cameris aut aulis privatis domibus, sed duntaxat in ecclesiis, in quibus sunt ad hoc fontes specialiter deputati, aliquos (nisi regum vel principum, quibus valeat in hoc casu deferri, liberi exstiterint, aut talis neccessitas emerserit, propter quam nequeat ad ecclesiam absque periculo propter hoc accessus haberi) audeat baptizare. Qui autem secus praesumpserit, aut suam in hoc praesentiam exhibuerit, taliter per episcopum suum castigetur, quod alii attentare similia non praesumant.'

[16] Cambrai, 1 October 1317 (*Veterum scriptorum* VII, 1345) (The Cambrai synodal collection in BnF, MS lat. 1592 has the exact same statute but records it as one added to the Cambrai synodal in 1321 [fol. 26r, col. 2]); Orléans, 1320, *Veterum scriptorum* VII, 1289; Arras, n.d. (second half of the fifteenth century), *Concilia Germaniae* VIII, 246–7.

[17] St-Brieuc, 17 October 1421, Pocquet, 23: 'In morte priusquam ad ecclesiam et fontem baptismatis portari posset, baptizet prius persona puerum eciam si solus pater esset presens sub forma prescripta et hoc facere doceant sacerdotes in vulgari, nam sine baptismo morientes numquam videbunt Deum facie ad faciem sicut *Salvator noster asserit, nisi quis renatus fuerit ex aqua et spiritu sancto non poterit intrare in regnum celorum*, tales sic debiles potest sacerdotes in domo baptizare, et filios principium, sine eo quod ad fontes ecclesie deferantur, sed eis hoc facere jus de ceteris interdicit.'

[18] Soissons, n.d. (thirteenth century), *Veterum scriptorum* VIII 1538; Tréguier, *c.* 1334, *Thesaurus* IV, 1097; Chartres, *c.* 1355–68, Jusselin, 80; St-Brieuc, 1421, Pocquet, 23.

[19] See for example: Paris, *c.* 1196–1208, Pontal, p. 54; Rouen, *c.* 1231–5, Bessin, II, 53–4; Coutances, n.d. (thirteenth century), Mansi XXV, 30–1; Bayeux, 1300, Mansi, XXV,

pronouncement is part of the first legislation studied here, the great synodal collection of Paris (*c.* 1196–1208), whose direction to priests to 'instruct the laity, . . . (even the women), fathers and even mothers how to baptize children in dire necessity' becomes the model for legislation across Europe.[20] In the earliest synodal legislation, midwives are not singled out for particular mention and even in later legislation, where midwives are mentioned, instructions continued to be given to teach all the laity the baptismal formula.[21]

The first legislation mentioning midwives and emergency baptism specifically is from a 1311 Paris synod. The opening part of statute reiterates basically the text from previous synods, reminding priests that baptism is an important sacrament which should be done carefully and correctly, and it orders the priests to teach their parishioners how to perform an emergency baptism. This statute ends with a short statement saying that 'on account of this there should be in every vill skilled midwives sworn to perform emergency baptism'.[22] Instructions for diaconal visitations are included in an edition of the 1365 Meaux synodal collection. Midwives were needed in every parish, the legislation declares, because of the perils of childbirth. These midwives were to be carefully selected and sent to the bishop's court, where they were

61; Orléans, n.d. (before 1314), *Veterum scriptorum* VII, 1274; Reims, *c.* 1328–30, Gousset, II, 539; Tréguier, *c.* 1334, *Thesaurus* IV, 1097–8; Meaux, n.d. (*c.* 1346), *Thesaurus* IV, 892; Chartres, n.d. (*c.* 1355–68), Jusselin, 80. Some statutes also remind the priest to instruct the laity to sprinkle or pour water upon the child during the saying of the baptismal formula (Paris, n.d., after 1311, Harlay, *Synodicon*, p. 33; St-Brieuc, 1421, Pocquet, 22–3).

[20] Paris, *c.* 1196–1208, Pontal, p. 54: '[D]oceant frequenter sacerdotes, laicos baptizare debere pueros in necessitate (etiam mulieres) patrem etiam et matrem in summa necessitate.' This synodal collection was highly influential, not just throughout northern France where it is the progenitor of several important synodal collections (including the Angevine collection known as the *Synodal de l'Ouest* and the earliest Cambrai synodal books), but also throughout Europe. For more on the history of French synodal legislation, see J. Avril, 'Naissance et évolution des législations synodales dans les diocèses du Nord et de l'Ouest de la France (1200–1250)', *Zeitschrift der Savigny-Stiftung Kanonistische Abteilung* 72 (1986), 152–249; O. Pontal, *Les statuts synodaux*, Typologie des sources du Moyen Âge occidental, fasc. 11: A-III.1 (Turnhout, 1975).

[21] For example, see below, n. 22, or Arras, n.d. (second half of fifteenth century), *Concilia Germaniae* VIII, 245–6.

[22] *Synodicon*, ed. Harlay, p. 33: 'Item, caveat quilibet Curatus et Sacerdos circa Sacramentum Baptismi, quod ipse Baptismus cum honore et reverentia celebretur, et cum magna cautela, et praesertim in prolatione verborum in quibus virtus Sacramenti consistit, verba distincte proferendo, scilicet; *Ego baptizo te in nomine Patris et Filii et Spiritus sancti, amen.* Et quod saepe Sacerdotes parrochianos suos doceant, ut quando puer in summa necessitate baptizandus fuerit, ille qui baptizabat nomen imponat puero, et tunc dicat aquam effundendo distincte et ordinate formam verborum praedictorum verbis latinis vel Gallicis, sine interpositione aliorum verborum, et cum debito ordine, *Ego baptizo te in nomine Patris*, etc. et propter hoc sint in singulis villis obstetrices peritae et super hoc juratae.'

to obtain a 'certificate' of approval after an examination and an oath-taking ceremony. The parish rector was to keep records on these midwives who were in his parish.[23] Here it is unclear whether the ecclesiastical officials are concerned about the physical dangers that could threaten both the infant and mother in addition to the spiritual perils which awaited the fragile and possibly dying newborn. But in both the Meaux and Paris legislation, there is a recognition that the midwives should be the focus of ecclesiastical attention in the struggle to improve pastoral care. How systematic these 'licensing' or oath-taking procedures were is unclear, nor is it clear exactly what was examined by ecclesiastical authorities beyond knowledge of how to perform correctly an emergency baptism. Other sources beyond the ecclesiastical legislation have yielded, so far, only a little concrete evidence about how this midwifery system worked. In visitation records for the archdeaconry of Josas from the late fourteenth century, A. Saunier has found evidence that female parishioners selected the midwife for their area under the auspices of the curate and parish churchwardens. Once again no qualifications are specified, although it is clear that the archdeacon sees these midwives as holding a position which requires them to take an oath and obtain a certificate or license from his court or the Official's court in Paris.[24] Saunier notes, however, that this way of selecting and regulating midwives was far from systematic. At times midwives appear to be 'spontaneously generated', since the archdeacon only insists on some midwives' regulation long after the community's de facto recognition of their skills and abilities.[25]

While stressing that midwives should learn the proper baptismal form, the

[23] Meaux, 1365, *Thesaurus* IV, 929: 'Item, propter pericula quæ circa partus mulierum sæpe eveniunt, diligenter inquirat et faciat quod in unaquaque parochia una sit obstetrix jurata aut duæ juxta parochiæ multitudinem, et ad hanc eligendam et procurandum quod eligatur cogant matricularios ecclesiæ per citationem officii, si opus sit, ipsamque electam ad curiam mittant indilate, ut examinetur, et juret, ut moris est, litterasque approbationis a curia obtineat, et de ejus electione rescribat, aut rescribi injungat per ecclesiæ rectorem.'

[24] Saunier, 'Visiteur', 46. The *Registre des causes civiles de l'officialité épiscopale de Paris, 1384–1387*, ed. J. Petit (Paris, 1919) includes a single entry of a midwife taking her oath of office ('Amelota, uxor Symonis Maupertuis de Villanova Regis, juravit fideliter exercere in dicta villa officium obstetricis, etc., et admissa ad dictum officium' [c. 1]). P. Biller mentions that in the fourteenth century there is evidence of 'sworn' midwives practising also in Rouen and Rheims (P. Biller, 'Childbirth in the Middle Ages', *History Today* 36 [August 1986], 42–9 [p. 43]), while in the fifteenth century there are records of midwives practising in Lille (Petrelli, 'Regulation', p. 281). Editor's note: Biller took his data from Jacquart, *Milieu médical*, p. 48 and n. 3, who notes five 'sworn' midwives from Paris in the fourteenth century and two from Reims; Rouen was a mistake.

[25] Saunier, 'Visiteur', 46. This 'spontaneous generation' fits with Green's provisional definition of the medieval female medical practitioner as being often a woman who 'actively "sells" her craft to her community or that the community itself makes that recognition and comes to her for healing': Green, 'Documenting', p. 336.

other legislation on midwives and emergency baptism has little concern about the actual regulation of midwives. In the edition of the Reims council of 1408 edited by Mansi, one of Jean Gerson's sermons has been excerpted for the edification of the clergy. Gerson stresses, among other matters, the importance of making sure that everyone knows how to administer baptism correctly; otherwise, midwives (or other lay people) could end up baptizing an infant incorrectly.[26] This council also has a checklist of concerns for a visiting diocesan official to use when he toured the parishes. One matter on this list was to make sure that the local midwives understood the correct way to perform a baptism.[27] In the fifteenth century, legislators from Arras and Tournai included in their synodal statutes instructions that parish priests were to instruct midwives how to perform an emergency baptism correctly. The Tournai legislation also asks that priests teach these 'midwives and women' how to assess whether a birthing situation is indeed a true emergency.[28]

As the Tournai legislation establishes, ecclesiastical officials did express some concern about midwives possibly overextending their authority and baptizing 'unnecessarily', but this concern was expressed not just about midwives, but about any lay-performed baptism. Diocesan statutes from the mid-fourteenth-century synods of Chartres and Meaux firmly reminded parents that they were only allowed to perform a baptism in 'greatest necessity'.[29] And many synodal collections instruct the parish priest to question the parents closely, if the infant should survive, after the lay-performed baptism. If the priest finds that no irregularities occurred in the

[26] Council of Reims, 1408, Mansi XXVI, 1064: 'Sic obstetrices aut laici baptizare quandoque putantes parvulos, de quorum morte dubitant, forma debita et a Christo instituto non utuntur.'

[27] Council of Reims, 1408, Mansi XXVI, 1070: 'Item, circa baptismum dum puer est baptizatus ab obstetrice, qualem se habet, et doceatur.

Item, si obstetrices sciunt unam formam baptizandi in parochia sua; et super hanc paterenter obstetrices interrogari, et doceri, quod hæc est forma, spargendo aquam super puero; *Enfant je te baptise au nom du Pere et du Fils et du Saint Esprit*. Amen.'

[28] Arras, n.d. (second half of fifteenth century), *Concilia Germaniae* VIII, 246: 'Item præcipimus singulis curam animarum habentibus, quatenus instruant matronas obstetrices, qualiter tantum impellente necessitate, pueros habeant baptizare, videlict sub hac forma, et non alia, sive lingua laicali, sive latina: *Ego baptizo te in Nomine Patris, et Filii, et Spiritus Sancti. Amen*. Et faciant cum trina immersione in aqua.'

Tournai, 4 October 1481, Le Groux, p. 82: '⟨O⟩bstetrices et mulieres quid et qualiter in casu necessitatis circa dictum sacramentum agendum sit instruant.'

[29] Chartres, *c*. 1355–68, Jusselin, 80: 'Ut pater vel mater non baptisent pueros suos nisi in summa necessitate.' Meaux, *c*. 1346, *Thesaurus* IV, 892: 'Doceant etiam sacerdotes patrem et matrem posse baptizare in maxima et summa necessitate, aliter autem non.' In the early fifteenth century, Agnes la Chauvelle was brought before an archdeacon's official in Chartres and fined for an unnecessary baptism: M. W. Labarge, *Women in Medieval Life: A Small Sound of the Trumpet* (London, 1986), p. 81.

baptism, he is to complete the ceremony at the parish church, 'supply[ing] what is lacking, namely the bit of salt and the touching of the ear with saliva . . . [and then] over the font, without the immersion, [the priest should perform] the rest of ceremony'.[30] This recapturing of the baptismal moment was done, thirteenth-century Coutances legislation claims, not because the lay baptism failed to grant salvation, but to 'augment the virtue' of the hastily performed lay ceremony.[31] If irregularities in the emergency baptism were found or suspected, the priest was to perform a conditional baptism. No one could be baptized twice, but it was important to ensure that all Christians were validly baptized for both reasons of personal salvation and Christian communal integrity. By the Carolingian era, in response to concerns over anomalous situations, the conditional baptismal formula ('If you are baptized, I do not baptize you, but, if you are not yet baptized, I baptize you, etc.') had been developed and its practice was further confirmed by Alexander III.[32] Many of the northern French synodal collections contain statues instructing priests to perform a conditional baptism if there are concerns over the lay-performed baptism.[33]

One of the occasions when an emergency baptism was to be performed was after a caesarean section. In the Middle Ages this operation only came about if the labouring mother should die before giving birth and the fetus was thought still to be alive within her body. They were essentially desperation operations to bring out the infant in order to baptize him or her. Both R. Blumenfeld-Kosinski and P. Sigal note that the first medieval mention of caesarean sections is not in medical literature, but rather in

[30] '⟨S⟩uppleatur quod deest, scilicet pabulum salis et aurium linitio cum salvia . . . et super fontes, sine immersione omnia fiant, que solent fieri' (Angers, Pontal, pp. 140, 142).

See also for example, Synod of Paris, Pontal, p. 56, and *PL* 212, 59; Orleans, *c.* 1314, *Veterum scriptorum* VII, 1272–5; Meaux, *c.* 1346, *Thesaurus* IV, 842; Cambrai, n.d., before 1260, Boeren I, p. 133; Cambrai, 1287/1288, Boeren II, pp. 132–3; Cambrai, *c.* 1300–7, *Veterum scriptorum* VII, 1292 and BnF, MS lat. 1592, fol. 55r, col. 1; and Tournai, 1366, Le Groux, pp. 3–4.

[31] Coutances, n.d. (thirteenth century), Mansi XXV, 30–1: 'non quantum ad salutem, sed quoad augmentum virtutum'.

[32] X 3.42.2 (Friedberg II, 644): 'De quibus dubium est, an baptizati fuerint, baptizantur his verbis praemissis: "Si baptizatus es, non te baptizo, sed, si nondum baptizatus es, ego te baptizo, etc."'

[33] Angers, Pontal, pp. 140, 142; Rouen, *c.* 1231–5, *Concilia Rotomagensis*, ed. Bessin, II, 54; Le Mans, 1247, *Veterum scriptorum* VII, 1371–2; Cambrai, before 1260, Boeren I, p. 133; Cambrai, *c.* 1300–7, *Veterum scriptorum* VII, 1292–3; Bayeux, 1300, Mansi XXV, 61; Paris, after 1311, *Synodicon*, ed. Harlay, pp. 33–4; Reims, *c.* 1328–30, Gousset II, 539; Orléans, *c.* 1314, *Veterum scriptorum* VII, 1274–5; Tréguier, *c.* 1334, *Thesaurus* IV, 1097–8; Meaux, *c.* 1346, *Thesaurus* IV, 892–3; Chartres, *c.* 1355–68, Jusselin, 80; Tournai, 1366, Le Groux, pp. 3–4.

Two synodal texts instruct the priest to speak the conditional formula aloud and in French so that the laity present at the ceremony will understand that no one can be baptized twice: Chartres, *c.* 1355–68, Jusselin, 80; Reims, *c.* 1328–30, Gousset, II, 539.

synodal legislation, starting with the synod of Paris.[34] Not only are caesarean sections mentioned in various synodal collections examined for this essay, but the statutes giving directions on how to perform such operations are often placed in the sections dealing with baptism. Clearly caesareans were deemed important, not as medical operations that might save the physical life of an infant, but as spiritually life-saving procedures. Blumenfeld-Kosinski has assumed that the ecclesiastical legislation on caesareans was directed specifically at midwives, and while it does not seem unlikely that midwives did perform many caesareans, none of the legislation examined offers any clear clues on who was expected to perform this operation. All that is ever given are a series of laconic instructions on how to proceed. One is to make sure that mother is quite dead, but the fetus is alive. Some statutes recommend that one hold the corpse's mouth open (so that the fetus may continue to receive fresh air) and then perform the operation. The child, if alive, should be baptized immediately, but if it is dead it should be buried outside the cemetery.[35] The focus is on trying to grant the infant the possibility of salvation, not on the problem of who might perform the caeserean or the baptism.

This examination of the synodal and conciliar legislation of northern France during the late Middle Ages shows that midwifery in the period was neither a gathering of ignorant women in need of professional medical enlightenment nor a cabal of female medical practitioners who were being systematically oppressed by a hostile Christian church. It seems likely from the ways in which the Church set out to professionalize this group that they were recognized for holding the necessary medical knowledge to assist in births according to the medical norms of the time. The legislation also clearly demonstrates that midwives were becoming increasingly recognized as an important part of pastoral care, required both to recognize emergency births as they occurred and to be able to perform emergency baptisms as the situation required. A careful examination of midwifery in this period requires an analysis of why the Church saw a crucial pastoral role for midwives and how they brought them into a system of regulation and licensing.

[34] Blumenfeld-Kosinski, *Not of Women Born*, pp. 26–7, and Sigal, 'La grossesse,' p. 34.

[35] Synod of Paris, Pontal, p. 72; Soissons, n.d. (thirteenth century), *Veterum scriptorum* VIII, 1545; Cambrai, n.d. (before 1260), Boeren I, 133; Cambrai, *c.* 1287–8, Boeren II, 133; Cambrai, *c.* 1300–7, *Veterum scriptorum* VII, 1293; Orléans, *c.* 1314, *Veterum scriptorum* VII, 1282; Rouen, 1311, Bessin, II, 84; Reims, *c.* 1328–30, Gousset II, 544; Meaux, n.d. (*c.* 1346), *Thesaurus* IV, 897; Tournai, 1366, Le Groux, p. 4; Reims, 28 April 1408, Mansi XXVI, 1072; St-Brieuc, 21 October 1421, Pocquet, p. 24.

Credulous Midwives and Sorcerous Ones

Anxiety over guaranteeing the creation of correct Christian identity spills over into a fear about the instability of Christian identity. Can the laity, including midwives, be trusted to perform a baptism correctly? Are those baptized in an emergency baptism truly Christian? How can one identify a correctly baptized Christian from an incorrectly baptized one? These worries about the permeable borders of the Christian community are also revealed in the earliest legislation that I found on midwives. In a Sens council from the early thirteenth century there is a canon which 'orders under the pain of excommunication that no Christian wet-nurse should nourish the son of a Jew nor should Christian midwives attend the childbed of Jewish women'. The fear here is the fear of seduction, that is, that the good, but incredulous Christian midwife or wet-nurse will be induced to believe the falsehoods propagated by their Jewish employers.[36]

The difficulty in identifying the cultural significance of the midwife is evidenced in the debate around the issue of witchcraft and midwives. Greilsammer in her article on the history of midwifery in the low countries examines synodal legislation from the northeastern French dioceses of Cambrai and Tournai, pointing out that 'as early as the first half of the thirteenth century, in the older statutes of Cambrai, mention is made of "sortilegia in sacramentis" among the cases reserved to the bishop'. She reads this as a clear message that the Church was openly concerned about the 'religious orthodoxy' of midwives and their possible sorcerous intentions.[37] 'Sortilegia in sacramentis' is mentioned as one of the sins that should be reserved for the bishop, not just in the Cambrai legislation mentioned by Greilsammer, but in many of reserve case listings in many of the synodal and conciliar collections from all over northern France.[38] There is, however, no stated connection between such *sortilegia* and midwives in any legislation. In legislation from Soissons and Nantes priests are warned not to allow mothers to keep the baptismal chrismale (chrism-cloth) or christening clothing because they might use to perform some sort of

[36] Sens, *c.* 1212–13, Mansi XXII, 850: 'Statuimus sub poena excommunicationis ne nutrix Christiana nutriat filium Judæi, et ne Christianæ obstetrices intersint puerperio Judæarum, nec alii Christiani eis serviant, ne per superficialem legis suæ probabilitatem, quam prave exponendo prætendunt, servientes Christianos secum commorantes in suæ incredulitatis inducat baratrum.' (This archdiocesan legislation was promulgated as additions to the original synod of Paris collection.)

Chartres, *c.* 1355–68, contains a similar legislation to this canon, forbidding Christian women from being servants and nursemaids in Jewish households, but it does not mention midwives (Jusselin, 85).

[37] Greilsammer, 'Midwife', pp. 307–8.

[38] See for example, Countances, n.d (thirteenth century), Mansi XXV, 43; Cambrai, 1277, Boeren I, p. 401; Bayeux, 1300, Mansi XXV, 71.

magic.[39] Other statutes warn priests to keep an eye on the chrism and sacred oil to prevent their use as magical aids.[40] That legislators were aware of the possibility of sacramental abuse is clear, but it is not evident from the legislation that there was concern about midwives performing such actions. Rather, as we have seen above, the concern was over whether midwives understood when to perform an emergency baptism and how to perform one.[41]

Conclusion

For the most part, northern French ecclesiastical legislators situated the midwife within their concerns about the baptism and maintaining a proper Christian identity. The insistence on the need for infant baptism, and the central position that this sacrament occupied in the Church's views on individual salvation and recognition within the Christian community of the living and dead, helped to establish tensions between the ecclesiastical authorities' desire to control this initiation rite and their need to ensure that all were safely inside the fold. Teaching the laity how to baptize correctly was an acknowledgment that the more important issue was ensuring that all members of the Christian community were properly initiated members of the community. By the fourteenth century legislators from dioceses in central and eastern regions of northern France were issuing instructions about how to baptize correctly specifically to midwives, whose occupation guaranteed that they would be likely to encounter those anomalous situations that so worried Church authorities.

This raises two interesting questions that further research on medieval midwives might answer. The first is whether ecclesiastical concern over baptism helped to create a 'professional' class of midwives, and the second is whether this professionalization of midwifery can be geographically traced: did it spread out from more demographically dense regions (such as the Île-de-France) to less populated areas of France? Certainly Saunier suggests that a parish midwife in the archdeaconry of Josas occupied an official position, which was validated through elections, exams, oaths and letters of commissions. In addition, Saunier has noted that the population density of a given

[39] Soissons, n.d. (thirteenth century), *Veterum scriptorum* VIII, 1539, and Nantes, *c.* 1320, *Thesaurus* IV, 954.

[40] See for example, Synod of Paris, Pontal, p. 56; Soissons, n.d. (thirteenth century), *Veterum scriptorum* VIII, 1538; Coutance, n.d. (thirteenth century), Mansi XXV, 31; Cambrai, before 1260, Boeren I, 133–4; Orléans, before 1314, *Veterum scriptorum* VII, 1274; Reims, *c.* 1328–30, Gousset II, 539; Chartres, *c.* 1355–68, Jusselin, 80.

[41] What is true about legislation on magic, is also true about legislation that lists abortions and the use of potions of sterility (contraceptives) as reserved cases for the bishop. The legislation gives no indication whether midwives or any other group of people should be viewed as the usual suspects in these cases. For a sample of reserve case listing, see above, n. 38.

region is the most important factor in determining whether a parish has access to a recognized midwife.[42] Reading the legislation carefully also reveals that while ecclesiastical legislators were worried about how to bring emergency baptisms within their notions of what a normal baptism should be, they were not overtly concerned about midwives as sources of witchcraft. Further research on midwifery in published and unpublished church court records, visitation records, synodal legislation, confessor manuals, miracle stories, and other such material should develop a more complex understanding of the role of the midwife in medieval society than is currently provided.

[42] Saunier, 'Visiteur'.

Medicine for Body and Soul: Jacques de Vitry's Sermons to Hospitallers and their Charges[1]

Jessalynn Bird

This article contextualizes Jacques de Vitry's advice to hospitallers and their patients in his *Sermones ad status* and *Historia occidentalis*, valuable sources for the history of medieval hospitals published here in a companion appendix. Jacques' opinions reflect the training in moral theology which he and the future Innocent III received in Peter the Chanter's circle in Paris. By the late twelfth century, the lucrative study and practice of medicine and law also flourished in Paris. Although popes and reformers, including Jacques' colleague Robert of Courson, attempted to restrict those responsible for pastoral care to the liberal arts course preparatory to theological studies, medicine and theology were not innately inimical disciplines.[2] Medical scholars and theologians, most of them clerics in lower orders, used similar dialectical and exegetical techniques. For example, master Giles of Corbeil, responsible for bringing Salernitan medicine to Paris, supported the moralists' agenda for the reform of the clergy, adding medical justification to their criticism of mandatory clerical celibacy.[3]

While acknowledging the validity of the medical vocation, Jacques and other monastic and moral theologians opposed the unbridled application of dialectic from the old Aristotelian corpus and the naturalist *Weltanschauung* of the recently translated *libri naturales* and their Arabic commentators to matters they felt were best governed by biblical, patristic, and legal authorities. Observation and argumentation might supplant rather than supplement textual authorities; the sciences might challenge rather than complement the theological imperatives necessary for spiritual salvation. Jacques reminded students that Greek and Arabic astrology, if unglossed by theological

[1] I would like to thank Peter Biller for inviting me to contribute this essay and providing expert criticism and helpful suggestions, Andrew Satchell for his advice on secondary literature, and the Fulbright association and the Thouron family for their financial support.

[2] S. Ferruolo, *The Origins of the University: The Schools of Paris and their Critics, 1100–1215* (Stanford, 1985), pp. 126, 142–3, 181–2, 184, 195, 206, 234, 243, 302–4; O'Boyle, *Art of Medicine*, pp. 11, 45–9; Baldwin, *Peter the Chanter*, I, 84–7 and nn. 146–9 in II, 59; Paris (1213) ii.20, iii.20 and Rouen (1214) ii.22, lvi in Mansi XXII, 831, 838, 910–11, 916.

[3] Baldwin, *Peter the Chanter*, I, 41 and 83; O'Boyle, *Art of Medicine*, pp. 9–19, 99–102, 115–24, 264–8 and n. 56 on p. 48; D. Jacquart, 'Medical Scholasticism', in *Western Medical Thought*, pp. 197–240 (pp. 197, 205–12, 215 and n. 25 on p. 381).

authorities, could lead to the spiritually hazardous belief that the planets determined human physiology and moral behavior, rather than the orthodox view that heavenly bodies merely influenced humans' humoral compositions and predilections for certain vices.[4] Medical treatment focussed on physical welfare could also hinder the soul's salvation. The Paris moralists disparaged doctors who recommended rest, eating, and even fornication to balance the body's humors rather than spiritually salutary vigils, fasting, labour, and self-mortification. Some fed their patients' specious hopes for recovery so that they eschewed the spiritual medicine of confession and extreme unction.[5] Their concerns influenced the Fourth Lateran Council (1215), which warned doctors to address a disease's moral aetiology before its physical symptoms.[6]

Modern debates concerning power, disease, poverty and the marginal have dominated the history of hospitals and leper houses, leading Saul Brody and Françoise Bériac to claim that theologians formed social conceptions of leprosy by uncritically transmitting medical lore in their sermons and treatises, thereby persuading ecclesiastical and secular authorities to segregate lepers, medically defined as virulently contagious, from the general populace.[7] In fact, theologians, preachers and confessors often appropriated medical theories and imagery in their role as spiritual physicians,[8] but adapted their messages to appeal to or confront popular and learned opinion.[9] Jacques de Vitry played upon leprosy as a metaphor for sin,[10] medical descriptions of types of leprosy, and assumptions concerning its contagiousness, reflecting and inverting popular and learned conceptions in order to transfer the revulsion and social shunning generally reserved for lepers to sin. While leprosy was contagious and disfiguring, it could lead to conversion and salvation, sentiments reflected in Jean Bodel's *Congés*.[11] Jacques also joined contemporary statutes and confessors' manuals in justifying the regulation of sexual behaviour within marriage by medical theories: sexual relations during pregnancy and menstruation inflicted

[4] *Sermo ad scolares*, no. 16, in Pitra, pp. 365–72 (p. 368); Jacquart, 'Medieval Scholasticism', pp. 233–4, 237–8.

[5] *H.occ.* 4 (p. 82); *Sermo ad scolares*, no. 16, in Pitra, p. 370; Agrimi and Crisciani, 'Charity and Aid', pp. 179–81.

[6] C. 22, in *COD*, pp. 245–6.

[7] Brody, *Disease*, pp. 23–5, 58–9, 64–8, 73, 81–3; Bériac, *Lépreux*, pp. 102–5, 175–7. Contrast Touati, *Maladie*, pp. 21–51.

[8] Bériac, *Lépreux*, pp. 102–5; P. Anciaux, *La théologie du sacrement de pénitence au XIIe siècle* (Louvain and Gembloux, 1949), pp. 169–72; Bériou and Touati, *Voluntate dei*, pp. 58–9, n. 71.

[9] Peter the Chanter, *Summa de sacramentis et animae consiliis*, ed. J.-A. Dugauquier, AMN 4, 7, 11, 16, 21 (1954–67), §§ 268, 274, pp. 284, 287, 296; Peter of Corbeil in Le Grand, *Statuts*, pp. 191–3.

[10] Brody, *Disease*, pp. 107–34, 142–6; Bériac, *Lépreux*, p. 102; Touati, *Maladie*, pp. 105–8.

[11] *Sermones in epistolas et evangelia dominicalia totius anni*, ed. D. a Ligno (Antwerp, 1575), pp. 672, 783–4; Brody, *Disease*, pp. 89–92; Touati, *Maladie*, pp. 127–75; Bériou and Touati, *Voluntate Dei*, especially pp. 14–15.

leprosy or deformity upon the unborn.[12] Just as some modern religious groups used the medical model for the sexual transmission of AIDS to reinforce their moral ban on premarital intercourse, so Jacques and other theologians commandeered popular and medical associations of leprosy, lust and venereal disease in sermons, reminding young men that they risked contracting leprosy from prostitutes.[13]

The Paris masters also reacted to contemporary demographic and economic changes, formulating a 'theology of the poor' in response to the inflation and famine which struck the Paris area in the late twelfth century. Previously reserved for regular religious who renounced personal possessions, or used to contrast the powerless to the powerful, the term 'pauper' now also signified the materially destitute as objects of charity, reflecting the efforts of twelfth-century religious movements, prelates, popes, and theologians to ensure that the indigent were integrated into Christendom as a spiritual and social *status*.[14] While Robert of Courson's hopes that an ecumenical council could mandate compulsory poor relief were disappointed in 1215, Innocent III founded the hospital of Santo Spirito in Sassia as an example to bishops and their cathedral chapters, whom he and the moralists claimed were failing in their duty as the needy's first recourse.[15] The Paris circle warned secular and regular ecclesiastical officeholders to regard their church's revenues as the poor's patrimony and urged secular rulers to initiate almsgiving and force the rich to feed the impoverished during famines. Their advice paralleled Philip Augustus's measures and a gradual shift in the provision of charity from monastic houses and cathedral chapters to lay almsgiving.[16]

When masters and sermonizers addressed the new commercial elite, they advised them to maintain mental detachment from legitimately-acquired goods by surrendering surplus possessions to the regular religious or the involuntarily poor who, as objects of mercy, enabled the rich to earn salvation.[17] Although less meritorious than charitable works in life,

[12] Jacquart and Thomasset, pp. 185–90; Touati, *Maladie*, pp. 110–27; Bériac, *Lépreux*, pp. 118–19; Robert of Flamborough, *Liber poenitentialis* iv.226, v.285–8, ed. J. J. Firth (Toronto, 1971), pp. 236–8, 197–8, App. B, p. 297; *Sermo ad coniugatos*, no. 66 in Douai, Bibliothèque Municipale, MS 503, fols. 416v–417v.

[13] Jacquart and Thomasset, pp. 185–90; Touati, *Maladie*, pp. 115–17; Bériac, *Lépreux*, pp. 51–6, 119–20; Brody, *Disease*, pp. 52–8, 129–32, 169, 181–3, 185; *Sermo ad pueros et adolescentes*, no. 74, in Douai MS 503, fols. 436v, 437v; Paris (1213), Add. (missing numeration) in Mansi XXII, 854; Paris (1208), in Pontal, c. 88, p. 200.

[14] Mollat, *Pauvres*, pp. 9–21, 106–10, 129–42, 147–57; articles by M. Mollat, L. K. Little, J. Leclerq, and J. Batany in *Études*, ed. Mollat, I, 11–30, 35–43, 447–59; II, 469–86.

[15] Baldwin, *Peter the Chanter*, I, 236–7 and 317; II, 172–3 and 255–6; Longère, 'Pauvreté'; Paris (1213) iv.6, Mansi XXII, 840; *H.occ.* 30 (pp. 151–4). For Innocent, see n. 54 below.

[16] M. Mollat, 'Hospitalité et assistance au début du XIIIe siècle', in *Poverty in the Middle Ages*, ed. D. Flood (Werl, 1975), pp. 41–8.

[17] J. Bird, 'Reform or Crusade? Anti-Usury and Crusade Preaching during the Pontificate of Innocent III', in *Innocent III and his World*, ed. J. C. Moore (Aldershot,

testamentary almsgiving joined the endowment of anniversary masses and prayers as a means of truncating the departed's posthumous purgation; *exempla* depicted the torments awaiting executors who delayed or embezzled charitable bequests.[18] Jacques' estate-specific elegies in a sermon for the bereaved stress the primacy of charity for all classes, as do his *Sermones ad status*, which urge artisans and the working poor to repair the destitute's apparel and houses, and secular clergymen and the powerful to aid legally and financially the oppressed and afflicted.[19]

Whether motivated by civic pride and individual prestige, desire to provide the shelter which hospices offered to travellers, or pangs of guilt and fear concerning the poor they exploited by morally dubious money-lending and a commercial economy, merchants supported urban hospitals as individuals and members of confraternities.[20] While the Paris masters agreed that almsgiving was more painful than fasting, prayer, or bodily discipline for the avaricious, they fretted that merchants and usurers would use socially honourable charitable donations to avoid making shameful and individual restitution to those harmed by their business practices. Gifts to religious houses enabled the donor to believe that he benefitted from the house's prayers and provided access to the Christian burial, prayers, and masses denied him by bishops and priests who excommunicated or refused absolution to malefactors until they made reparations. In council canons and sermons the Paris moralists warned religious institutions to screen donations – better to let themselves and the needy perish than wittingly accept anything derived from usury, theft, or rapine. Their teaching influenced many from the Flanders-Brabant region, who so abhorred illicit profit that they renounced their relations' wealth and served the poor and abject in hospitals and leper houses, including Jacques' spiritual muse, Mary of Oignies, who ate wild herbs rather than accept tainted gifts.[21]

Jacques and other moralists were ideally poised to observe and influence contemporary religious movements. As theology masters, *scolastici*, bishops and members of cathedral chapters, they shaped the local clergy through disciplinary actions, preaching, and teaching. Many tapped into the Premonstratensian and Cistercian orders' intellectual and activist networks, while

1999), pp. 165–86; *Sermo ad dolentes*, no. 45, Trento, Biblioteca comunale, MS 1670, fol. 94ra–b; Longère, 'Pauvreté', pp. 260–72; Rubin, *Charity and Community*, pp. 84–5.

[18] *Die* Exempla *von Jakob von Vitry*, ed. G. Frenken (Munich, 1914), no. 56, p. 125; *Sermo ad dolentes*, no. 45, Trento MS 1670, fols. 91ra–93ra; Crane, nos. 114–15, pp. 52–3.

[19] *Sermo ad dolentes*, no. 46, Trento MS 1670, fols. 93vb–94rb; *Sermo ad artifices mechanicos*, no. 62, Douai MS 503, fols. 404v–406v; *Sermones ad potentes et milites*, nos. 51–3, fols. 374r–382r; *H.occ.* 3 (pp. 79–81); *VA* 24 (*PL* 205, 90).

[20] Imbert (1982), pp. 51–2; J. H. Mundy, 'Charity and Social Work in Toulouse, 1100–1250', *Traditio* 22 (1966), 203–87; S. Epstein, *Wills and Wealth in Medieval Genoa 1150–1250* (Cambridge, MA, 1984), pp. 149–50, 178–9, 185–6, 192–5.

[21] Bird, 'Reform or Crusade?' esp. pp. 169–81; Bonenfant, 'Hôpitaux', 16, 21, 23; *Sermo ad hospitalarios*, no. 40, Trento MS 1670, fol. 84ra–b; Hugh of Floreffe, *Vita Ivettae reclusae Hugi*, ed. G. Henschenius, AA SS January 1 (Antwerp, 1643), pp. 868–87.

others were appointed crusade preachers and legates by Innocent III and his successors. As a Paris master, reform preacher, canon regular at Oignies in Flanders-Brabant, bishop of Acre, auxiliary bishop of Liège (1227–9), and cardinal of Tusculum (1229–40), Jacques joined a network of Paris-educated reformers involved in pastoral care, preaching the crusades, and the reform of religious houses, who shaped local and papal policies in collusion with contacts from the episcopate, papal curia, and various religious orders.[22]

Jacques' letters, sermons, and *Historia Iherosolimitana* reflect the moralists' conviction that these activities could spiritually renew Europe. Through prayers, confession, sermons and the mass, the laity could lead a quasi-monastic life; mental devotion could transform the labours inherent to each *status* and occupation into a penance equal to the monastic profession. However, concerned that the proliferation of quasi-regular observances might result in abuses and hypocrisy, the moralists insisted that the status of the regular religious be reserved for those who vowed poverty, chastity and obedience and adopted a recognized rule. In order to maintain discipline and prevent misuse of religious privileges, internal reform mechanisms, including statutes, rules, chapter meetings, and annual or triennial general meetings, must be supplemented by conciliar legislation and visitation and reform by papal representatives, bishops, or their delegates.[23]

Jacques' *Historia occidentalis* (*c.* 1219–21), written shortly after the Fourth Lateran Council's decrees selectively confirmed the reform initiatives of Innocent III and the Paris circle, records his personal observation of current religious movements while calling for a continuing reform of all social orders,[24] as do his *Sermones ad status*, edited during his cardinalate (1229–40).[25] His sermons to the poor and afflicted, pilgrims, the sick and lepers, those serving and managing hospitals, their donors, and affiliated confraternities represent an edited amalgam of his preaching in hospices and hospitals during his wide travels in Europe and the Near East. His sermons and history reflect the exhortations hospital personnel encountered in weekly chapters, when their rule and statutes were read, or heard from reforming episcopal or papal delegates. Like the latter, Jacques judged hospitals by their ability to reform themselves and their adherence to a rule

[22] J. L. Bird, 'Heresy, Reform and the Crusades in the Circle of Peter the Chanter, c.1187–c.1240' (unpublished D.Phil. dissertation, University of Oxford, 2001).

[23] J. Bird, 'The Religious's Role in a Post-Fourth-Lateran World: Jacques de Vitry's *Sermones ad Status* and *Historia Occidentalis*', in *Medieval Monastic Preaching*, ed. C. Muessig (Leiden, Boston and Cologne, 1998), pp. 209–30 (pp. 222–7).

[24] B. C. Cannuyer, 'Le date de rédaction de l'Historia Orientalis de Jacques de Vitry (1160/70–1240), évêque d'Acre', *Revue d'histoire ecclésiastique* 78 (1983), 65–72. I am preparing an English translation of the *Historia occidentalis* for the University of Liverpool Press.

[25] Jean Longère is currently editing the *Sermones ad status*. For now, see the lacunae-ridden edition in Pitra, pp. 344–465, and the literature cited in C. Muessig, 'Paradigms of Sanctity for Thirteenth Century Women', in *Models of Holiness in Medieval Sermons*, ed. B. M. Kienzle (Louvain-la-Neuve, 1996), pp. 85–102.

and statutes.[26] His plans for the social and religious roles of hospitals and leper houses, their personnel and patients were shared by some bishops, communes and reformers intent on regulating new religious groups. Although lay-persons originally staffed many leper houses and hospitals, in the late twelfth and early thirteenth centuries they were increasingly categorized as regular religious, accorded similar privileges and required to follow a recognized rule.[27]

Jacques includes the entire spectrum of hospitaller institutions in his history. For the charitable work performed by hospices or hospitals shifted in organization and ethos in response to religious life's evolving forms and goals. While bishops, cathedral chapters and Benedictine monasteries had long maintained hospices as part of their emulation of the early church's communal life and ownership, the monastic and canonical orders founded by the *Wanderprediger* in the late eleventh and early twelfth centuries sought to combine greater isolation from worldly concerns with pastoral care for the laity and extended participation in the religious life to previously excluded groups. Stressing poverty and manual labour rather than liturgy, they devoted more resources to charitable work, staffing hospices in areas of wilderness. However, a dramatic increase in the urban poor led some bishops and canonical orders to oversee new hospices, while lay confraternities and wealthy individuals founded independent and quasi-regular hospitals.[28] The Augustinian rule's adaptability suited this charitable mission, and many hospitals' written rules or oral customs were inspired by it and the statutes of notable local houses. Some, such as the hospitallers of the Holy Spirit, those of St John in Jerusalem, the Antonine and Trinitarian orders, and the abbeys dependent upon St Jacques du Haut-Pas and Roncevaux organized into canonical congregations with a formal rule and statutes, papal privileges, and exemption from episcopal authority.[29] Because hospitals of all stripes often clashed with parish clergy over the provision of spiritual services and parishioners' alms, bishops resented the privileges of the hospitaller orders and attempted to visit and regulate independent hospitals.[30] However,

26 Bonenfant-Feytmans, 'Organisations', 44–5.

27 Paris (1213), iii.9, and additions in Mansi XXII, 836, 854; J. Avril, 'Le IIIe concile de Latran et les lépreux', *Revue Mabillon* 60 (1981), 21–76; Bériac, *Lépreux*, pp. 233–59, balanced by Bériou and Touati, *Voluntate dei*, especially pp. 5–9, 18–19, 21–2.

28 *H.occ.* 20–4 (pp. 128–39); Imbert (1982), pp. 15–66; Mollat, *Pauvres*, pp. 53–8, 62–9, 75, 87, 111–16, 121–9; Imbert (1947), pp. 58–62, 74–95, 233–44; J.-M. Bienvenu, 'Fondations charitables laïques au XIIe siècle: l'exemple de l'Anjou', in *Études*, ed. Mollat, II, 563–9. For the Flanders-Brabant region, see Bonenfant, 'Hôpitaux', 3–44, and Spiegeler, *Hôpitaux*, pp. 46, 89–99.

29 *H.occ.* 29 (pp. 149–50); E. N. Rocca, 'Ospedali e Canoniche Regolari', in *La vita comune del clero nei secoli XI e XII*, Miscellanea del Centro di Studi Medioevali 3.1 (Milan, 1962), pp. 16–25; Le Grand, *Statuts*, pp. v–viii, 97, 111; J. C. Dickinson, *The Origins of the Austin Canons and their Introduction into England* (London, 1950), pp. 163–96.

30 Imbert (1947), pp. 142–5, 278–80; Le Grand, 'Maisons-Dieu et léproseries', 83–4, 90, 152–3; Spiegeler, *Hôpitaux*, pp. 105–10.

despite Jacques' reservations regarding the military orders' misuse of their privileges, confirmed by his experience as a crusade preacher and legal wrangles with them as bishop of Acre, he praised their military prowess and hospital work in his *Historia orientalis* and addressed two sermons to their fighters. His advice to hospitallers was meant to include members of the military orders who staffed hospitals in Europe and the Near East.[31]

Some independent hospitals lacked written rules and did not acknowledge episcopal oversight. Their numbers increased during the thirteenth century as urban governments assumed the management of hospitals and professional confraternities founded institutions reserved for their own members.[32] Jacques and other reformers wanted to prevent ill-disciplined quasi-regulars obtaining the privileges due to the regular religious, and claimed that hospitals of this ilk failed to meet the minimum criteria for religious institutions. True discipline demanded a rule and obedience to a superior, not a fraternal organization. Private possessions must be renounced; their retention undermined communal life, voluntary poverty, and detachment from the world. While Jacques praised the Order of Santiago for obtaining a papal dispensation which allowed its fragile lay members to remain married, he criticized exclusive 'religious' establishments such as the chapters of secular 'canonesses' in Flanders-Brabant, where most lived in a secular manner without sufficient safeguards for their chastity.[33]

The quasi-regular beguines and the early Humiliati and Franciscans were also attracted to hospitals as a form of lay-driven devotion which combined contemplation with an apostolic involvement in the world. The dividing line between private charity and hospitals was a thin one; devout lay-persons and quasi-regulars often involved themselves in hospital work as members of confraternities, *conversi/ae* or low-level servants, exercised private austerities and charitable acts, or transformed their homes into small hospitals. The sisters of the Hôtel-Dieu of Angers were admitted expressly to aid female servants (*pedissecae*) in nursing and feeding the infirm with the aid of clerical and lay brethren who were not otherwise occupied with spiritual services or the administration of hospital property.[34] Jacques' sermons to hospitallers

[31] *Historia orientalis* 64–6, ed. F. Moschus (Douai, 1597), pp. 111–23; *Sermones ad fratres ordinis militaris*, nos. 37–8, in Pitra, pp. 405–21; discussion of quaestors below.

[32] Le Grand, *Statuts*, pp. 1–2; Bonenfant-Feytmans, 'Organisations', 43–4; Mollat, 'Hospitalité', pp. 41–3, 47–8; M.-L. Windemuth, *Das Hospital als Träger der Armenfürsorge im Mittelalter* (Stuttgart, 1995), pp. 88–112.

[33] *H.occ.* 26, 31 (pp. 141–2, 156–8) for privileges, see Bonenfant, 'Origines de l'Hôpital Saint-Jean. Son importance', in *Annales de la Société Belge d'Histoire des Hôpitaux* 3 (1965), 57–78 (p. 66); Imbert (1947), pp. 74–96.

[34] *H.occ.* 28 (pp. 144–6); Ep. I, ed. R. B. C. Huygens (Leiden, 1960), pp. 75–6; Bird, 'Religious' Role', pp. 225–7; Risse, *Mending Bodies*, p. 152; A. Forey, 'Women and the Military Orders in the Twelfth and Thirteenth Centuries', in *Military Orders and Crusades* (Aldershot, 1994), article IV, 63–91 (pp. 67–9); G. G. Meersseman, *Dossier de l'ordre de la Pénitence au XIIIe siècle* (Fribourg, 1961); Le Grand, *Statuts*, §§ 8–10, pp. 24–5 (Angers).

invoke the personal ministry of Christ, St Martin, Thibaud count of Champagne and a devout matron who cared for a leper in her own home to shame hospitaller personnel who delegated the care of the sick entirely to hired servants. Humble tasks help foster compassion and the recognition of human infirmity; the stench they endure now is a penance which helps them to escape hell.[35]

However, Jacques cautioned male hospital personnel not to become too familiar with *sorores* and *conversae*. Platonic affection could become physical attraction, and male and female patients ought to be segregated and treated by their own sex.[36] Some hospital statutes prohibited young or attractive women from being admitted as *sorores* or hired as servants. Brothers were forbidden to talk with either group except in public about house business, and many hospitals provided for separate dormitories, refectories and disciplinary chapters and severely punished those caught 'fornicating'.[37] However, female *conversae*, oblates, and recluses continued to attach themselves to male religious houses and scarce resources often meant that it was difficult to maintain segregated living spaces. Robert of Courson's legislation urged male religious houses not to admit young or suspect women unless separate accommodation were possible. Even then, women ought not to be accepted for the sake of blood relation or donations, but for their usefulness to the house's work.[38]

Jacques' history and sermons were written while reforming bishops were zealously implementing Fourth Lateran's stipulation that new religious orders adopt a recognized rule by continuing to impose variations of the Augustinian rule upon hospitals and leper houses in their dioceses. The Paris moralists' theories regarding bishops' duty to visit and correct non-exempt religious houses in their dioceses were summarized in the legislation of the Paris master Robert of Courson, whom Innocent III appointed legate in France to hold provincial councils in preparation for the Fourth Lateran Council (1215). Robert reinforced episcopal rule-making by requiring hospitals or leper houses with sufficient resources for their personnel to live communally to adopt a fitting rule, religious garb, and the three monastic vows.[39] His statutes for the reform of religious houses, hospitals, and leper

[35] No. 39, Trento MS 1670, fol. 81ra; no. 40, fol. 84ra; Crane, nos. 94–5, pp. 43–5.

[36] No. 40, Trento MS 1670, fol. 84ra; see Crane, nos. 100–1, pp. 46–7.

[37] *H.occ.* 22, 29 (pp. 134–5, 147); Le Grand, *Statuts*, §§ 4, 6, pp. 8–9 (Hospital of St John); §§ 37–8, 47, 52, pp. 29, 31, 32 (Amiens/Montdidier); §§ 30–7, 54–7, 65, pp. 48, 51–2 (Hôtel-Dieu in Paris); Paris (1213) iii.1, iii.3, in Mansi XXII, 831.

[38] Forey, 'Women', pp. 66–92; Paris, iii.14, in Mansi XXII, 837.

[39] Bonenfant-Feytmans, 'Organisations', 32, 37, 43, 45; Le Grand, *Statuts*, pp. xii and 1–5; cf. Imbert (1947), pp. 212–16, 268–9; Paris (1213) iii.9, in Mansi XXII, 835–6. However, I disagree with some of Bonenfant-Feytmans's conclusions. She felt that the reformers' efforts reflected an attempt to unite all hospital congregations into one order, which foundered when Innocent III blocked the formation of new orders at the Fourth Lateran Council. Honorius III proved more flexible and pushed for regulation by bishops, resulting in a bloom of

houses reflected the rules composed by bishops linked to the Paris circle and influenced the *content* of statutes adopted by hospitals in Flanders-Brabant and Northern France after the Fourth Lateran Council (1215), as bishops and hospital officials drew upon recent conciliar work, the customs of houses successfully adapted to local conditions, and rules imported from famous institutions.[40]

Jacques' history commends hospitals disciplined by bishops in northern France and Flanders-Brabant who employed Paris moralists, including the Hôtel-Dieu of Paris, overseen by the bishop of Paris and his cathedral chapter. Many theologians became canons at Notre Dame, including Peter the Chanter and Robert of Courson, and both bishop and chapter persistently regulated the hospital personnel's religious life and managed the Hôtel-Dieu's property, initiating a massive rebuilding programme in the late twelfth century. Its benefactors included Peter of Corbeil, the Paris-educated archbishop of Sens, and Stephen of Nemours, bishop of Noyon and brother of Peter of Nemours, bishop of Paris. Both men legislated for hospitals in their dioceses, as did Stephen, dean of Notre Dame, who imposed a rule upon the Hôtel-Dieu in Paris between 1217 and 1221.[41] Jacques maintained his ties to these bishops and masters, created by a common education and collaboration in reform projects and various crusades, while he was writing his sermons and history.[42]

Jacques also lauded episcopally-supervised hospitals in Tournai, Brussels, and Liège.[43] Among these, the hospital of Saint-Jean in Brussels is an outstanding example of a successful episcopal reorganization of an independent hospital founded by a charitable confraternity in emulation of the confraternity of the Holy Spirit in Cologne. Although the confraternity's lay members did not personally serve the indigent and sick, they soon claimed the privileges of regular religious. In return for papal protection, Innocent III demanded they live as such, and by 1211, Jean de Béthune, bishop of Cambrai had imposed a rule on the hospital's personnel after consulting men experienced in regulating the religious,

rule-making *c.* 1220. A simpler explanation is that reforming bishops were temporarily busied by the crusade project, and returned to rule-making after it was safely launched.

40 This model should replace the older thesis that the rule of the hospital of Saint John either directly or indirectly formed the basis of most hospital rules in Europe. Le Grand, *Statuts*, pp. ix–x, xi–xix, 1–2; M.-Th. Lacroix, *L'Hôpital Saint-Nicolas du Bruille (Saint-Andre) à Tournai de sa fondation à sa mutation en cloître (c. 1230–1611)*, 2 vols. (Louvain-la-Neuve, 1977), I, 112–29, 146, 157–8; Imbert (1982), pp. 55–61; Risse, *Mending Bodies*, pp. 148–52; n. 39 above.

41 Robert had also been a canon at Noyon. See L. Brièle and E. Coyecque, *Archives de l'Hôtel-Dieu de Paris, 1157–1300* (Paris, 1894), pp. x–xii, xiii, xv, xix–xxi, 16, 19, 37, 130, 134; Baldwin, *Peter the Chanter*, I, 6 and 19; Hinnebusch, p. 278; Bonenfant-Feytmans, 'Organisations', p. 30; Le Grand, *Statuts*, pp. xiii and 43–53, 191–3.

42 Jacques de Vitry, *Lettres*, ed. Huygens, eps. II, IV, VII, perhaps also I and VI.

43 *H.occ.* 29 (pp. 150–1).

perhaps the same moralists who influenced Hugh Pierrepont, bishop of Liège.[44]

Hugh also took an unusually pro-active role in regulating religious houses in his diocese, spurred on by the Paris masters he employed, including John of Nivelles and John of Lirot, canons in Liège linked to Jacques through a common Paris education and their work in pastoral care, the promotion of the crusades, the reform of monastic life, and the oversight of religious women.[45] John of Lirot and Nivelles acted as mediators for the leper house of Cornillon, and may have persuaded Julienne, an orphan oblate there, to resist the leper house's takeover by prebendaries.[46] John of Nivelles helped reorganize several hospitals dependant on the cathedral chapter of Saint-Lambert and the monasteries of Val-Saint-Lambert and Saint-Laurent, and may have influenced the imposition of the Augustinian rule upon the burghers staffing the hospital of Saint-Christophe.[47] While a canon of St Nicholas at Oignies, Jacques also became one of Hugh's familiars, accompanying him to the Fourth Lateran council. He later served as an auxiliary bishop and executor of Hugh's will. His praise for Liège's hospitals almost certainly included Saint-Matthieu, founded by Hugh in 1204.[48] John of Nivelles witnessed several of Hugh's decisions affecting this hospital's property and relations with Val-Saint-Lambert,[49] and donors followed the Paris circle's teaching that usurped tithes must not be given directly to religious houses in return for prayers, but first ought to be restored to the bishop of the diocese to which they had originally belonged.[50]

Jacques' sermons to hospitallers and their charges illustrate the methods moralists used to persuade both groups to reform themselves and adopt their ideal social and religious roles. He praises hospitallers for renouncing the world, adopting the religious habit and a frugal lifestyle, and devoting themselves and their possessions to spiritual and physical works of mercy. Using mercantilistic imagery familiar to the artisan, burgher and noble

[44] P. Bonenfant, *Cartulaire de l'hôpital Saint-Jean de Bruxelles (actes des XIIe et XIIIe siècles)* (Brussels, 1953), introduction and no. 10, p. 19, 'Hôpitaux', 19–21, 27–9, 45, and 'Origines', 57–78; Bonenfant-Feytmans, 'Organisations', 35–7; Lacroix, *L'hôpital Saint-Nicolas*, I, 113; Le Grand, *Statuts*, pp. ix, xviii.

[45] C. Renardy, *Les maîtres universitaires dans le diocèse de Liège: Repertoire biographique (1140–1350)* (Paris, 1981), nos. 481, 496, pp. 355–7, 362–3; *H.occ.* 10 (p. 103); E. W. McDonnell, *The Beguines and Beghards in Medieval Culture* (New Brunswick, 1954), pp. 40–7, 156.

[46] Renardy, *Maîtres*, pp. 356, 362; Spiegeler, *Hôpitaux*, pp. 114–16, 122–3, 159.

[47] Renardy, *Maîtres*, pp. 361–2; Spiegeler, *Hôpitaux*, pp. 113, 121; É. Poncelet, *Actes des princes-évêques de Liège: Hugues de Pierrepont, 1200–1229* (Brussels, 1941), no. 86, p. 92 and no.105, p. 109.

[48] Bonenfant-Feytmans, 'Organisations', 34–5; Renardy, *Maîtres*, p. 138; S. Bormans, E. Schoolmeesters and É. Poncelet, *Cartulaire de l'Eglise Saint-Lambert de Liège*, 6 vols. (Brussels, 1893–1933), I, 139–41, no. 87; Poncelet, *Actes*, pp. 92, 109, 198.

[49] Poncelet, *Actes*, no. 86, p. 92 (1211) and no. 105, p. 109 (1212).

[50] Poncelet, *Actes*, no. 105, p. 109 (1212); Third Lateran (1179), c. 10 in *COD*, p. 217; Fourth Lateran (1215), c. 61, in *COD*, p. 262.

classes, he reassures donors and hospital personnel that their charitable work converts transitory riches into heavenly treasure and earns them participation in the Church's prayers and masses and eternal life, in contrast to the merciless, whom Christ will condemn at the last judgement.[51] As one of the various satisfactions imposed for committing sin, works of mercy formed an intrinsic part of the penitential system and could literally save souls. Jacques' audience, composed of hospitallers, donors and members of charitable confraternities, was familiar with these concepts from the sermons which hospital quaestors preached when collecting alms.

However, Jacques attacks these preachers' warped interpretations of the authorities commonly cited in papal or episcopal letters granted to them. These letters offered a partial remission of enjoined penance as a reward for individuals' generosity in almsgiving. While grudgingly conceding that these partial indulgences were valid, the Paris circle excoriated quaestors who oversimplified the complex penitential process and exploited their audiences' desire to circumvent doing penance.[52] Unlike quaestors who lauded almsgiving as an automatic route to salvation, Jacques emphasizes that God respects motives and devotion more than the amount given; alms ought to be given in secret, not ostentatiously to win human praise. He tries to guard his audience from a formulaic and materialistic correlation of the quantity of almsgiving with that of penance deleted by reminding them of man's dual composition, body and soul. Although they can earn heaven by refreshing the bodies of the poor on earth, spiritual works of mercy are even more commendable, including an exemplary life, preaching, and exhortation which free those imprisoned in sin, the spiritual 'burial' of a regular religious dead to the world or the corpses of sins interred through confession and penance.[53] Jacques' opinions on almsgiving were reflected in the works of his contemporaries, including Thomas Chobham, Peter the Chanter, Robert of Courson and Innocent III, and diffused to the populace through sermons.[54]

The human objects of these charitable works were united in their physical inability to work and lack of social status. The Paris circle faced the task of redressing the social problem of the destitute and afflicted and spiritually ministering to them as groups and as individuals. Their *ad status* sermons and confessors' manuals reflect a concern for identifying the special circumstances each *status* faced, the sins they were prone to commit, and the means of salvation available to them. Their sermons to the sick and poor stressed that God used bodily afflictions to punish sinners and convert those he loved from sin, inflicting suffering on earth to spare them the agonies of

[51] No. 39, Trento MS 1670, fols. 80ra–b, 81va–b; Longère, 'Pauvreté', 262–3.

[52] No. 40, Trento MS 1670, fol. 82ra; *H.occ.* 10 (103–6).

[53] No. 40, Trento MS 1670, fols. 82ra, 83ra. Compare the carefully guarded papal letters of indulgence granted to quaestors. See Fourth Lateran Council (1215), c. 62, in *COD*, p. 263; de Angelis, *Innocenzo III*, p. 37; Pressutti, nos. 4182, 4244.

[54] Bolton, 'Hearts'. I am writing articles on the Paris moralists' treatment of indulgences and quaestors.

purgatory or hell. In contrast, the incorrigible remained materially prosperous until the last judgement. Jacques urged his audience not to despair of doing penance for their sins or anger God by murmuring and blasphemy, but to win his favour and furnish a good example to others through patient endurance, prayers and praise. The sufferings inherent to their *status* safeguarded against the vices of pride, avarice, and attachment to the world, and if borne with the proper spirit, could become a powerful form of penance similar to the voluntary poverty practiced by regular religious, leading to the spiritual amelioration of the sufferers themselves, the rich who gave to them, and the hospitallers who cared for them.[55] The physical hardships endured by the unhealthy, destitute, and pilgrims helped to detach them from the world, leading Jacques to cluster these groups closer to the regular religious in his *Sermones ad status* than those whose professions or social duties precluded contemplation. In contrast, his sermons to hospitallers and to the rich and powerful present the abject as human shells for the suffering Christ, dwelling upon their deformities and the possibility of contagion to stress the charitable's heroism.[56]

For once the voluntary poverty and humility previously regarded as the exclusive preserve of the regular religious were extended to those remaining in their lay *status*, a greater respect for the world and the active life led to a new esteem for the body, and hospitals combined spiritual and physical care.[57] Some historians claim that hospitals did not attempt to cure the sick, but simply warehoused them until they spontaneously healed or died.[58] However, while the hospital of St John in Jerusalem was exceptional in its maintenance of surgeons and four full-time physicians, other elements of its medical care were widely copied in European hospitals, including the restoration of the body's humoral balance through bed-rest, diets tailored to the ailing's sex and illness, nursing care, and a strict attention to hygiene, including bathing and shaving.[59] Jacques exhorts

55 *Sermones ad leprosos et alios infirmos*, nos. 41–2, ed. Bériou and Touati in *Voluntate dei*, pp. 101–16 (pp. 102–7, 111–12), 117–28 (pp. 121–2, 123–6); *Sermones ad pauperes et afflicti*, Trento MS 1670, fols. 87va–91ra; Crane, nos. 108–11, pp. 50–2; Agrimi and Crisciani, 'Charity and Aid', pp. 172–5; Longère, 'Pauvreté'; Touati, *Maladie*, pp. 35–7, 102–4, esp. p. 102 n. 79; Bériac, *Lépreux*, pp. 89–117, 123–34; Brody, *Disease*, pp. 61, 101, 103–6, 147–89.

56 Touati, *Maladie*, pp. 50–1 and works cited on p. 51 n. 91; Bériou and Touati, *Voluntate dei*, pp. 24–9, 31, 38–41, 43–5, 50–2, 63, 70–2. For Jacques' *Sermones ad status*, see A. Forni, 'Giacomo da Vitry, predicatore e «sociologo»', *La Cultura* 18 (1890), 34–89, esp. pp. 45, 59–69; J. Longère, *Oeuvres oratoires des maîtres parisiens au XIIe siècle: Étude historique et doctrinale*, 2 vols. (Paris, 1975), I, 368–71.

57 Agrimi and Crisciani, 'Charity and Aid', pp. 178, 187–8.

58 For the debate, see E. J. Kealey, *Medieval Medicus: A Social History of Anglo-Norman Medicine* (Baltimore and London, 1981), p. 83; Horden, 'Discipline of Relevance', 306–7; and the articles by S. Edgington and C. Tell in *The Military Orders*, ed. M. Barber (Aldershot, 1994–), II, *Welfare and Warfare*, ed. H. M. Nicholson, pp. 27–41.

59 Kedar, 'Twelfth-Century Description', pp. 11, 21, 23–4; Le Grand, *Statuts*, §§ 1–2, 9, pp. 12–14.

hospitallers to keep beds and buildings clean so that their patients' sufferings are not exacerbated by filthy surroundings.[60] He also castigates hospital personnel who practice charity without consideration of their patients' physical health. When the simple poor and infirm labouring under an acute fever or another 'hot' illness ask for rich foods like wine and meat, some brothers and sisters give it to them, aggravating their condition. Servers must withhold foods they know to be 'contrary', although they are excused if they err from simple ignorance.[61] The hospital at Amiens allowed patients a lengthy convalescence to avoid instantaneous relapses,[62] and although most hospitals could not afford to permanently retain physicians, some such as Saint-Jean of Brussels allowed them to be called at the patient's expense in the case of a *particularis infirmitas*.[63] Other hospitals employed physicians by the early thirteenth century, and one surgeon named Hubert donated his services to the personnel and patients of the Hôtel-Dieu in Paris for his spiritual health and in appreciation for the hospitals' aid in renting a house.[64]

However, in all hospitals, the first line of treatment for bodily illness was reconciliation with God, and spiritual healing and preparation for death by confession and enjoined penance preceded bed-rest and medical treatment. Jacques' sermons to the leprous and sick confirm the primacy of spiritual therapy and were probably meant to be delivered in hospitals.[65] Most hospices possessed a chapel, where masses and liturgical prayers performed in sight of the patients' beds generated suffrages for the souls of the hospital's inmates, personnel, and donors. The patients' prayers not only fulfilled their end of the social and religious contract by saving their benefactor's souls, but represented one of the few forms of penance available to them in their weakened state, penance necessary for the divine healing of body and soul.[66] This was particularly true of the permanent residents of leper houses, who were treated as regular religious and participated in the house's liturgy and

[60] No. 39, Trento MS 1670, fol. 81ra; no. 40, fol. 84ra.

[61] No. 40, Trento MS 1670, fol. 83rb; Rubin, *Charity and Community*, p. 71; Le Grand, *Statuts*, §§ 16, 21, p. 46 (Hôtel-Dieu in Paris); § 14, p. 56 (St-Julien); § 34, p. 40 (Amiens); § 9, pp. 24–5 (Angers); Trinitarian Rule (1198), in *The Trinitarians' Rule of Life*, ed. J. J. Gross (Rome, 1983), §§ 16–17, p. 12.

[62] Le Grand, *Statuts*, §§ 34, 36, p. 40.

[63] Bonenfant, 'Hôpitaux', 27–8.

[64] Kedar, 'Twelfth-Century Description', pp. 20–1; Brièle and Coyecque, *Archives*, no. 143, pp. 62–3 (1221), n. 57 above. For treatment in leper houses, see Kealey, *Medieval Medicus*, p. 105; Touati, *Maladie*, pp. 173–5; Risse, *Mending Bodies*, pp. 188–9; Bériac, *Lépreux*, pp. 259–62.

[65] Nos. 41–2, in Bériou and Touati, *Voluntate dei*, pp. 101–2, 117–20, 126–8.

[66] Kedar, 'Twelfth-Century Description', 19; Spiegeler, *Hôpitaux*, pp. 193–6; Le Grand, *Statuts*, § 14, pp. 10–11; § 6, p. 15 (Hospital of St John); § 7, p. 24 (Angers); § 24, p. 46 (Hôtel-Dieu in Paris); Imbert (1947), pp. 145–7; n. 70 below. Patients could also contribute materially through begging or duties in the hospital (Kealey, *Medieval Medicus*, pp. 97–8, 100–1).

general duties.[67] Burials, masses, and prayers for the dead served the patients' souls and spiritually rewarded the hospitals' donors and personnel.[68]

The needy's role as intercessors meant that theologians and canonists sought to categorize them into the deserving and undeserving.[69] Thomas Chobham warned the poor not to beg if they could earn their daily bread through manual labour. Beggars must seek only daily necessities, shun deceit, and earn the alms given them by praying for their benefactors.[70] The well-travelled Jacques knew that many hospices' denizens included prostitutes and thieves who robbed ingenuous pilgrims and travellers and that some preferred begging their bread to earning it.[71] Some hospitallers balked at literally following the gospel injunction to give everything to the impoverished. Although many hospitals' rules required them actively to seek out the poor and accept all for whom the house possessed resources,[72] Hôtel-Dieux often referred the chronically ill, including lepers and sufferers from ergot, to specialist institutions and turned away freshly mutilated criminals and those capable of mendicancy or manual labour.[73] Jacques urges them to trust that God will provide, and offers some pragmatic guidance derived from theological and canonical debates on prioritizing charity. If their resources permit, they must give to all the needy. Otherwise they ought to select the most destitute, humble, and righteous who will pray for them, rejecting the dishonest and blasphemous, including actors, vagabonds, and ribalds who will squander their alms on drink and dice. Although the rich allow just indigents to perish and support entertainers' scurrilous songs and blasphemies, when hospitallers give to sinners they should do so because they are human beings, not to support their sins.[74]

[67] Le Grand, *Statuts*, pp. xxv–xxviii, 184–9; Kealey, *Medieval Medicus*, pp. 97–8, 107–116; Risse, *Mending Bodies*, pp. 186–8; P. Bonenfant, 'L'ancienne léproserie Saint-Pierre à Bruxelles', *Annales de la Société Belge d'Histoire des Hôpitaux* 3 (1965), 85–98 (p. 88).

[68] *Sermo* no. 39, Trento MS 1670, fol. 81va–b; Le Grand, *Statuts*, §§ 6, 14, pp. 10–11, 15 (St John in Jerusalem); §§ 1–4, 57–8, pp. 21–3, 33 (Angers); § 16, pp. 37–8 (Hôtel-Dieu of Amiens); §§ 19–20, 69–70, pp. 46, 52–3 (Hôtel-Dieu in Paris); Trinitarian rule (1198), ed. Gross, §§ 37–9, p. 15.

[69] Mollat, *Pauvres*, pp. 137–8, 141–2; Rubin, *Charity and Community*, pp. 68–70.

[70] Thomas Chobham, *Summa Confessorum* art. 7, dist. 2, q. VIa, ed. F. Broomfield, AMN 25 (1968), p. 297.

[71] No. 40, Trento MS 1670, fols. 82vb–83va; *Sermo ad peregrinos*, no. 50, Douai MS 503, fol. 372r; *Sermo ad pauperes et afflictos*, no. 44, Trento MS 1670, fol. 91ra; Crane, no. 112, p. 52.

[72] No. 39, Trento MS 1670, fols. 81ra, 81va; Le Grand, *Statuts*, §§ 5, 16, pp. 23, 25 (Angers); § 14, pp. 10–11 and §§ 3–5, 9, pp. 14–15 (St John in Jerusalem); Kedar, 'Twelfth-Century Description', pp. 18, 24–6; Bolton, 'Hearts', p. 139.

[73] Agrimi and Crisciani, 'Charity and Aid', p. 190; Bonenfant, 'Hôpitaux', 27; Le Grand, *Statuts*, §§ 5–6, 13–14, pp. 23–5 (Angers); Kealey, *Medieval Medicus*, p. 89; Spiegeler, *Hôpitaux*, pp. 47–8.

[74] No. 40, Trento MS 1670, fol. 83ra–b; Crane, nos. 77, 97–8, pp. 35, 45–6; Rubin, *Charity and Community*, pp. 69–70; J. W. Baldwin, 'The Image of the Jongleur in Northern France around 1200', *Speculum* 72 (1997), 635–63, and *Peter the Chanter*, I, 198–204.

However, unbounded charity demanded ceaseless expenditure, while liturgy for donors and self-perpetuation as an institution required assured revenues. Founders, resources, and affiliations influenced a hospital's functions, and the daily life of hospital personnel could vary greatly. An oblate at the leper house of Cornillon, St Julienne read theology and undertook the care of the ill as a voluntary penance. Yet in the penurious leper houses where Ivette of Huy and Mary of Oignies and her husband served as *conversi/ae*, the struggle for subsistence meant little spare time for liturgical services.[75] Prosperity brought its own problems. Prebendaries, oblates, and confraters gave donations with the condition that they were provided for during their lifetime.[76] For a congeries of motives drove lay participation in hospital work, including compassion, private penance, familial prestige and security, and community need. Hospices' charitable work sometimes became a social security network for those of modest means in ill health or old age.[77] Hospitals glutted with religious personnel risked becoming priories devoted to liturgical intercession; those which accepted oblates or were founded by burghers or artisans often became exclusive rest homes for donors or members of a confraternity or guild. Jacques and other reformers feared that individuals' desire for financial security or sustenance would blight 'proper' penitential and devotional motives for entering religious houses and undermine hospital discipline.[78] In order to combat the diversion of resources from the care of the infirm and poor, Robert and his episcopal allies limited the number of hospital personnel and demanded that prebendaries and oblates follow the house's rule or be expelled, forfeiting the possessions donated at their entry.[79]

Jacques savaged those who adopted the outward trappings of a religious regular, yet caused scandal and dissension by rebelling against discipline implemented by superiors and prelates. Their failure to disengage from the world manifested itself in their acceptance of donations tainted by usury, simoniacal entry into a religious house through social pressure, blood

For Innocent III's discriminating charity in Rome, see Bolton, 'Hearts', esp. pp. 128–9, 136–7.

[75] Spiegeler, *Hôpitaux*, pp. 157–60 and *vitae* cited.

[76] Imbert (1947), pp. 281–3.

[77] J. H. Mundy, 'Charity and Social Work in Toulouse, 1100–1250', *Traditio* 22 (1966), 203–87; Forey, 'Women', pp. 63–91. For charity's full spectrum, see Spiegeler, *Hôpitaux*, pp. 38, 46–8, 89–99, 195–7; J. W. Brodman, *Charity and Welfare: Hospitals and the Poor in Medieval Catalonia* (Philadelphia, 1998).

[78] *H.occ.* 29 (p. 149); Dickinson, *Austin Canons*, pp. 145–8; Bonenfant, 'Hôpitaux', 25–6, 29–30; Bonenfant, 'Origines', 59–60.

[79] Spiegeler, *Hôpitaux*, pp. 159–60, 151; Paris (1213) iii.9, in Mansi XII, 835–6; Bonenfant, 'Origines', 70. Despite the opposition of local echevins and burghers, Robert of Courson supported the attempts of the provost of the chapter of Saint-Martin to regulate an unruled lay-founded hospital in Ypres following a council he held at Reims (1213). See E. Feys and A. Nelis, eds., *Les cartulaire de la prévôte de Saint-Martin a Ypres*, 2 vols. (Ypres, 1880–84), I, 27–9, nos. 78, 89–90, and II.i, 60, no. 80; Bonenfant, 'Hôpitaux', pp. 25–6.

relation or gifts, and retention of private possessions.[80] Contemporary episcopally-dictated hospital statutes, the councils of Robert of Courson, and the Fourth Lateran Council (1215) combatted these abuses by requiring hospital personnel to take the three monastic oaths, installing internal and external means of discipline and correction,[81] banning simoniacal entry and private property, and demanding that no one be accepted as a brother or sister unless he or she could minister to the infirm or manage the hospital's possessions.[82]

The retention of personal possessions and simoniacal entry were linked to hospitals' financial insecurity. While the Chanter's circle recognized that religious orders often demanded gifts from new members from ignorance or poverty, particularly leper houses faced with the long-term care of entering lepers, the statutes of reformed hospitals followed Robert of Courson in demanding humiliating penances or expulsion for personnel found with private possessions. Those discovered with them at death forfeited the church burial, prayers, and masses which helped release their souls from purgatory.[83] These statutes also regulated the reception and accounting of gifts and bequests, and the careful management of a hospital's resources; even the quality and quantity of their personnel's food and clothing was to be contingent on diverting as few resources as possible from the care of the needy.[84] Jacques reprimands the Trinitarians for investing in property to secure future revenues. Motivated by fears for the future and trusting that the austerities of their regular life suffice for salvation, they are hoarding the alms their quaestors collect rather than immediately expending them on charitable work as their donors intended.[85]

[80] *H.occ.* 4 (p. 83); no. 40, Trento MS 1670, fols. 82va–b, 83va.

[81] Paris (1213) ii.10, xii and Rouen (1214) ii.13, in Mansi XXII, 828, 829, 908; Le Grand, *Statuts*, §§ 1–2, 58–65, 68, pp. 43–4, 51–2 (Hôtel-Dieu in Paris); §§ 5–6, 8–9, 21–7, 45–50, pp. 36–9, 41–2 (Amiens); §§ 45–52, 55, pp. 30–2, 32–3 (Angers); Trinitarian rule (1198), ed. Gross, §§ 20–4, 29–30, pp. 12–14.

[82] Paris (1213), ii.1, ii.27, iii.6, Add.i, and Rouen (1214) ii.1, xxx, in Mansi, XXII, 825–6, 833, 844–5, 905–6, 911; Fourth Lateran (1215), cc. 63–6, in *COD*, pp. 264–5; Spiegeler, *Hôpitaux*, pp. 161–3, 165; Le Grand, *Statuts*, §§ 1–4, pp. 35–6 (Amiens/ Montdidier); §§ 6, 16, pp. 55–6 (Saint-Julien); §§ 4, 7, 9, p. 44 (Hôtel-Dieu in Paris); §§ 15, 17, pp. 25–6 (Angers).

[83] Paris (1213), iii.9, in Mansi XXII, 835–6; Le Grand, *Statuts*, § 13 p. 10 (St John in Jerusalem); § 49, p. 42 (Amiens); § 62, pp. 51–2 (Hôtel-Dieu in Paris); §§ 21–2, p. 26 (Angers); A. Forey, 'Recruitment to the Military Orders (Twelfth to mid-Fourteenth Centuries)', in *Military Orders and Crusades*, article II, 139–171 (pp. 155–7); Bériac, *Lépreux*, pp. 224–30; J. Lynch, *Simoniacal Entry into the Religious Life from 1000–1260: A Social, Economic and Legal Study* (Colombus, 1976); Baldwin, *Peter the Chanter*, I, 121 and 172–3, 176, 181, 191, 193.

[84] No. 40, Trento MS 1670, fol. 82va–b; Le Grand, *Statuts*, §§ 9, 29–34, 36, 41, 54, 56, pp. 25, 27–8, 29–30, 32–3 (Angers); §§ 25–9, 48, 53, pp. 47–8, 50, 51 (Hotel-Dieu in Paris); §§ 36–40, 43, pp. 40–1 (Amiens).

[85] *H.occ.* 25 (pp. 139–41). Jacques refers to the rule drafted by the Trinitarians' founder, the Paris master John of Matha, in consultation with the bishop of Paris and the

Jacques urges hospital brothers who stockpile clothing and bedding while Christ's poor shiver naked in their hospices to trust that God will provide, reminding them that liturgical prayers are useless without works of mercy.[86]

Jacques also reprimands hospitallers for their unscrupulous fund-raising techniques. Their quaestors exploit the hospitallers' image as regular religious and dispensers of charity to extort alms from the faithful through various deceptions, cultivating beards and other outward markers of the religious life,[87] and displaying fake relics. Because their ultimate aim is profit, not their audience's spiritual health, they promise salvation and partial-indulgences to all donors and accept tainted money from usurers and other criminals. They abuse and misinterpret genuine letters of indulgence, forge and steal others, preach in others' jurisdictions without authorization, and squander donations on gambling, feasting, and whoring. Prelates and monasteries must not allow them to preach, grant them letters of indulgence, or use their dirty money for building churches or charity work.[88]

Although A. Bonenfant-Feytmans believed that Jacques was criticizing the early friars' mendicancy, he was actually addressing a much wider problem.[89] The Paris circle used anti-vice preaching to move their audiences to contrition and self-reform, often manifested by taking the cross or giving alms to the crusade. Because the moralists' techniques were similar to the methods of unscrupulous quaestors, they risked being branded as charlatans. Jacques' history acknowledges that although the Paris-educated Fulk of Neuilly preached primarily to bring sinners to repentance, his alms-raising for a new parish church and the crusade gave rise to popular suspicions of peculation. He attempts to divert criticism to those preaching in order to obtain money or, as alleged in the case of Pierre de Roissy, fame and benefices.[90] Because the penance preacher and the quaestor differed largely

abbot of St Victor. It incorporated many of the reforms promoted by the Paris moralists (ed. Gross, pp. 9–15).

86 No. 39, Trento MS 1670, fol. 80va–b; Crane, nos. 92–3, pp. 72–3; Le Grand, *Statuts*, § 23, pp. 46–7 (Hôtel-Dieu in Paris); § 11, p. 25 (Angers); Paris (1213) ii.4–5, iii.13, in Mansi XXII, 826–7, 837.

87 Beards were worn by the brothers of many hospitaller orders and also served as one of the markers of apostolic 'sanctity' sported by wandering preachers: Caesar, *Dialogus* iv.10, ed. Strange, I, 181–3; Trinitarian rule (1198), ed. Gross, § 40, p. 15.

88 *H.occ.* 10 (pp. 103–6); no. 40, Trento MS 1670, fol. 83va; *Sermo ad theologos et ad praedicatores*, no. 19, Douai MS 503, fol. 293r; V. L. Kennedy, 'Robert of Courson on Penance', *Mediaeval Studies* 7 (1945), 290–336 (pp. 330–1).

89 Bonenfant-Feytmans, 'Organisations', 38–9. On the contrary, Jacques praises the friars' penance preaching (Bird, 'Religious' Role', pp. 219–22). The mendicants, like any preacher originating outside of the diocesan clergy, were criticized for infringing upon parochial jurisdiction and pandering to their audiences to obtain alms. They responded by separating their preaching from their begging (Pressutti, no. 2250).

90 *H.occ.* 8–10 (pp. 94–106).

in intangible motives, Odo of Sully, bishop of Paris, Robert of Courson, and other legislators tied to the Paris circle passed statutes restricting quaestors' activities, which were confirmed by the Fourth Lateran Council.[91] Its cautions echo Jacques' critiques and letters from Innocent III and Honorius III which warned the faithful of those impersonating genuine hospitaller quaestors and rebuked the Antonine, Hospitaller and Templar orders for employing unqualified and unscrupulous alms-collectors and abusing the privileges granted them.[92]

In conclusion, Jacques' history and sermons to hospitallers and their patients are valuable sources for the organization of charity and testify to the impact of lay involvement in this sphere as part of the larger revolution in religious movements in the late twelfth and early thirteenth centuries. They illustrate reformers' attempts to ensure that charitable donations were not squandered in overhead costs but actually aided the poor for whom they were intended, and demonstrate the success of Paris reformers and bishops in imposing reforms upon hospitals in northern France and Flanders-Brabant as part of their efforts to channel lay-led religious movements into acceptable forms. Finally, they illuminate the links between the social and theological realms and the mechanics of the dialogue between the popular, learned and theological spheres on the 'proper' relationship of the spiritual and temporal, of body and soul.

91 Paris (1208), §§ 61, 68, 92 and additions, §§ 40–2, ed. Pontal, I, 74 and 76, 86, 164, 166; Paris (1213) i.8–9, Add.ix, and Rouen (1214) i.9–10, in Mansi XXII, 821, 846, 901; Fourth Lateran (1215), c. 57, c. 62, in *COD*, pp. 261, 263–4.

92 H. J. Nicholson, *Templars, Hospitallers and Teutonic Knights: Images of the Military Orders, 1128–1291* (Leicester, 1993), p. 29; *PL* 214, 419–20 (1198). For the Antonites, see Windemuth, *Hospital als Träger*, p. 61; Pressutti no. 4435 (1223).

Texts on Hospitals

Translation of Jacques de Vitry, *Historia Occidentalis* 29, and Edition of Jacques de Vitry's Sermons to Hospitallers[1]

Jessalynn Bird

This chapter contains an annotated translation of chapter 29 of Jacques' *Historia occidentalis* and a transcription of his sermons to hospitallers based on two manuscripts.[2] I have added capitalization and punctuation, although I have not standardized spellings or listed slight variants in wording or case. Jacques' indebtedness to Peter the Chanter's *Verbum Abbreviatum* is indicated in the footnotes.

On the hospitals of the poor and leper houses[3]

There are, moreover, other congregations without estimate or fixed number throughout all the western regions, ⟨composed⟩ of men and women who renounce the world and live according to a rule in leper houses or hospitals for the poor, ministering to the destitute and infirm devoutly and with humility. They live, however, as a community according to the Rule of St Augustine without any private possessions and in obedience to one superior, and once they have taken the habit of a regular, they vow perpetual continence to the Lord.

In addition, the men and the women sleep and eat separately, with every precaution and ⟨complete⟩ chastity. As much as the pursuit of hospitality and ministry to Christ's poor permit, they do not neglect hearing the canonical hours, day and night. In houses where there is a larger convent and a more numerous congregation of brothers and sisters, they frequently gather in chapter to correct the failings of the delinquent or for necessary and honest

[1] I would like to thank Robert Kraft, Grover Zinn, Philip Rusche, Daron Burrows and Peter Biller for their help in identifying the citations in nn. 107 and 195–6 below.

[2] Trento, Biblioteca comunale, MS 1670 (F55) and Douai, Bibliothèque municipale, MS 503. Jean Longère and Carolyn Muessig kindly recommended these manuscripts to me.

[3] *H.occ.* 29; pp. 146–51.

business. Furthermore, they often have readings from the holy scriptures read out to them in the refectory while they are refreshing their bodies and in other set places and determined hours while they observe silence.[4] The infirm men and healthy guests whom they admit into their houses are required to eat and sleep separately from the women.

Their chaplains minister to the indigent and invalids in spiritual matters, instruct the ignorant with the word of divine preaching, console the faint-hearted and feeble, and exhort them to long suffering and actions of thanks with every humility and devotion.[5] By night and day, they continually celebrate the divine offices in a common chapel so that all the infirm can hear them from their beds. They also assiduously and sollicitously hear the ailing's confessions, supply them with extreme unction and other sacraments, and give a fitting burial to the dead.

These ministers of Christ are sober, frugal, and extremely rigorous and austere to themselves and their bodies, yet as much as they are able, they supply necessities to the needy and infirm with a ready spirit and hearts overflowing with compassion. The more abject they are in the Lord's house upon the way, the more exalted position they will attain in their ⟨eternal⟩ homeland.[6] Because they frequently endure so many of the sick's filthinesses and the nearly intolerable assault of ⟨various⟩ stenches, inflicting injury upon themselves for Christ's sake, I believe that no other kind of penance is comparable to this holy martyrdom, precious in God's sight.[7] The Lord will transform the ordures of these squalors, which they use like manure to fertilize their minds for bearing fruit, into precious stones and instead of a stench there will be a sweet fragrance ⟨in heaven⟩.[8]

However, this holy and God-beloved rule of hospitality and religion of hospitals is so corrupted in many places and houses and is, as it were, reduced wretchedly to nothing, that this base and execrable congregation of reprobate men displeases not only those who more fully perceive their wickedness, but also reeks in God's sight. Under the guise of hospitality and the cloak of piety, they have become quaestors, and through lies, deceptions, and every means which they possess they churlishly extort monies. Feeding themselves, they care nothing for the needy, except when they use them as a pretext to wring alms from the faithful, proffering a little to the poor and infirm, so that by this fraudulent kind of hunting, their crafty traffickers and cunning hucksters acquire many things. In fact, those who distribute a pitiful amount to the destitute in order to receive more and seek riches under the pretext of alms ought to be reckoned hunters rather than benefactors. So beasts, birds, and fish are snared; a morsel of food is placed

[4] *Rule of St Augustine*, in *PL* 32, 1379.3.

[5] *Rule of St Augustine*, *PL* 32, 1384.11.

[6] Psalm 83. 11. Jacques uses the scriptural *domus domini* (Lord's house) to allude to *domus dei*, a common title for hospitals which received the poor, sick and travellers.

[7] Psalm 115. 15.

[8] Isaiah 3. 24.

on the hook to reel in sacks of money. These men so importunately and disrespectfully and anxiously solicit alms that, destroying the reverence due to them as regular religious, they render themselves contemptible. St Jerome says against them: 'It is better to have nothing to give, than impudently to solicit so that you can give.'[9]

Indeed many hospitals shamefully acquire many things through bearded brothers who outwardly feign many things in hypocrisy, or through mercenary and mendacious chaplains unafraid to deceive simple people and put their sickle into another's harvest,[10] or through letters of indulgence which they abuse out of lust for base profit. We will not even speak of those who, unafraid to use false letters and stolen bulls to their perdition, incur the heinous crime of forgery. Those things which they dishonourably collect, they expend even more scandalously 'in orgies and drunkenness'[11] and devote themselves secretly in their haunts to other shady practices. Although they are not ashamed to do these things, we nonetheless blush to recite them at present.

Retaining nothing of their instituted regulations or purity of their order except the outward habit, virtually all of them are received ⟨into their houses⟩ through simoniacal intervention. Those who so dishonourably entered, even more shamefully imitate those already dwelling there, in murmuring and dissension, in quarrels and insurrections, in idleness and dissolution, in ⟨locked⟩ coffers and retention of private possessions, in lairs and foul things and every kind of vileness, without affection, without mercy, without trust.[12] While they make up well-accoutred beds for men's eyes, they are empty of the poor and ill, arranged sheerly for ostentation and deception. Houses of hospitality and piety are transformed into dens of robbers, prostitutes' brothels, and the synagogues of Jews.[13]

However, this sort of pestilential corruption and abominable hypocrisy does not infect all hospitals. In fact, there are some regular congregations and outstanding religious houses or hospitable chapters which do not lack the zeal of charity, the unction of piety, the ornament of decency, and the rigour of discipline. Some such are the hospitals of the Holy Spirit in the city of Rome,[14]

[9] Jerome, *Epistulae* 52, ed. I. Hilberg, CSEL 54 (1910), p. 440, lines 3–5.

[10] Deuteronomy 23. 25.

[11] Romans 13. 13.

[12] Romans 13. 13; 1. 31.

[13] Luke 19. 46.

[14] After Guy of Montpellier founded a hospital which served pilgrims, the ill and poor, pregnant women, and orphans, his order soon spread widely in the Midi and was approved by Innocent III in 1198. Guy and his brethren were invited to staff the hospital of Santo Spirito in Sassia as part of Innocent's papal charity programme in Rome (*H.occ.*, App. C, p. 282 and n. 25, pp. 149–50; references to key documents in de Angelis, *Innocenzo III*, and Bolton, 'Hearts', and '"Received in His Name": Rome's Busy Baby Box', in *Innocent III: Studies on Papal Authority and Pastoral Care* (Aldershot, 1995), article XIX, 153–67; rule published in *PL* 217, 1129–58, and more recently by P. de Angelis, *Regula sive statuta hospitalis Sancti Spiritus: La più antica*

and of St Sampson in the city of Constantinople,[15] and the head house of ⟨the order of⟩ St Anthony,[16] and the hospital of St Mary of Roncevaux at the entrance to Spain,[17] and some other hospitals which please God and are very necessary for the poor, pilgrims, or the infirm. Moreover, in Paris[18] and Noyon[19] in France, in Provins in Champagne,[20] Tournai in Flanders,[21] Liège

regola Ospitaliera di Santo Spirito in Saxia (Rome, 1954) and A. Francesco la Cava, *Regulae S. Spiritus: Regola dell'Ordine Ospitalerio di S. Spirito* (Milan, 1947).

15 An ancient Byzantine *xenodochium* famous for its professional staff of physicians and nurses. Jacques probably learned of it from returning crusaders who had captured Constantinople in 1204. Innocent took the hospital under papal protection in 1208, although it was later absorbed by the Templar order (*H.occ.*, p. 150 n. 1); T. S. Miller, 'The Sampson Hospital of Constantinople', *Byzantinische Forschungen* 15 (1990), 128–30, and *The Birth of the Hospital in the Byzantine Empire* (Baltimore and London, 1985), pp. 141–66, 172–3, 185–9, 192.

16 Gaston of Dauphiné founded a lay confraternity dedicated to St Anthony in La-Motte-Saint-Didier near Vienne, which staffed a hospice serving travellers and those afflicted with St Anthony's fire, a disfiguring condition which struck those eating ergot-infected grains. Although a local Benedictine priory initially oversaw their work, by the later twelfth century they had become a far-flung independent hospitaller order. A branch was established in Acre during Jacques' episcopate there (*H.occ.*, App. C, pp. 281–2; M.-L. Windemuth, *Das Hospital als Träger der Armenfürsorge im Mittelalter* (Stuttgart, 1995), pp. 53–65; A. Mischlewski, *Grundzüge der Geschichte des Antoniterordens bis zum Ausgang des 15. Jahrhunderts* (Cologne and Vienna, 1976), ch. 1.

17 Founded in Navarre in 1131 to protect pilgrims to Compostella from the harsh conditions of the mountain passes and brigands, Roncevaux spawned a congregation of dependent hospitals (*H.occ.*, App. C, p. 280; Mollat, *Pauvres*, pp. 116–17).

18 Jacques probably meant the Hôtel-Dieu in Paris, although there were many hospitals and leper houses in the city and diocese of Paris. See *H.occ.*, App. C, p. 279 and p. 150 n. 4; Le Grand, 'Maisons-Dieu et léproseries', especially pp. 51, 54–9. On the Hôtel-Dieu in Paris, see E. Coyecque, *L'Hôtel-Dieu de Paris au Moyen Age: Histoire et documents*, 2 vols. (Paris, 1889–91); A. Chevalier, *L'Hôtel-Dieu de Paris et les soeurs Augustiniennes (650 à 1810)* (Paris, 1901), pp. 40–84; and the bibliography listed by Bonenfant-Feytmans, 'Organisations', 27.

19 Perhaps the Hôtel-Dieu of St John or the leper house founded in Noyon (*H.occ.*, App. C, p. 278 and p. 150 n. 4).

20 The Hôtel-Dieu in Provins near Jacques' birthplace of Vitry in Champagne was founded to serve those travelling to the region's famous fairs and boasted the famously generous Thibaud VI of Champagne as a patron. The hospital was dependent upon the chapter of Saint-Quiriace, whose canons ministered to the ill. Henry of Champagne soon translated it from its original location to the palace of the countesses of Brie and Champagne. He also founded a hospital dedicated to the Holy Spirit for the indigent, widows and children in the late twelfth century. (*H.occ.*, App. C, p. 280 and p. 150 n. 5; A.-C. Opoix, *Histoire et description de Provins*, 2nd edn [Provins and Paris, 1846], pp. 322–3, 331–2; Bonenfant-Feytmans, 'Organisations', 32–3; Le Grand, *Statuts*, p. xiv and 'Maisons-Dieu et léproseries', p. 120.)

21 Tournai boasted three hospitals and two leper-houses by the late twelfth century (*H.occ.*, p. 150 n. 5, and App. C, p. 284). For the episcopal hospital in Tournai and the statutes of Walter, bishop of Tournai (1220–52), see Bonenfant-Feytmans, 'Organisations', 33; Lacroix, *L'hôpital Saint-Nicolas*, I, 113; Le Grand, *Statuts*, pp. xxi, xvii; Bonenfant, 'Hôpitaux', 27–9.

in Lotharingia,[22] and Brussels in Brabant,[23] there are hospices of piety and houses of decency, outbuildings of sanctity, convents of virtue and religion, refuges for paupers, aid for the wretched, consolations for the mourning, sustenance for the starving, sweetness and soothing for the ailing.[24]

Sermo ad hospitalarios et custodes infirmorum thema sumptum ex ⟨p⟩salmo.[25]

Beatus qui intelligit super egenum et pauperem. In die mala liberabit eum dominus.[26] *Longos fac funiculos tuos et clauos tuos consolida ad dexteram et leuam penetrabis et semen tuum gentes hereditabit et ciuitates desertas inhabitabit.*[27] Uerba sunt Ysaias LIIII ad doctores de uirtute uerbi dei. Per funiculum quidem predicatio intelligitur, qua ligari debemus ne ad malum curramus. De hoc funiculo in Eccl. dicitur X [*sic*]: *Funiculus triplex difficile rumpitur,*[28] idest predicatio triplex que prouocat ad amorem, incutit timorem, infert pudorem. Debet ergo predicator huiusmodi funiculos longos facere predicationem propagando. Auditor uero hos funiculos longos facit dum ea que in predicatione dicuntur non detractat sed magis addit, ut si ammoneatur pauperem pascere, ipse insuper uestit; si ammoneatur in cibo quadragesimali ieiunare, ipse in pane et aqua ieiunat. De hoc funiculo dicitur in Iob XL: *An extrahere poteris leuiathan hamo et fune ligare linguam eius?*[29] Hamo enim uerbi d⟨e⟩i extrahuntur peccatores de faucibus diaboli cuius lingua, que sibilat et uenenum infundit suggerendo, funiculo predicationis ligatur ut eis non noceat qui sane doctrine acquiescunt. Clauos autem appellat propheta uerbi pungitiua et commotiua, de quibus in Eccl. in fine: *Uerba sapientis quasi stimuli et quasi claui in altum defixi.*[30] Uerba autem commotiua debemus consolidare idest ne excidant firmiter memorie commendare ad dexteram et leuam penetrando. Acutis enim uerbis timoris debemus penetrare corda peccatorum, qui per leuam, et

[22] These included the hospitals of St Christopher (pre-1183), Saint Matthieu (1203), and the *leprosarium* of Mont Cornillon (pre-1176); Spiegeler, *Hôpitaux*, p. 99.

[23] For Brussels' boom in hospitals and *leprosaria*, see *H.occ.*, p. 150 n. 6 and App. C, p. 278; P. Bonenfant, 'Hôpitaux et bienfaisance publique dans les anciens Pays-Bas des origines à la fin du XVIIIe siècle', in *Annales de la Société Belge d'Histoire des Hôpitaux* 3 (1965), 3–98; Bonenfant-Feytmans,'Organisations', 35 nn. 62–3.

[24] Psalm 9. 10, Matthew 5. 5, Luke 6. 21.

[25] Pitra no. 39, in Trento MS 1670, fols. 79vb–81vb and Douai MS 503, fols. 343r–345v. The title in the Douai manuscript explicitly applies the sermon to hospitallers (a category which perhaps included lay confraternities staffing hospitals) and the *sorores* and *fratres* who served some institutions: *Sermo ad hospital⟨ari⟩os et fratres religiosos et sorores custodes infirmorum thema sumpta ex psalterio.*

[26] Psalm 40. 2.

[27] Isaiah 54. 2–3.

[28] Ecclesiastes 4. 12.

[29] Job 40. 20.

[30] Ecclesiastes 12. 11.

uerbis amoris corda iustorum, qui per dexteram intelliguntur, et semen uerbi d⟨e⟩i firmiter plantare in cordibus auditorum ut hereditate⟨m⟩ gentis domino acquirimus q⟨ue⟩ ciuitates deserte appellantur quia a gratia, domino, et a bonis operibus derelicte. Has autem ciuitates inhabitat qui peccatores conuertiendo bonis operibus eos exornat. Orate igitur dominum ut funiculis uerborum d⟨e⟩i hodie corda nostra domino firmiter astringantur. Quam adherere deo bonum est ut unus spiritus efficiamini cum ipso.

Beatus qui intelligit super egenum et pauperem et cetera. Hoc est quod in euangelio dominus ait, Matt. V: *Beati misericordes quia ipsi misercordiam consequentur.*[31] Unde Psalmus: *Ego sicut oliua fructifera ⟨in domo Dei⟩ speraui in misericordia dei.*[32] Qui enim per misericordie opera uelut oliua non fructificat, frustra in misericordia domini sperat. Teste enim Iacobo II: *Iudicium sine misericordia ei qui non facit misericordiam.*[33] Misericordia siquidem uia est hominis ad d⟨eu⟩m et dei ad hominem. Misericordia enim d⟨eu⟩m traxit de celo ad terram, sicut scriptum est, *propter miseriam inopum et gemitum pauperum nunc exurgam dicit dominus,*[34] ut scilicet, ueniam in carnem [*sic*] pugnaturus contra diabolum. Misericordia hominem de exilio reduxit ad patriam. D⟨e⟩i enim filius inclinauit se ut nos erigeret, humiliauit se ut nos exaltaret, in se reconcilians iu⟨stiti⟩a summa.[35] Ut igitur misericordiam ad proximos habeamus, d⟨e⟩i largitatem diligenter attendamus, ut non sit auarus in miserendo qui expertus est misericordie in d⟨e⟩o. *Iocundus enim homo qui miseretur et comodat, disponet sermones suos in iudicio*[36] qui miseretur cord⟨e⟩ compaciendo et iniurias dimmittendo, odientes se diligendo, ore pro persecutoribus orando, indoctos instruendo, pusillanimes consolando, inquietos corripiendo, duros et rebelles ex caritate increpando, opere pascendo esurientem, potando sitientem, uestiendo nudum, uisitando infirmum, recipiendo peregrinum, redimendo captiuum, sepeliendo mortuum.[37]

Qui igitur predictis modis miseretur proximo accomodat d⟨e⟩o. Unde in Parabolis XIX: *Feneratur domino qui miseretur pauperis et uicissitudinem suam reddet ei.*[38] *Centuplum* enim *accipiet* in presenti, idest bona spiritualia q⟨ue⟩ centuplo bonis temporalibus sunt maiora et omnium bonorum q⟨ue⟩ in ecclesia d⟨e⟩i fiunt participationem et insuper *uitam eternam* in futuro.[39] Unde Augustinus in persona domini: *Habuisti me largitorem, fac me debitorem ut habeam te feneratorem,*[40] non solum autem fenerator d⟨e⟩o sed proximo. Unde in Ecc⟨lesiastico⟩ XXIX: *Qui facit misericordiam fenerator ⟨est⟩ proximo suo,* quia multiplicius redibit quam impendatur *et qui preuale⟨a⟩t manu*

[31] Matthew 5. 7; cf. *VA* 103 (*PL* 205, 285–6).
[32] Psalm 51. 10.
[33] James 2. 13.
[34] Psalm 11. 6.
[35] The previous two words are unclear in both manuscripts.
[36] Psalm 111. 5.
[37] Cf. Matthew 25. 34–46.
[38] Proverbs 19. 17.
[39] Matthew 19. 29.
[40] Augustine, *Sermones*, no. 123, in *PL* 38, 686.43–4.

mandata seruat.[41] Manu non tamen ore mandatam seruat excellenter, quia miseria oleum est supernatans sicut scriptum est Iacob. II: *Misericordia superexaltat iudicium.*[42] *Qui* igitur *miseretur et commodat disponet sermones suos in iudicio.*[43] Opera enim misericordie in iudicio allegabunt pro eo, dicente domino Matt. XXX [*sic*]: *Esuriui et dedisti mihi manducare.*[44] Et Apoc. XIIII: *Opera enim* iustorum *sequentur eos* sicut opera impiorum persequentur iniustos.[45] Teste utique Ambrosio: *Sola misericordia comes est defunctorum.*[46] Unde dominus in iudicio opera misericordie pre ceteris esse remuneraturum promittit, sicut scriptum est Matt. XXV: Percipite *regnum. Esuriui enim et dedistis mihi manducare.*[47] Opera uero misericordie omissa uel eorum omissionem comminatur se pre ceteris operibus condempnaturum, sicut scriptum est eodem capitulo: *Ite maledicti in ignem eternum. Esuriui enim et non dedistis mihi manducare.*[48] Unde in psalmo: *Et super ipsos tonabit in celis*[49] et in Ecc⟨lesiastico⟩ XXIII: *Domine pater et dominator uite mee ne sinas me cadere in* illa exprobatione.[50]

Ad hoc autem mundo renuntiastis et habitum religionis assumpsistis ut non solum uestra sed uos ipsos operibus misericordie impendatis ut scilicet Christum in membris suis omni die reficiatis preeligentes abiecti esse in domo domini, idest in hospitali,[51] quam habitare in tabernaculis peccatorum. Matt. III [*sic*]: Unde et uobis facientibus *uoluntatem patris qui est in celis.*[52] Spiritualiter dicitur quod estis mater Christi eo quod Christum in membris suis pascitis et nutritis, implendo in uobis quod scriptum est in Matth⟨eo⟩ VI: *Nolite thesaurizare uobis thesauros in terra ubi erugo et tinea demolitur, ubi fures fodiunt et furantur. Thesaurizate autem uobis thesauros in celo.*[53] Omne quidem terrenum uel erugine consumitur ut metalla, uel putredine et uermibus ut uestes, uel a furibus et raptoribus tollitur ut lapides preciosi et alie possessiones. In hiis ergo omne genus auaricie reprehenditur. Et spiritualiter autem per eruginem[54] intelligitur superbia q⟨ue⟩ decorem uirtutum obfuscat, per tineam inuidia q⟨ue⟩ studium bonum et bone conuersationis uestimenta lacerat, per fures heretici et demones qui incautos seducunt et omnem spiritualem possessionem tollunt.

41 Ecclesiasticus 29. 1.
42 James 2. 13.
43 Psalm 111. 5.
44 Matthew 25. 35.
45 Apocalypse 14. 13.
46 Ambrose of Milan, *Expositio evangelii secundam Lucam* 7 in CSEL 14 (1957), p. 255, lines 1270–1; cf. *VA* 98 (*PL* 205, 278–9).
47 Matthew 25. 34–5.
48 Matthew 25. 41–2.
49 I Kings 2. 10.
50 Ecclesiasticus 23. 1.
51 See n. 6 above.
52 Matthew 7. 21.
53 Matthew 6. 19–20.
54 Douai, MS 503: rubigine.

Hii autem qui pauperes pascere renuunt Marc. XI assimilantur ficui in qua Christus non nisi folia inuenit. Et quia Christo esurienti non dedit manducare, maledicta est ab eo et continue desiccata.[55] Qui enim Christum in paupere non pascunt maledicti sunt et ab omnis humore gratie desiccantur. Teste utique Salomone in Parab⟨olis⟩ XXI: *Qui obturat aurem suam ad clamorem pauperis, ipse clamabit et non exaudietur.*[56] Propterea in Ecc⟨lesiastico⟩ dicitur XXIX: *Propter mandatum assume tibi pauperem et propter inopiam eius ne dimittas eum uacuum. Perde pecuniam propter fratrem et amicum et ne abscondas eam sub lapide in perdicionem.*[57] Propter mandatum et non causa uane laudis reficere debemus pauperes. Teste q⟨ui⟩dem Augustino: *Cum causa iactantie pauper reficitur etiam ipsum misericordie opus in peccatum uertitur.*[58] Mandatum autem est dare indigentibus, Luc. VI [*sic*]: Unde *date et dabitur uobis.*[59] Si dare est in mandato uel precepto, transgressor est qui pauperi non uult dare. Matt. XVI: Sicut autem qui perdit animam suam in hoc seculo in uitam eternam custodit eam,[60] ita qui perdit pecuniam a se alienando et aliis errogando. Frumentum si conseruas perdis, si seminas renouas. Ita est de elemosina et de pecunia erogata. Eccl. XXIX: *Qui non est abscondenda sub lapide in perdicionem,*[61] idest, sub cordis duritia uel ad litteram, non est abscondenda in terra.

Qui autem elemosinas nomine pauperum recipiunt et eas prout unicuique opus est pro posse suo non diuidunt, Ioh⟨anne⟩s XII: Similes sunt Iude proditori qui ad opus pauperum loculos portabat et eas furto asportabat.[62] Propterea Ieronimus ait: *Ecce fame torqueor et tu iudicas quantum uentri meo satis sit? Aut diuide statim quod acceperis, aut, si timidus largitor es, dimitte largitorem, ut sua ipse distribuat.*[63] Sicut autem ex officio tenemini pascere esurientes, ita et potare sitientes. Si uinum dare non potes, da calicem aq⟨ue⟩ calide qu⟨em⟩ si non habueris, da calicem aq⟨ue⟩ frigide[64] qu⟨em⟩ si nec frigidam, da bonam uoluntatem cum scriptum sit, Luc. VI: *Omni petenti te tribue.*[65] Teste enim Gregorio: *Ante dei oculos numquam manus uacua est a munere, si archa cordis repleta est bona uoluntate.*[66] Si ergo non habemus exterius unde elemosinam tribuamus; de nobis metipsis faciamus. Qui enim compatitur tribuit elemosinam de seipso quod plus est quam facere elemosinam de suo. Si autem habes unde subuenias et non subuenis prout necessitas pauperum exigit

55 Mark 11. 13–14, 20–1.
56 Proverbs 21. 13.
57 Ecclesiasticus 29. 13.
58 Isidore of Seville, *Sententiarum libri tres* iii.9, in *PL* 83, 733.38–40. There is a similar but not identical passage in Augustine, *Contra mendacium* vii.18, ed. J. Zycha, CSEL 41 (1900), p. 489, line 14.
59 Luke 6. 38.
60 Matthew 16. 25.
61 Ecclesiasticus 29. 13.
62 John 12. 4–6; for this paragraph, see *VA* 47, 104 and 106 (*PL* 205, 151–2 and 286–90).
63 See n. 9 above.
64 Cf. Matthew 10. 42.
65 Luke 6. 30.
66 Gregory the Great, *XL homeliarum in euangelia* I.v.3, in *PL* 76, 1094.11–13.

quantum in te est occidisti. Eccl. V: Hee sunt *diuicie conseruate in malum domini sui.*[67] Unde in libro Sapientie XIIII: *Creature dei facte sunt in odium et temptationem hominum et in muscipulam insipientium*[68] qui, scilicet, male utuntur eis uel male retinent contra necessitatem afflictorum.

Non solum autem pascere et potum dare sed et uestimentis nudos tenemini operire, sicut scriptum est Ysa. LVIII: *Cum uideris nudum operi eum et carnem tuam ne despexeris.*[69] Teste autem Gregorio: *Qui misereri uult proximo, a se trahat necesse est originem miserendi.*[70] Carnem autem nostram in paupere despicimus cum oculos a paupere auertimus et eum nudum relinquimus uel propter nuditatem eum tanquam uilem contempnimus. Econtra Iob ait XXXI: *Si despexi pereuntem eo quod non haberet indumentum et absque operimento pauperem si non benedixerunt mihi latera eius et de uelleribus ouium mearum calefactus est.*[71] Et Tobias ait V [*sic*]: *Noli auertere faciem tuam ab ullo paupere.*[72] Ita enim fiet ut non auertatur a te facies domini. Frustra quidam manus ad dominum in oratione leuat qui eas pro posse suo ad pauperes non extendit, et in euangelio dicitur Luc. III, *qui habet duas tunicas det unam non habenti.*[73] Martinus supererogauit qui unum pallium diuidens medietatem pauperi dedit. Aliquando etiam cum precepisset unam tunicam dari pauperi et uidisset quod nimis esset uilis et manicas curtas et quasi detruncatas haberet, ita quod brachia pauperis non operiret, ipse clam uocato tunica quam indutus erat illi dedit et tunicam pauperis induit. Cumque missam celebraret manus suas in altum eleuaret ne brachia sua nuda populo apparerent subito manicas deauratas que brachia sua usque ad manus tegerent, additas a domino, curtis manicis tunice respexit.[74] Econtra quidam fratres hospitalium multas tunicas et calidas pelles habere uolunt, et Christi pauperes in hospitali nudi remanent ⟨et⟩ frigore cruciantur, cum tamen gratia pauperum multa possideant pro quibus sustentandis fideles elemosinas hospitalibus prebuerunt.

Aliquando autem quandam nobilem mulierem uidi que, cum esset in ecclesia tempore hyemali, quedam paupercula mulier post tergum suum gemebat pre angustia frigoris. At illa cepit cogitare quod pelliceum quo induta erat daret illi pauperi mulieri. Sed multum graue erat ei missam relinquere nec poterat expectare donec celebrata fuisset missa, cum mulier nuda frigore cruciaretur. Unde uocata illa duxit eam seorsum, ascendens turrim seu campanile ubi campane ecclesie dependebant, et dato pelliceo mulieri ad ecclesiam inferius est reuersa. Finita autem missa capellanus secreto accessit ad eam dicens: 'Domina, quo perrexistis quando recessistis

[67] Ecclesiastes 5. 12.
[68] Wisdom 14. 11.
[69] Isaiah 58. 7; Jacques is drawing on *VA* 131 (*PL* 205, 325–6).
[70] Gregory the Great, *Moralia in Iob* XIX.xxiii.38, in *PL* 76, 122.37–8.
[71] Job 31. 19–20.
[72] Tobias 4. 7.
[73] Luke 3. 11.
[74] Crane, no. 92, pp. 42 and 173.

ab ecclesia? Sciatis quod nec unum uerbum potui dicere cum essem in secreto misse donec fuistis reuersa'. Ex quo patet quantum deo placeat nudum uestiri qui mulieri sancte, que cum cordis angustia missam reliquerat, totum residuum reseruauit.[75] Carnem igitur nostram ne despeximus. Scriptum est enim Iob IV: *Uisitans speciem tuam non peccabis.*[76] Dicitur quod sol ideo obscuratus est in morte Christi quia dominum suum nudum uidere erubuit et tu non confunderis Christum in paupere nudum uidere. In actibus autem apostolorum legimus IX quod adueniente Petro circumsteterunt eum uidue flentes et ostendentes tunicas et uestes quas faciebat illis Dorcas. Unde et a morte meruit suscitari.[77] Cum autem de conceptu uere compassionis nasci soleat elemosina, auaricia tanquam mulier uenefica partum iugulat ne in lucem prodeat. Iohannes III: *Qui enim uiderit fratrem suum necessitatem habentem et clauserit uiscera sua ab eo non est caritas dei in eo.*[78]

Nunc autem de illa specie misericordie que hospitalitas dicitur uideamus a qua spiritualiter hospitalarii nominantur. Teste autem apostolo XII ad Hebreos per hanc quidam d⟨e⟩o placuerunt angelis in hospitio receptis[79] et Petrus ait preterea IIII: *Hospitales inuicem sine murmuratione.*[80] Ad h⟨oc⟩ autem spiritualiter ex ordine uestro obligati estis et astricti ut hospitalitatem sectantes dicere ualeatis cum Iob XXXI: *Foris non mansit peregrinus et hostium meum uiatori patuit.*[81] De Loth autem legimus a Gen. XIX quod in uespere sedebat ad portam ciuitatis ut hospites inuitaret[82] et Iohannes in epistola tercia in fine reprehendit Diotrepem qui fratres non recipiebat[83] et in libro Sapientie in fine de Egyptiis qui inhospitales erant dicitur: *Ista paciebantur secundum suas nequitias.*[84] Alii quidem ignotos non recipiebant aduenas, alii bonos hospites in seruitudinem redigebant et, Iosue II, Raab meretrix quia exploratores hospitio recep⟨it⟩, merito hospitalitatis soluta est a peccatis et adiuncta est populo dei.[85] Igitur secundum consilium Salomonis in Eccl. XI: Mittatis *panem* uestrum *super transeuntes aquas,*[86] idest super peregrinantes de loco ad locum transeuntes et post multa tempora inuenietis illum, scilicet in retributionem iustorum. IIII Reg. IIII. Sunamitis mulier tenuit Helyseum ut eum in hospicio reciperet et suscitauit dominus filium eius a morte.[87] Et Iohannes in epistola tercia ait ad Gaium.[88] *Karissime fideliter agis quidquid*

[75] Crane, no. 93, pp. 42–3 and 173.
[76] Job 5. 24.
[77] Acts 9. 36–42.
[78] I John 3. 17.
[79] Hebrews 12. 22; for this paragraph, compare *VA* 129 (*PL* 205, 324–5).
[80] I Peter 4. 9.
[81] Job 31. 32.
[82] Genesis 19. 1.
[83] III John 1. 9.
[84] Wisdom 19. 12.
[85] Joshua 2. 3–21.
[86] Ecclesiastes 11. 1.
[87] IV Kings 4. 8–37.
[88] III John 1. 5.

operaris in fratres et hoc in peregrinos ab eis enim nullam expectamus retributionem sed a solo d⟨e⟩o qui ait, Matt. XXX, *hospes eram et collegistis me.*[89] Et Ysa. ait LVIII: *Egenos uagosque induc in domum tuam.*[90] Exemplo igitur discipulorum dicentium Luc. XXIIII: *Mane nobiscum domine quoniam aduesperascit et inclinata est iam dies* et tenuerunt eum.[91] Non solum inuitandi sunt hospites sed tenendi et trahendi et secundum possibilitatem dom⟨us⟩ non in lectis sordidis aut fetidis sed in stratis honestis et bene compositis colligendi. Ad hoc enim ministros et ancillas, conuersos et conuersas in hospitalibus habere debetis ut sordes abluant et lectos mundos conseruent. In quibusdam autem locis plures moriuntur fetore et aeris corruptione quam proprii corporis egritudine.

Nunc autem de uisitatione pauperum infirmorum et captiuorum subiungamus, de qua in euangelio Matt. XXV: *Infirmus eram uel in carcerem et uisitastis me.*[92] Et Iacobus ait I: *Religio munda et immaculata apud deum hec est uisitare pupillos et uiduas in tribulatione eorum.*[93] Et Iob ait V: *uisitans speciem tuam non peccabis* idest homines fragiles tibi similes.[94] In Exodo autem dicitur X quod, factis tenebris in Egypto, *nemo fratrem suum uidit*. In tenebris enim sunt qui a fratribus infirmis oculos auertunt et eos uisitare nolunt.[95] Et in Ecc⟨lesiastico⟩ dicitur VII: *Non te pigeat uisitare infirmum.*[96] Ex hoc enim in dilectione firmaberis. Non solum enim per ministros sed per uos ipsos debetis uisitare infirmos et eis ministrare manibus propriis leuando, portando, et ad lectos reportando. H⟨e⟩c enim ualde placent d⟨e⟩o. Expedit quidem modicum fetorem sustinere ut fetorem inferni ualeatis euadere. Hec enim humilitatis officia multum prouocant ad compassionem et ad infirmitatis nostre cognitionem. Unde cum dominus solo imperio infirmos et leprosos posset curare, propria tamen manu propter humilitatis exemplum tangebat illos.

Et de beato Martino legimus quod osculatus est leprosum qui continuo mundatus est a lepra, et de Theobaldo bone memorie, quondam comite Campanie, dicitur quod unctum secum portabat et sotulares cum uncto manu propria pauperibus dabat, ut sic ad compunctionem et deuotionem atque humilitatem prouocaretur et ut pauperes affectuosius pro ipso orarent, attendentes in tanto uiro tante humilitatis obsequium.[97] Ille autem, uir nobilis deo deuotus licet secularis, consueuerat uisitare leprosum quemdam extra

[89] Matthew 25. 35.
[90] Isaiah 58. 7.
[91] Luke 24. 29.
[92] Matthew 25. 36.
[93] James 1. 27.
[94] Job 5. 24.
[95] Exodus 10. 21–23.
[96] Ecclesiasticus 7. 39.
[97] Cf. *VA* 107 (*PL* 205, 290). On St Martin of Tours (d. 397), see C. Stancliffe, *St Martin and his Hagiographer* (Oxford, 1983). On Count Thibaud of Champagne (d. 1152), see ch. 7 above, nn. 15 and 35, in this chapter n. 20 above, and Baldwin, *Peter the Chanter*, I, 236–7, 255–6.

uillam que Sezenna uocaretur. Accidit quod moriretur leprosus. Cum autem post aliquantum tempus comes reuerteretur ad uillam memoratam descendit more solito uisitaturus leprosum extra uillam, in domuncula in qua habitare solebat leprosus. Quo reperto, quesiuit ab eo quomodo esset illi. Qui ait: 'Bene per gratiam dei nunquam mihi melius fuit.' Expectantibus autem militibus et seruientibus extra domum leprosi, uenerunt quidam ciues de uilla predicta domino suo occurrentes et quesierunt a militibus ubi comes esset. Qui dixerunt: 'Loquitur cum leproso qui in illa domuncula commoratur.' At illi dixerunt: 'Mortuus est leprosus ille, jam mensis preteriit ex quo sepeliuimus eum in cymiterio talis ecclesie.' Cum autem comes exiret dixerunt illi: 'Quare in uanum borastis? Leprosus ille dudum mortuus est et sepultus.' At ille ualde ammirans et ad domunculam leprosi reuertens non inuenit illum, uerumtamen magnam sensit odoris suauitatem et ita dominus illi ostendit quantum grata habeat opera pietatis. Raro enim uel nunquam inuenimus quod homines pii et benigni licet seculares et peccatores malo fine uitam terminarent sed tandem a domino uisitantur. Econtrario impii et crudeles et sine affectione homines frequenter morte pessima solent spiritum exalare. De primis Cornelius centurio, de secundis exemplificat Herode.[98]

Noui quandam nobilem dominam que ualde compaciebatur infirmis et maxime leprosis. Uir autem ejus miles, potens et nobilis a Deo, abhominabatur leprosos, quod eos uidere non poterat nec eos infra septa domus sue intrare permittebat. Quadam die, cum leprosus quidam extra domus ambitum ante portam clamaret, quesiuit domina si manducare aut bibere uellet. Cui ille: 'Ecce his crucior uehementissimo solis ardore, non manducabo neque bibam nec aliquod a te seruicium recipiam, nisi tuleris me in domum tuam.' Cui illa: 'Numquid nosti dominum meum quantum abhorreat leprosos et ipse redire debet, quia diu est quod iuit uenatum. Si te inueniret in domo sua forsitan et me et te occideret.' Illo autem non acquiescente sed gemente et plorante, mulier nobilis non potuit planctus ejus sustinere sed propriis brachiis ipsum in domum suam portauit. Cumque rogaret ut refectionem reciperet, nullo modo acquiescere uoluit, nisi prius in propria camera uiri sui et in lecto ejus domina ipsum ferret, ibi enim desiderabat quiescere antequam manducaret. Cumque illa sicut tota spiritu pietatis et compassionis affluebat gemitus et lacrimis leprosi ferre non posset, tandem uicta precibus eum in lecto suo quiescere fecit, puluinar suum sub capite ejus subponens et coopertorio grisio corpus leprosi tegens. Et ecce uir ejus de uenatione fatigatus rediens ait uxori, 'Aperi cameram illam ut dormiam et requiescam. Estus quidem magnus erat.' Cumque illa stupefacta et tremens, et de morte leprosi magis quam de sua metuens, nesciret quid faceret et aliquantulum tardaret, dominus cum magna indignatione thalamum ingrediens, post modicum tempus ad uxorum regressus ait: 'Modo benefectisti que lectum meum optime preparasti, sed miror ubi tales species aromaticas reperisti quibus tota camera ita respersa est odore suauitatis quod uisum et

[98] Crane, no. 94, pp. 43–4 and 173–4; Acts 10. 1–30; Mark 6. 14–28; Acts 12. 1–23.

mihi quod fuerim in paradyso.' Quo audito mulier, que non nisi mortem expectabat, ingressa camera ita inuenit, sed leprosum non reperit. Que pre ammiratione et miraculi magnitudine cuncta per ordinem marito suo narrauit. At ille ualde compunctus, qui prius uelut leo fuerat, mansuescere cepit uelud agnus, et meritis uxoris sue ita ad Deum conuersus ducere cepit uitam non minus religiosam quam uxor.[99]

Ecce quam acceptum est deo officium uisitandi infirmos et incarceratos qui scilicet in carcere egritudinis detinentur uel etiam in carcerem materiali et compedibus captiui tenentur quos uisitare debemus corporaliter ad eos eundo, consolando et reficiendo et si ualemus a carcere et morte eripiendo. Iuxta illud: *Domine, quis similis tui?* Et respondens ait, *Eripiens inopem de manu fortiorum eius.*[100] Et Iob ait XXIX: *Conterebam moles iniqui et de dentibus eius predam auferebam.*[101] Et iterum ait XXIX: *Auris audiens beatificabat me et oculos uidens testimonium reddebat mihi eo quod liberassem pauperem uociferantem et pupillum cui non erat adiutor. Benedictio perituri super me ueniebat et cor uidue consolatus sum.*[102] De amicis autem Iob I legimus quod eum uisitare uenerunt in graui infirmitate[103] et Thobias I: *pergebat per omnes qui erant in captiuitate et monita salutis dabat eis.*[104] Refert beatus Gregorius de Paulino Nolatie [*sic*] episcopo, quod cum omnia expendisset pro captiuorum redemptione tandem seipsum captiuum uendidit ut liberaret filium cuiusdam uidue. Unde postquam aliquantulum in capitiuitate seruiuit conuertet dominus cor tyranni ut eum liberaret et meritis eius omnes liberati sunt qui cum eo captiui tenebantur.[105]

Sepultura insuper mortuorum qu⟨e⟩ spiritualiter ad uestrum pertinet ministerium ualde commendatur in scripturis. Unde angelus ad Thobiam IX: *Quando orabas cum lacrimis et sepeliebas mortuos ego obtuli orationem tuam domino.*[106] De beato etiam Antonio legimus quod duobus leonibus obsequentibus, cum ferramenta non haberet quibus terram apereritque, Paulum primum heremitam sepeliuit et Zozimas, uno leone adiuuante, sepeliuit corpus Sancte Marie Egyptiace.[107] Multum autem prodest inspiciendo et sepeliendo mortuos ⟨et⟩ nouissi⟨m⟩a sua recordari. Teste enim Ecc⟨lesiastico⟩ VII: *Melius est ire ad domum luctus quam ad domum conuiuii.*[108] In illa enim

99 Crane, no. 95, pp. 44–5 and 174–5; cf. *VA* 129 (*PL* 205, 325).

100 Psalm 34. 10; compare this paragraph to *VA* 98, 104 and 131 (*PL* 205, 280, 287 and 326).

101 Job 29. 17.

102 Job 29. 11–13.

103 Job 2. 11.

104 Tobias 1. 15.

105 Gregory the Great, *Dialogorum* III.i.1–8, ed. A. de Vogüé and P. Antin, 2 vols., Sources Chrétiennes 260, 265 (Paris, 1979–80), I, 256–64, lines 1–94. Gregory attributes the story to Paulinus of Nola (353–431).

106 Tobias 12. 12.

107 Jerome, *Vita Sancti Pauli* 16, in *PL* 23, 27.21–28.18; Sophronius, *Vita S. Mariae Aegyptiacae* 26, trans. Paul the Deacon, in *PL* 73, 688–9; see n. 104 above. Jacques borrows directly from *VA* 132 (*PL* 205, 326).

108 Ecclesiastes 7. 3.

finis cunctorum ammonetur hominum et uiuens cogitat quid futurum sit. Uisitare igitur debetis speciem nostram in speculo mortuorum et sepeliendo mortuos et persequendo corpora eorum usque ad locum sepulcri et pro animabus eorum domino supplicando. Cum ergo beatitudo promittatur hiis qui intendunt super egenum et pauperem,[109] ordo uester ordo beatitudinis merito p⟨otes⟩t dici et religio pietatis de qua apostolus ait Paulus ad Thimotheum IIII: *Exercitatio corporis ad modicum ualet pietas uero ad omnia.*[110] Ualde igitur preciosa est h⟨ec⟩ medicina qu⟨e⟩ ualet contra omnes anime egritudines cum nulla sit medicina q⟨ue⟩ ualeat expellere cunctas corporis infirmitates. Non solum autem pietas contra omnes spirituales infirmitates prodest, sed, teste insuper apostolo Paulo ad Thimotheum, eodem capitulo, *promissionem habens uite q⟨ue⟩ nunc est et future,* idest duplicis uite, gratie scilicet et future.[111] Iuxta illud Matt. XIX: *centuplum accipiet et uitam eternam possidebit.*[112] Unde legimus quod quidam episcopus cum predicaret in ecclesia quod centuplum reciperent qui omnia que haberent pauperibus erogarent, quidam diues hoc audiens ualde commotus est et compunctus et omnia que habuit in manu episcopi dedit. Episcopus uero omnia pauperibus erogauit. Patre autem mortuo, filii episcopum in causam traxerunt bona paterna repetentes; qui cum reddere non posset inspiratum est ei ut filiis responderet: 'Eamus ad patrem uestrum'. Cum igitur ipsum de tumulo extraxissent, inuenerunt in manu eius cartam, in qua scriptum erat quod non solum pecuniam, quam dederat in manu episcopi, sed insuper centuplum recipisset. Quod uidentes filii episcopum absoluerunt.[113] Uos igitur fratres karissimi et sorores qui non solum uestra sed et uos metipsos ad usum pauperum tribuistis si in sancto proposito et in operibus pietatis perseueraueritis, recipietis premium quod *oculos non uidit nec in cor hominis ascendit* [114] quod uobis retribuet dominus uester Ihesus Christus qui uiuit et regnat per omnia secula seculorum. Amen.

Item sermo ad hospitalarios et custodes infirmorum thema sumpta ex Parabol⟨is⟩ XVI capitulo.[115]

Misericordia et ueritate redimitur iniquitas et in timore domini declinatur a malo.[116] Deut. XVII: *In ore duorum aut trium testium stabit omne uerbum.*[117] Duo testes ueraces et fideles qui numquam mentiuntur nec aliquid fallunt sunt duo

[109] Matthew 5. 7.
[110] I Timothy 4. 8.
[111] I Timothy 4. 8.
[112] Matthew 19. 29; cf. *VA* 108 (*PL* 205, 291–2).
[113] Crane, no. 96, pp. 45 and 175.
[114] I Corinthians 2. 9.
[115] Pitra no. 40, Trento, MS 1670, fols. 81vb–84rb and Douai, MS 503, fols. 345v–348v.
[116] Proverbs 16. 6.
[117] Deuteronomy 19. 15 (see also 17. 6).

testamenta, uetus scilicet et nouum quorum auctoritate omnia uerba sua doctor ecclesiasticus debet confirmare. Tres etiam testes dicuntur, lex et proph⟨et⟩e atque euangelium. Hii testes in causa d⟨e⟩i producuntur contra peccatores et contemptores uerbi dei. In quorum persona Iob ait X: *instauras testes tuos contra me.*[118] Multi autem hos testes eo audire nolunt quia operibus eorum contrarii sunt, sicut in libro Sapientie II de uiro iusto et doctore ueritatis dicunt reprobi: *Contrarius est operibus nostris et inproperat nobis peccata legis.*[119] *Factus est nobis in traductionem cogitationum nostrarum. Grauis est nobis etiam ad uidendum.*[120] Ipsi quidem nec uidere nec audire uolunt eos qui mala eorum reprehend⟨un⟩t. Sed quomodo sustinebunt uerbera qui non possunt sustinere uerba? Alii autem audiunt sed uerba in opera non conuertunt. Quam miseri qui panem masticant et ita pigri sunt quod transglutire nolunt. Sed mures ueniunt et fauces eorum perforantes extrahunt panem ex ore ipsorum. Mures quidam infernales, idest demones, panem eis auferunt quam manducare ceperunt et cum gaudio receperunt. Sicut scriptum est Luc. VIII: *Uenit diabolus et tollit uerbum de corde ipsorum.*[121] Unde Augustinus: *Placent uobis uerba, ego quero facta. Nolite me contristare prauis moribus uestris quia delectatio mea non est in hac uita nisi bona uita uestra.*[122]

Quidam enim similes sunt puero qui gallici uocant chamion, qui multas nutrices lactendo exhaurit et tamen non proficit nec ad incrementum peruenit sed uentrem durum h⟨abe⟩t et inflatum. Corpus autem eius non producitur ad incrementum.[123] Quidam etiam quando contra peccata sua audiunt loqui notant alios et non sibi attribuunt, nec attendunt se tales esse quales audiunt, sicut symia que credebat se esse pulcram et, respiciens in speculo uidit figuram turpissimam, nec credere poterat se esse talem, sed circa se respiciebat si talem uideret figuram. Uos autem fratres quod duorum aut trium testium testimonio audientis absque dubitatione credatis et uerba in opera conuertatis.

Misericordia et ueritate redimitur iniquitas et cetera,[124] in Parab⟨olis⟩ XIII: *Redemptio enim anime uiri proprie diuicie*[125] dum scilicet de propriis bonis fac⟨it⟩ elemosinam. Unde dictum est Nabugod. IIII: *Elemosinis redime peccata tua.*[126] Opera enim caritatis et pietatis delent peccata sicut scriptum est. *Caritas operit multitudinem peccatorum*[127] et in Parab⟨olis⟩ dicitur XXI: *Munus absconditum extinguet iram et donum in sinu indignationem maximam,*[128] quando scilicet

[118] Job 10. 17.
[119] Wisdom 2. 12.
[120] Wisdom 2. 14–15.
[121] Luke 8. 12.
[122] Augustine, *Sermones de Uetere Testamento* 17, ed. C. Lambot, CCSL 41 (1961), p. 243, lines 183–5.
[123] Cf. Crane, no. 308, pp. 129 and 268.
[124] Proverbs 16. 6; compare what follows to *VA* 104–6, 108 (*PL* 205, 286–91).
[125] Proverbs 13. 8.
[126] Daniel 4. 24.
[127] I Peter 4. 8.
[128] Proverbs 21. 14.

elemosina sit in secreto et non in ostentatione.[129] Et in Ecc⟨lesiastico⟩ dicitur III: *Ignem ardentem extinguit aqua et elemosina resistit peccatis*[130] et in Thobia dicitur IV: *Elemosina ab omni peccato et a morte liberat et non patitur animam ire in tenebris*[131] et in euangelio dicitur Luc. XI: *Date elemosinam et omnia munda sunt uobis*,[132] quod intelligendum est quando homo a seipso incipit, ut prius s⟨ibi⟩ det elemosinam quam alii, et prius sui quam alterius misereatur. Unde in Ecc⟨lesiastico⟩ dicitur XXX: *Miserere anime tue placens sibi deo et contine et congrega cor tuum in sanctitate.*[133] Qui enim placere uult d⟨e⟩o in aliis faciat misericordiam quod prius incipiat a se ipso continendo cor suum in sanctitate ut stabilis sit in bono et congregando ut cordis euagationem non habeat sed cogitationes suas ad d⟨eu⟩m restringat. Teste autem Augustino, *Qui ordinate uult elemosinam dare, a se ipso debet inchoare*, ut scilicet sit quasi lignum fructiferum Gen. I, *cuius semen sit in semetipso super terram.*[134]

Cum autem duplex sit misericordia, una corporalis alia spiritualis, una uisibilis scilicet alia inuisibilis, quanto melior est anima quam corpus, tanto spiritualis melior est corporalis. Per hanc enim corpus reficitur aliquando moriturum, per illam reficitur anima in eterno uictu. Elemosina spiritualis est pascere famelicum pane uerbi d⟨e⟩i. *Non* enim *in solo pane* materiali *uiuet homo.*[135] Ysa. LVIII et ideo debemus *panem esurienti frangere*,[136] quod est diuinas scripturas exponere. Dare etiam debemus sitienti potum sapientie salutaris Parab. XVIII: *aqua* enim *profunda uerba ex ore uiri.*[137] Unde Ierem. II: *Prohibe guttur tuum a siti.*[138] Uestiendus est nudus uirtutum et sancte conuersationis uestimentis de quibus in Apoc. dicitur XVI: *Beatus qui custodit uestimenta sua ne nudus ambulet.*[139] Recipere debemus hospites in corde nostro per dilectionem et ad domum ecclesie pro posse nostro reducere. Sicut scriptum est, Ysa. LVIII: *Egenos uagosque induc in domum tuam.*[140]

Uisitandi sunt infirmi qui peccatorum egritudine detinentur, iuxta illud Matt. IX: *Non est* sanis *opus medico sed male habentibus*[141] uisitandi sunt et liberandi captiui qui in carcere diaboli et in tenebris peccatorum sunt reclusi. De quo carcere Psalm. ait: *Educ de carcere animam meam*[142] et Ysa. ait LXI: *Spiritus domini super me eo quod unxerit me ut predicarem captiuis indulgentiam et*

[129] Cf. Matthew 6. 4.
[130] Ecclesiasticus 3. 33.
[131] Tobias 4. 11.
[132] Luke 11 .41.
[133] Ecclesiasticus 30. 24.
[134] Genesis 1. 11; Augustine, *Enchiridion ad Laurentium de fide, spe et caritate* xx.76, ed. M. Evans, CCSL 46 (1969), p. 90, lines 27–8.
[135] Deuteronomy 8. 3, Matthew 4. 4, Luke 4. 4; cf. *VA* 101 (*PL* 205, 284–5).
[136] Isaiah 58. 7.
[137] Proverbs 18. 4.
[138] Jeremiah 2. 25.
[139] Apocalypse 16. 15.
[140] Isaiah 58. 7.
[141] Matthew 9. 12; *VA* 131 (*PL* 205, 326).
[142] Psalm 141. 8.

clausis apertionem.[143] Sed et spiritualiter mortuos sepelimus dum peccata nostra per penitentiam regimus et ab oculis domini abscondimus ne uideat illa ad uindictam. *Beati enim quorum remisse sunt iniquitates et quorum tecta sunt peccata.*[144] Unde in Deut. XXI precepit dominus quod cadauer hominis suspensi in patibulo *non permaneat in ligno sed eadem die sepeliatur.*[145] Celeriter enim debemus peccatum per confessionem sepelire ne mali exempli fetore terra ecclesie corrumpatur. Mortuus insuper spiritualiter sepelitur dum homo religiosus et mundo mortuus in religione absconditur. Unde apostolus Coloce. III: *Mortui estis et uita uestra abscondita est cum Christo*[146] et Iob III de talibus ait: *Gaudent uehementer cum inuenerint sepulcrum.*[147]

Sunt insuper alie species elemosine spiritualis et misericordie. Est enim misericordia ignoscens, misericordia parcens, et aliquid de pena relaxans, misericordia corripiens, misericordia intercedens. De misericordia ignoscente scriptum est: *Dimittite et dimittentur uobis.*[148] Maius quidem est iniuriam tacendo fugere quam respondendo superare. Unde ad Hephesios IIII: *Omnis amaritudo et ira et indignatio et clamor et blasphemia tollatur a uobis cum omni malicia. Estote benigni, compacientes, misericordes, donantes inuicem sicut deus donauit uobis in Christo.*[149] De misericordia parcente et aliquid de pena relaxante, inferimus exempl⟨um⟩ summi iudicis qui semper punit citra merita et remunerat super merita. Plerumque enim culpa est totam culpam persequi. Iustitia enim semper habere debet misericordiam sibi adiunctam. Iustitie quidem ueritas in seueritatem et crudelitatem uertitur nisi misericordie dulcedine condiatur. De misericordia corripiente dicitur. *Corripiet me iustus in misericordia,*[150] et apostolus ad Galath. VI: Si *preoccupatus fuerit homo in aliquo delicto, uos qui spirituales estis huiusmodi in spiritu lenitatis instruite* uel corripite.[151] Et Augustinus ait, *Corrigite arguendo, consolamini alloquendo, exemplum prebete uiuendo.*[152] De misericordia intercedente scriptum est. *Pater ignosce eis quia nesciunt quid faciunt.*[153] Et Moyses in Exodo, *aut dimitte eis aut dele me de libro tuo.*[154] Cum igitur tot sint species spiritualis misericordie semper homo a se ipso debet inchoare Eccl. XIIII: *Qui* enim *sibi nequam est bonus erit.*[155] Qui sibi crudelis est, quomodo aliis misericors esse poterit? Unde necesse est fratres ut ab omni peccato animas uestras custodiatis. Ualde enim

[143] Isaiah 61. 1.
[144] Romans 4. 7.
[145] Deuteronomy 21. 23.
[146] Colossians 3. 3.
[147] Job 3. 22.
[148] Luke 6. 37; cf. VA 98–102 (*PL* 205, 278–86).
[149] Ephesians 4. 31–2.
[150] Psalm 140. 5.
[151] Galatians 6. 1.
[152] Augustine, *Enarrationes in Psalmos*, psalm 50, par. 1, ed. E. Dekkers and J. Fraipont, 3 vols., CCSL 38–40 (1956), I, 600, lines 20–1.
[153] Luke 23. 34 (paraphrase).
[154] Exodus 32. 31–2.
[155] Ecclesiasticus 14. 5.

crudelis est qui animam suam occidit. Ualde enim fatuus est qui alienum mortuum luget et de morte propria non dolet. Unde oportet ut prius uobis subueniatis quam aliis. Offerens enim non placet a munere sed munus ab offerente. Unde in Gen. dicitur IIII: *Respexit dominus ad Abel et ad munera eius.* Prius respexit ad Abel quia iustum uidit, unde eius oblatio d⟨e⟩o placuit. *Ad Cayn autem et ad munera eius non respexit.* Licet enim recte obtulerit quia munera obtulit d⟨e⟩o, male tamen diuisit quia animam dedit diabolo.[156]

Nisi igitur uobis ipsis misereamini, quid proderit aliis misereri? Necque enim cibi parcitas aut uestis asperitas aut religionis austeritas aut barbe prolixitas prodesse poter⟨i⟩t nisi per ueram cordis contritionem et oris confessionem anima prius a peccatis purgetur. Si enim barba prolixa beatum faceret quam beatior hyrco foret.[157] Hec sunt signa religionis. *Iudei signa querunt,*[158] uos *autem* nolite *gloriari nisi in cruce domini nostri ihesu Christi* et mentis puritate in obedientia et cordis humilitate.[159] Sicut autem mare semper rebellat littori quo tenetur et cohercetur, ita in religionem quidam semper rebellant et se opponunt prelatis suis qui eos cohercent. Equi feroces et bestie siluestres eo q⟨uod⟩ similes quiescunt et iacent ⟨et⟩ mansuescunt.

Ue hiis qui in congregatione fratrorum aut sororum semper litigant et mansuescere nolunt qui dicere deberent sicut Abraham dixit ad Loth, Gen. XIII: *Non sit iurgium inter me et te fratres enim sumus.*[160] Etiam archa quidem Noe, leo contra agnum non rugiit, lepus canem non timuit [*sic*], coruus columbam non laniat. Supportare igitur oportet inuicem et maxime in religione in qua uix potest esse, quin mali cum bonis commorentur. Nam lilium est inter spinas, granum inter paleas, sathan inter filios d⟨e⟩i, Saul inter prophetas. In archa enim Noe, idest in claustro, est agnus cum lupo, columba cum strucione et coruo, munda cum immundis, et mitia cum feris et *in calatho* Iere. XXIIII: *ficus* bone ualde et male ualde.[161] Bonum est igitur linguam refrenare et linguosos sibilatio⟨nes⟩ superare. Teste enim Iere. XXIII: *Onus erit unusquisque* [*sic; recte*: *unicuique*] *sermo suus.*[162] Ergo qui silentium tenet a magno onere alleuiat⟨ur⟩. Teste utique apostolo secunda Thimoth. II: *Seruum domini non oportet litigare sed mansuetum esse ad omnes.*[163] Teste autem Ecc⟨lesiastico⟩ XXII: *Mittens lapidem in uolatilia deiciet illa sic qui conuiciatur amico dissoluit amicitiam*[164] quasi dicat sicut lapidis ictu uolatus auis dicitur enim conuicii uerbo uis amicitie dissoluitur et quam ut ait Ysa. XXXII: *Cultus iusticie est silentium.*[165] Habeatis silentium in ore ut non

[156] Genesis 4. 4–5.

[157] Douai, MS 503 varies significantly: Si quidem barbatum faceret sua barba beatum, immundi idcirco non esset sanctior hyrco.

[158] I Corinthians 1. 22.

[159] Galatians 6. 14.

[160] Genesis 13. 8.

[161] Jeremiah 24. 2.

[162] Jeremiah 23. 36.

[163] II Timothy 2. 24.

[164] Ecclesiasticus 22. 25.

[165] Isaiah 32. 17.

litigetis, scilicet teneatis silentium in corde ut non murmuretis. Quibusdam enim grauis est obedientia et religiosa statuta, de quibus Ysa. ait XXX: *Onus iumentorum austri.*[166] Hii sunt qui onerantur statutis religiosis et preceptis honestis murmurant enim deliciosi accusantes et causantes austeritatem religionis et dicentes cum reprobis iudeis, sicut legimus in Exo. XVI: *Cur induxit nos dominus in desertum ut occideret omnem multitudinem istam fame*[167] et Num. XI: *Sed et Moysi uisa est res intolerabilis iratusque est furor domini ualde.*[168]

Ecce quam periculosum est religiosis conqueri et murmurare pro temporalibus uel secularibus desideriis sicut Dathan et Abyron. Num. XVI: Qui moysi dixer⟨un⟩t *numquid parum est tibi quod eduxisti nos de terra que latte et melle manabat ut occideres nos in deserto.*[169] Quam miseri qui porros cepe idest allia Egypti[170] que lacrimas prouocant dulcia reputant, Ysa. V: *ponentes amarum dulce et dulce amarum,*[171] dum manna spirituale [*sic*] fastidiunt eo quod non uident illud sicut non uideri non [*sic*] curabant saporem, sed uidere uolebant speciem, sicut diuites qui uolatilia coram se coqui faciunt ut magis alliciantur. Non igitur in deserto delicata cibaria uel sumptuosa uestimenta requiratis. Qui autem uilibus indumentis erubescit preciosis gloriabitur. Dominus tuus pannis uilibus inuolutus fuit et nudus in cruce pependit. Tu grossis et abiectis ac ueteribus uestimentis erubescis, murmuras, et indignaris; dominus quidem in hac uita asinum corporis non curat exornare sed in futuro si bene seruie⟨ri⟩t ipsum exornabit et quatuor dotibus uelut phaleris decorabit. Philip. III: Quando *reformabit corpus humilitatis nostre configuratum corpori claritatis sue.*[172] Igitur iuxta consilium sapientis, Sap. I: *Custodite uos a murmuratione que nihil prodest et a detractione parcite lingue uestre*[173] et in eodem libro Sapientia dicitur I quod *spiritus sapientie licet benignus non liberabit maledictum a labiis suis*[174] idest peccatorem propter labia quantum labiis benedicat et oret d⟨eu⟩m. Et detractor quidem coquus est diaboli qui fac⟨it⟩ ei pulmentum in quo unus pon⟨it⟩ linguam maledicendo, alius cor consentiendo, alius aures libenter audiendo. Hec est diaboli galatina que h⟨ec⟩ omnia simil⟨iter⟩ fouare nouit. Propterea in Parabolis Salomon ait XXIII: *Noli esse in conuiuiis peccatorum,* qui scilicet sanguinem proximorum bibunt, *nec in commessationibus eorum,* quo carnes ad uescendum conferunt.[175] Multi enim abstinent a carnibus coctis qui tamen libenter uescuntur carnibus crudis. Unde Iere. XIX: *Unusquisque carnes amici sui comedet in obsidione in qua*

[166] Isaiah 30. 6.
[167] Exodus 16. 3.
[168] Numbers 11. 10.
[169] Numbers 16. 13.
[170] Numbers 11. 5.
[171] Isaiah 5. 20.
[172] Philippians 3. 21.
[173] Wisdom 1. 11.
[174] Wisdom 1. 6.
[175] Proverbs 23. 20.

concludent eos inimici eorum.[176] Ergo qui detrahit fratri a⟨liqui⟩d moribus[177] obsideretur et in Apoc. dicitur XVI: *Manducauerunt linguas suas pre dolore*[178] idest refecti sunt alter male sermone alterius pre inuidia et cordis malicia et in Eccl. dicitur X: *Si mordeat serpens in silentio nihilominus eo habet qui occulte detrahit.*[179] Ergo detractor serpens est, serpen⟨s⟩ enim habens morsum et linguam uenenosam. Sicut autem musce cadaueribus et immundiciis pascuntur sicut sanguisfuga ulceribus adheret sanguine corrupto impletur, ita detractor peccatis aliorum reficitur et detractionibus delectatur.

Patet igitur quod miser⟨er⟩i anime sue est a commotionibus et litibus, a murmuratione et detractione et aliis pestibus spiritualibus abstinere. De hac enim elemosina seu misericordia spiritualiter intelligitur quod in euangelio dicitur Luc. XI: *Date elemosinam et omnia munda sunt uobis.*[180] *Misericordia et ueritate redimitur iniquitas.*[181] Non enim prosunt opera misericordie nisi fiant debito modo et in ueritate, recta scilicet intentione, non causa iactantie uel laudis humane. Unde in Ecc⟨lesiastico⟩ dicitur XXIX: *Conclude elemosinam in sinu pauperis et hec pro te exonerabit ab omni malo.*[182] Ualde quidem efficax est realis oratio. In sinu dicit ut fiat elemosina in abscondito, sine iactantia et inani gloria. In sinu etiam secure seruamus bona q⟨ue⟩ ibi ponimus et securus est qui debito modo dat elemosinam quia non perdet retributionem. Indebito modo dant qui pauperum indigentiam non considerant. Unde Augustinus: Qui dat *ut careat tedio interpellantis, non ut reficiat uiscera indigentis* et rem et meritum perdit.[183] Indebite dat qui pauperem obiurgando exasperat. Unde in Eccl⟨esiastico⟩ IIII: *Declina pauperi aurem tuam sine tristicia et redde debitum tuum,* temporalem scilicet consolationem, *et responde pacifica in mansuetudine.*[184] Sine tristicia ut scilicet non contristes pauperem nec despicias. Nam etsi aliqua reprehensibilia in pauperibus uidemus non ob hec despicere uel relinquere eos debemus, quia plerumque quos infirmitas morum uulnerat medicina paupertatis sanat. Et quoniam de ipsis scriptum est Luc. XVI: *Cum defeceritis recipient uos in eterna tabernaculo*[185] teste Gregorio: *Si eorum amicitiis eterna tabernacula acquirimus, dantes procul dubio pensare debemus, quia patronis munera potius offerimus quam egenis ⟨largimur⟩.*[186] Cum mansuetudine igitur et benignitate pauperes et infirmos debetis tractare. Unde Ecc⟨lesiasticus⟩ IIII: *Animam esurientem ne despexeris et non exasperes pauperem in inopia sua*[187] et iterum XVIII: *Filii in bonis non des querelam et in*

[176] Jeremiah 19. 9.
[177] The previous two words are unclear in both manuscripts.
[178] Apocalypse 16. 10.
[179] Ecclesiastes 10. 11.
[180] Luke 11. 41.
[181] Proverbs 16. 6.
[182] Ecclesiasticus 29. 15; cf. *VA*, chs. 104–6 in *PL* 205, 286–90, esp. 288.
[183] Augustine, *Enarrationes in Psalmos*, psalm 42, par. 8; I, 481, lines 13–15.
[184] Ecclesiasticus 4. 8.
[185] Luke 16. 9.
[186] Gregory, *Moralia in Iob* XXI.xxix.29; *PL* 76, 207.22–5.
[187] Ecclesiasticus 4.2.

omni dato non des tristiciam uerbi mali nonne ardorem refrigerabit ros, sic et uerbum melius quam datum.[188] Et iterum in Ecc⟨lesiastico⟩ XLI: Erubesce *ab obfuscatione dati et accepti,*[189] datum obfuscat tristitia et acceptum in gratitudine. Teste autem eodem Ecc⟨lesiastico⟩ XVIII: *Stultus acriter improperat et datum indisciplinati tabescere facit oculos.*[190]

Quod dictum est contra illos qui dare differunt et indigentes expectare faciunt. Econtra Iob ait XXXI: *Si oculos uidue expectare feci.*[191] Teste autem Salomone in Parab⟨olis⟩ XXII: *Qui pronus est ad misericordia benedicetur.*[192] *Qui autem obdurat aurem suam ad clamorem pauperis faciendo scilicet fundam aurem afflictis clamabit tempore et non exaudietur.*[193] Unde in Ecc⟨lesiastico⟩ IIII: *Cor inopis ne adflixeris et non protrahas datum angustianti.*[194] *Qui cito dat bis dat.*[195] Seneca: *Quantum addis more tantum d'mis* [*recte*: *demere*] *gratie.*[196] Festinare igitur debetis et non esse pigri ad opera misericordie dum tempus habetis. Qui enim differt hodie forsan cras non dabit uel ministrabit, superueniente morte uel graui infirmitate. Unde Eccl. XIIII: *Ante mortem benefac amico tuo et secundum uires tuas exporrigens da pauperi.*[197] Ante mortem dic⟨it⟩ quia cessabunt opera misericordie ubi nulla inuenietur misericordia. *Quis enim franget panem esurienti*[198] u⟨b⟩i o⟨mne⟩s reficientur pane celesti, et ita de aliis operibus misericordie est intelligendum. Unde in hac uita est festinand⟨um⟩. Quod autem ait: *Secundum uires tuas exporrigens da pauperi.*[199] Hanc propter illos qui timid⟨e⟩ reseruant q⟨ue⟩ pauperibus erogare debent. Contra quos Salomon in Parabolis ait: *Qui iustus est tribuet et non cessabit.*[200] Unde et Tobias ait IIII: *Si multum tibi fuerit habundanter tribue. Si exiguum fuerit etiam exiguum libenter inpertire stude*[201] et d⟨eu⟩s e⟨n⟩i⟨m⟩ magis respic⟨it⟩ affectum quam effectum. Magis pensat ex quanto quam quantum datur, quod patet in uidua que duo minuta offerens plus omnibus alii dicitur obtulisse.[202] Pietas enim dantis condit elemosinam, non quantitas dati. Cum igitur manus domini non sit abbreuiata non debetis nimis pusillanimes aut meticulosi esse, nec bonos pauperum quibus indigent auare retinere. Exemplum enim habetis Iohannem Alexandrinum, a quo dictum est

188 Ecclesiasticus 18. 15–16.
189 Ecclesiasticus 41. 24.
190 Ecclesiasticus 18. 18.
191 Job 31. 16.
192 Proverbs 22. 9.
193 Proverbs 21. 13.
194 Ecclesiasticus 4. 3.
195 H. Walther, *Lateinische Sprichwörter und Sentenzen des Mittelalters*, 5 vols. (Göttingen, 1963–7), IV, 155, no. 23944.
196 Seneca, *De beneficiis* iii.5, ed. C. Hosius (Leipzig, 1850), p. 25 line 24.
197 Ecclesiasticus 14. 13; cf. *VA* 107 (*PL* 205, 290–1).
198 Isaiah 58. 7.
199 Ecclesiasticus 14. 13.
200 Proverbs 21. 26.
201 Tobias 4. 9.
202 Mark 12. 42–4; compare this paragraph to *VA* 98 and 104 (*PL* 205, 280 and 288, 291).

hospitale Sancti Iohannis. Hic enim in misericordie operibus affluebat quod quasi litem et pactum cum domino habuit ut, quicquid d⟨eu⟩s daret, illi totum pauperibus erogabat. Sicut autem d⟨eu⟩s illi dare non cessabat ita ille Christo in pauperibus reddere non tardabat; tandem in hoc tam pio et tam sancto conflictu Iohannes uictus fuit et deus uicit, qui tam copiose illi dedit quod quibus daret non inuenit,[203] sicut legimus de Moyse, Exo. XXXVI: quod *uoce preconis clamari facte ut nullus ultra offeret ad opus tabernaculi* eo quod plura quam necesse fuisset offerebant.[204] Pauci hodie inueniuntur sacerdotes qui dicant offerentibus, 'Suffic⟨it⟩, non est opus ut amplius offeratis.' De quodam autem heremita legimus quod cum fere nudus ambulasset quesitum est ab eo: 'Quis te spoliauit?' At ille: 'Codex iste euangelii, qui est preda celestis docens omnia pauperibus esse erogata.' Cum autem quidam obiceret ei dicens: 'Quomodo omnia dedisti qui illum adhuc habes?' Statim dedit et aliis, uendito euangelio, ait: 'Ipsum uerbum uendidi, quod omnia uendi docuit et pauperibus erogari.'[205]

Licet autem hylariter, festinanter, et habundanter secundum posse uestrum ministrare pauperibus debeatis, tamen in dando elemosinam et ministrando pauperibus discretionem habere debetis. Iuxta illud: *Sudet elemosina in manu tua donec inuenias iustum cui des.*[206] Omnibus quidem indigentibus dare debemus corporalem elemosinam si ualemus. Alioquin dand⟨um⟩ est domesticis fidei et inter hos magis indigentibus et inter illos magis iustis. *Oculi enim domini super iustos.*[207] Unde Eccl. XII: *Benefac iusto et inuenies retributionem magnam, benefac humili et ne dederis impio,*[208] ut scilicet de elemosinis nutriatur in sua impietate, sicut quidam hystriones quia propter scurrilitatem suam datur eis nolunt laborare sed uagi discurrunt et remanent in sua leuitate. Unde Tobias IIII: *Panem tuum et uinum super sepulturam iuste constitue et noli ex eo manducare et bibere cum peccatoribus.*[209] Gregorius: *Panem et uinum suum peccatoribus prebet, qui iniquis subsidia pro eo quod iniqui sunt impendit.*[210] Unde et nonnulli huius mundi diuites cum fame crucientur Christi pauperes effusis largitatibus nutriunt hystriones. Qui uero indigen⟨t⟩i et peccatori panem

[203] Crane, no. 97, pp. 45–6 and 175. St John the Almsgiver (d. 620), patriarch of Alexandria, was renowned for endowing hospices in that city. The order of the Hospitallers of St John, now known as the Knights of Malta, originated as a confraternity-founded hospital dedicated to this saint, which served poor and sick pilgrims in Jerusalem. See J.S.C. Riley-Smith, *Hospitallers: The History of the Order of St John* (London, 1999), ch. 7 above nn. 58–9, and K. Urwin, *The Life of St John the Almsgiver*, 2 vols. (London, 1980–1).

[204] Exodus 36. 6–7.

[205] Crane, no. 98, pp. 46 and 176; Luke 18. 22.

[206] Augustine, *Enarrationes in Psalmos*, psalm 102, par. 12; III, 1462, lines 10–11. Compare this paragraph to *VA* 47, 49, 104 (*PL* 205, 147–50, 153–6, 288).

[207] Psalm 33. 16.

[208] Ecclesiasticus 12. 3, 6.

[209] Tobias 4. 18.

[210] Gregory, *Regula Pastoralis* iii.20, ed. B. Judic, F. Rommel and C. Morel, 2 vols., Sources Chrétiennes 381–2 (Paris, 1992), II, 388, lines 81–8.

suum non quia peccator sed quia homo est tribuit, nimirum non peccatorem sed iustum nutrit, quia in illo non culpam sed natu⟨ra⟩m diligit. Melius igitur est dare humili et iusto pauperi qui oret pro uobis et tandem in eterna tabernacula uos ualeat recipere quam hystrionibus, trutannis, et ribaldis qui bibunt in tabernis et ludunt cum deciis. Sed nec tales qui inhoneste se h⟨abe⟩nt ⟨uel⟩ d⟨eu⟩m blasphemantes iurant, postquam noueritis, unquam in hospitalibus uestris recipiatis, ne tollatis *panem filiorum et detis canibus* et immundis.[211]

Sudet igitur *elemosina in manu uestra* ut floreat et fructificet donec inueniatis quibus et qualiter sit danda.[212] Unicuique autem secundum quod opus h⟨abe⟩t, non uni omnia, sed diuersis diuersa. Scriptum est enim *dispersit, dedit pauperibus.*[213] Necessaria enim dentur, non superflua, non delicata aut sumptuosa cibaria nisi in necessitate egritudinis. In hoc autem multi hospitalarii delinquunt quasi sub specie pietatis circumeuntes lectos infirmorum et querentes a singulis quid manducare aut bibere uelint. Simplices autem pauperes et infirmi secundum proprium appetitum, licet febri acuta uel alia calida egritudine laborent, carnes petunt et uinum. Unde plerumque plures moriuntur ex contraria dieta quam ex ipsa infirmitate. Non igitur scienter dare debetis contraria cibaria infirmis sicut nec frenetico gladium quo se perimeret dare uelletis. Ubi autem m⟨odum⟩ egritudinis et qualitatem diete ignoratis, credo quod habetis excusationem licit ex contraria dieta moriatur infirmus.

De hac autem largiendi et ministrandi discretione nos instruit Gregorius dicens: *Necesse est ut sollicite perpendant ne commissa indigne distribuant ne quedam quibus nulla, ne nulla quibus quedam, ne multa quibus pauca, ne pauca prebeant quibus impendere multa debuerant; ne precipitatione hoc quod tribuunt inutiliter spargant; ne tarditate petentes noxie crucient; ne recipiende hic gratie intentio subrepat; ne dationis lumen laudis transitorie appetitus extinguat; ne oblatum munus coniuncta tristicia obsideat; ne in bene oblato munere animus plus quam decet hylarescat; ne si quidquam cum totum recte impleuerint, tribuant, et simul omnia postquam peregerint, perdant.*[214] Ecce quam discretos et timoratos oportet esse beneficos et maxime hospitalarios. Unde postquam Salomon ait XVI: *Misericordia et ueritate redimitur iniquitas*, statim subiunxit, *et in timore domini declinatur a malo.*[215] Timere quidem debent et cauere, ut ait Gregorius: Ne *cogitatione tumida super eos ⟨se⟩ quibus terrena largiuntur, extollant; ne idcirco se meliores estiment, quia sustentari per se ceteres uident.*[216] Cum igitur illorum ministerio quibus accepta largiuntur considerant se esse constitutos, nequaquam eorum mentes tumor subleuet sed timor premat. Cumque omnia benefecerint dicant, serui inutiles sumus, quod debemus facere fecimus.

211 Matthew 15. 26; Mark 7. 27.
212 Cf. *VA* 48, 105 (*PL* 205, 150, 288).
213 Psalm 111. 9.
214 Gregory, *Regula pastoralis* iii.20; II, 384, lines 24–35.
215 Proverbs 16. 6.
216 Gregory, *Regula pastoralis* iii.20; II, 382, lines 7–9.

Ammonendi insuper *sunt* benefici, teste Gregorio, *ut sollicite custodire studeant, ne cum peccata commissa elemosinis redimunt adhuc redimenda committant, ne uenalem dei iustitiam estiment, si cum curant pro peccatis nummos tribuere, arbitrentur inulte se posse peccare.*[217]

Magna igitur in officio et ministerio uestro adhibenda est cautela ne in uno offendatis et totum ammittatis, ne aliquam proprietatem usque ad obolum unum retineatis. Licet enim proprium retentum distribuere pauperibus uel in usus uestros necessarios conuertere proponatis, spe inani seducti, nullo modo uobis salus esse poterit nisi omnia fratribus et sororibus communicetis et priori uestre resignetis.[218] Ieron⟨imus⟩: *Quomodo possumus aliena distribuere, qui nostra timide retinemus?*[219] Cauea⟨ti⟩s insuper ne aliqu⟨i⟩ ex certa conuentione in collegio uestro uelitis recipere, quod frequenter priores uestri laici consueuer⟨un⟩t facere, questum estimantes pietatem et ignorantes symonie labem. Qui enim sic recipiunt uel recipiuntur d⟨e⟩i ultionem non euadent, cum nullo modo sint in statu saluandorum. Sed nec pure recipiantur, licet nulla de pecunia uel terrena possessione fiat conuentio, qui propter diuitias uel preces carnales aut minas recusatis et contemptis pauperibus ad religionem admittuntur, presertim cum intentionis oculos principaliter ad d⟨eu⟩m non ha⟨beant⟩. Sitis igitur cauti et timorati ut timore d⟨eu⟩m ab omni malo declinetis.

Cauete super omnia ne elemosinas de usura uel de furto aut rapina scienter recipiatis, inquirentes diligenter exemplo Tobie II et dicentes: *uide⟨te⟩ ne furtim sit.*[220] Melius est enim fame mori quam huiusmodi cadauere uesci aut pauperes sustentare. De hiis autem qui huiusmodi morticinum comedunt in Parabolis Salomon ait IIII: *Comedunt panem impietatis et bibunt uinum iniquitatis.*[221] Cum tamen Ezech⟨iel⟩ dicat IIII: *Morticinum et immundum numquam intrauit in os meum.*[222] Et per Ysa. dominus ait LXI: *Ego dominus diligens iuditium et odio habens rapinam in holocaustum.*[223]

De sancto autem Furseio legimus quod cum anima egrederetur de corpore concurrerunt demones ipsum ante tribunal iudicis accusantes, et quia sancte conuersationis fuerat, non inuenerunt quid ei obicerent nisi quod aliquando capam a quodam feneratore acceperat et ita contra ipsum sententia imminebat. Sed angelis sanctis orantibus pro ipso decreuit dominus ut anima ad corpus rediret et penitentiam ageret. Unde quidam demonum ualde iratus animam feneratoris a quo receperat capam in faciem eius proiecit. Unde postquam suscitatus fuit omnibus diebus quibus uixit apparuit in facie eius combustio ex anima feneratoris igne gehennali succensa.[224] Nec tamen

217 Gregory, *Regula pastoralis* iii.20; II, 388, lines 89–94.
218 Cf. *VA* 53 (*PL* 205, 366–70).
219 Jerome, *Epistulae* 52; ed. Hilberg, p. 529, lines 15–16.
220 Tobias 2. 21.
221 Proverbs 4. 17.
222 Ezechiel 4. 14.
223 Isaiah 61. 8.
224 Crane, no. 99, p. 46; *VA* 50 (*PL* 205, 159). On St Fursey (d. 650), see Crane, p. 176.

credimus quod sanctus homo sciret capam illam ex fenore fuisse acquisitam, sed debui⟨sse⟩t diligenter inquirere sicut qui in macello carnes emunt utrum sit sana uel leprosa aut fetida diligenter attendunt.

Non solum autem elemosinas de usura uel rapina accipere non debetis sed nec de licite acquisitis nimis impudenter et proterue petere. Teste enim Iero⟨nimo⟩: *Melius est non habere quod tribuas quam impudenter petere* quod des.[225] Non igitur importune uos aliorum hospitiis ingeratis. Teste quidem Eccl⟨esiastico⟩ XXI: *Pes fatui facilis est in domo proximi.*[226] Non mittatis mercennarios et questuarios predicatores pro elemosinis per fraudes et mendacia et falsas promissiones acquirendis. De quibus in Ezech. XIII dominus conqueritur dicens, *uiolabant me ad populum meum propter pugillum ordei et fragmentum panis ut interficerent animas q⟨ue⟩ non moriuntur et uiuificarent animas q⟨ue⟩ non uiuunt.*[227] Et ita sunt de familia Phar⟨a⟩onis Exo. II, qui mares interfic⟨it⟩ et feminas reseruuat,[228] dicentes *bonum malum et malum bonum.*[229] Cum tamen dicat Ysaias V: *Ue qui iustificat impium pro muneribus.*[230] Et Micheas III: *Si quis non dederit in ore eorum quippiam sanctificant super eum prelium.*[231] In omnibus igitur cautelam habeatis et honestatem seruare studeatis.

Habeatis in quantum s⟨ib⟩i pot⟨est⟩ [*sic*] hospitalia munda et non fetida, mundas officinas et lectos non sordidos ad opus infirmorum sed mundos et honestos, ne fetore crucientur et afflictio afflictioni addatur. Sint ex una parte uiri infirmi quibus ministrent conuersi, ex alia parte uel in alia domo sint femine quibus ministrent mulieres seu conuerse. Non ponatis paleas iuxta ignem nec mulieres prope homines. Teste utique Iero⟨nimo⟩: *Periculose tibi ministrat cuius uultum frequenter attendis,*[232] et iterum ait, *Scio quosdam conualuisse corpore et animo egrotare cepisse.*[233]

Unde de quodam heremita legimus quod cum uellet matrem suam ultra flumen portare, manus suas pallio inuoluit. Cumque mater indignaretur dicens: 'Numquid mater tua sum?' respondit: 'Non mireris mater, caro enim mulieris ignis est.' Caueant igitur fratres conuersi ne cohabitent aut nimiam familiaritatem habeant cum sororibus conuersis uel cum aliis quibuscumque mulieribus.[234] Iero⟨nimus⟩: *Solus cum sola secreto et absque arbitro uel teste non sedeas.*[235] *Nulla securitas ⟨est⟩ uicino serpente dormire,*[236] sicut ⟨cum⟩ uiris femine

[225] Jerome, *Epistulae* 52; ed. Hilberg, p. 431, lines 4–5. Compare this paragraph to *VA* 46, 48 (*PL* 205, 146–7, 152–3).

[226] Ecclesiasticus 21. 25.

[227] Ezechiel 13. 19.

[228] Exodus 1. 16–22.

[229] Isaiah 5. 20.

[230] Isaiah 5. 23.

[231] Micah 3. 5.

[232] Jerome, *Epistulae* 52; ed. Hilberg, p. 423, lines 15–16.

[233] Jerome, *Epistulae* 52; ed. Hilberg, p. 423, lines 14–15.

[234] Crane, no. 100, pp. 46–7 and 176.

[235] Jerome, *Epistulae* 52; ed. Hilberg, p. 423, lines 3–4.

[236] Jerome, *Contra Vigilantium* 16; *PL* 23, 352.12–13.

habitent, uiscarium ⟨e⟩n⟨im⟩ d⟨ed⟩eri⟨n⟩t diaboli.[237] Non igitur uir religiosus de preterita castitate confidat nec dicat in corde suo, 'H⟨e⟩c soror ualde religiosa est et nichil turpe cogito, licet illam frequenter uideam uel etiam manum eius ex castitate tangam, et si continuo motus illicitos non sentiat [*sic, recte*: sentiam]'. In Parabolis XXVI: Ignorat tamen *quid crastina patiat dies.*[238] Huiusmodi enim affectiones cito conuertuntur in carnales. Unde caueat sibi et prouideat in futurum, exemplo hyrundinis, que cum esset cum aliis auibus et semen lini in agro a quodam rustico seminaretur dixit illis: 'Uenite et manducemus semen istud quia ex illo posset nobis malum prouenire.' At ille ceperunt hyrundinem irridere et dicere: 'Quid potest nobis hoc modicum semen nocere?' Quibus hyrundo: 'Quia mihi credere non uultis non remanebo uobiscum in agris sed acquiram mihi familiaritatem alicuius boni uiri, in cuius domo nidificare possim et morari.' Procedente tempore, semen in agro proiectum creuit in linum et collecto lino inde factum est rete in quo inciderunt aues ille inprouide que consiliis hyrundinis acquiescere noluerunt.[239] Uos autem fratres karissimi et sorores d⟨e⟩o deuote ab omni specie mali abstinere uos et ab insidiis et retibus diaboli uobis precaueatis ut misericordia et ueritate redimatur iniquitas et timore d⟨eu⟩m declinetis a malo ipso prestante qui uiuit et regnat per omnia secula seculorum.

[237] The previous phrase is unclear in both manuscripts.
[238] Proverbs 27. 1.
[239] Crane, no. 101, pp. 47 and 176.

Religion as Medicine: Music in Medieval Hospitals[1]

Peregrine Horden

Around the time that the Normans were settling into their newly-conquered kingdom, and Archbishop Lanfranc was establishing the earliest hospital for the poor in England,[2] the revered Persian mystic, al-Hujwiri, set down the following description of hospital practice in Byzantium:

> It is well known that in the hospitals of Rum they have invented a wonderful thing which they call *angalyun*; the Greeks call anything that is very marvellous by this name, for example the Gospel and the Books of Mani. The word signifies 'promulgation of a decree'. This *angalyun* resembles the gut strings [of a musical instrument]. The sick are brought to it two days a week and are forced to listen while it is being played, for a length of time proportionate to the malady from which they suffer; then they are taken away. If it is desired to kill anyone, he is kept there for a longer period until he dies . . . [euthanasia?] Physicians and others may listen continually to the *angalyun* without being affected in any way, because it is consistent with their temperament.[3]

Hujwiri was writing either somewhere in Iraq, or in Lahore, whither he was taken in captivity and where he ended his days within a few years after 1072.[4] His account appears unexpectedly towards the end of a treatise on Sufi mysticism. He purposes to illustrate the potentially dangerous effects of music on the uninitiated (here the patients; the physicians are the adepts). Hujwiri had travelled all around the Middle East, including Syria. He could have seen Christian charitable institutions within the 'land of Islam' or

[1] This paper was read in draft, to its lasting benefit, by Carole Rawcliffe and John Henderson, who both also allowed me to profit from their forthcoming publications. Emilie Savage-Smith gave unstinting assistance with Arabic. Rebecca Flemming advised authoritatively about late Antique Galenism. Surviving errors and perversities are, of course, my own.

[2] As distinct from a monastic infirmary. See A. Meaney, 'The Practice of Medicine in England about the Year 1000', in *The Year 1000*, pp. 221–37; N. Orme and M. Webster, *The English Hospital 1070–1570* (New Haven and London, 1995), pp. 19–23.

[3] Hujwiri, *Kashf al-mahjub*, abridged trans. R. A. Nicholson, *The Oldest Persian Treatise on Sufiism*, E. J. W. Gibb Memorial Series 17, 2nd edn (London, 1935), ch. 24, pp. 407–8 (modified, with the kind assistance of Emilie Savage-Smith).

[4] See also Dols, *Majnun*, p. 170.

received reports of Byzantine ones from travellers. There was, moreover, no need for him to invent such a striking example to make his point. As the remainder of his chapter on *sama'* (listening) shows, he had many anecdotes from closer to home at his disposal.

None the less, for all its specious authenticity the vignette is puzzling. The *angalyun*, which clearly derives from the Greek *euaggelion* (gospel), appears to have been Hujwiri's coinage.[5] In Persian dictionaries it is defined as silk of changing colour, a species of brocade so called because of the type of material in which Eastern Christians wrapped their gospel books; but that hardly illuminates Hujwiri's usage.[6] Nor is there anything in the patristic or Byzantine definition of *euaggelion* which could have prompted the assimilation of 'gospel' to 'decree' and, yet more improbably, to the books of Mani and instrumental 'gut strings'.[7] Some hint of what prompted this semantic virtuosity may emerge later on. For the moment, I should simply like to use Hujwiri's vignette as a way of opening up and delimiting a field of investigation. Whatever the veracity of his sources, Hujwiri conveys the perception that there was, in Byzantium, some affinity between cultic practice, prescribing for patients (the 'decree'?), and music – between religion and medicine. Still more to my point, he locates this affinity within a hospital.

This paper is about religion as medicine. It is, therefore, not about medicine as a metaphor within religious discourse, or the theology implicit in medical ideology, or the relations between churchmen and doctors.[8] It looks at a domain in which the distinction between medicine and religion is difficult, a domain to which terms such as 'ambiguity' and 'overlap' are more appropriate than 'tension', the detection of which has driven much of the subject's historiography.[9] To exemplify this ambiguous domain, the paper offers a broad-brush depiction of the use of music in medieval hospitals. It compares the three medical traditions that derived from that of Classical Antiquity – Islamic, Byzantine, and western European, with the emphasis on the last of the three – not from the vantage point of musicology or religious history so much as from that of a theory in which religion can, sometimes, be perceived as medicinal.[10]

5 There is no entry for it in *A Greek and Arabic Lexicon: Materials for a Dictionary of the Medieval Translations from Greek into Arabic*, ed. G. Endress and D. Gutas (Leiden 1992–).

6 F. Johnson, *Dictionary: Persian, Arabic, and English* (London, 1852), p. 179; F. Steingass, *Persian–English Dictionary* (London, 1892), p. 115, both s.v. *anqalyun*. See also L. Ibsen al Faruqi, *An Annotated Glossary of Arabic Musical Terms* (Westport, CT, 1981), p. 4. I owe these references to Emilie Savage-Smith.

7 *A Greek Patristic Lexicon*, ed. G. W. H. Lampe (Oxford, 1961), and *Greek Lexicon of the Roman and Byzantine Periods*, ed. E. A. Sophocles (Boston, 1870), s.v. *euaggelion*.

8 Cf. for example Ziegler, *Medicine and Religion*.

9 Amundsen, *Medicine, Society, and Faith*.

10 I have drawn encouragement from ethnographic accounts of medico-religious healthcare systems to which music is central: e.g. S. M. Friedson, 'Dancing the Disease: Music and Trance in Tumbuka Healing', in *Musical Healing in Cultural Contexts*, ed. P. Gouk (Aldershot, 2000), pp. 67–84.

I

Until recently, that project would have kicked against the pricks. Medical historians have understandably identified their subject more or less with the history of doctors – elite 'dead white male' doctors at that. Such men were responsible for most of the evidence of medical thought and practice that survives from the Middle Ages. Through it, they speak to us of their zeal for Aristotelian learning, their concern for professional respectability, and their growing authority in matters previously left to the determination of laymen, such as the diagnosis of leprosy or sanctity.[11] Of course, the cultural and social history of medical scholasticism is an essential topic for medievalists.[12] But its pursuit should not entail that we view the medieval medical world solely in the way that the scholastics' literary legacy invites. Partly as a result of the accomplishments paraded in that legacy, partly (I assume) because of our own inescapable awareness of how modern biomedicine proceeds, we tend to privilege diagnosis and active treatment over prognosis and regimen.[13] It takes an effort of will, not to mention considerable patience in searching the evidence, for a medical historian to offer a narrative of a medieval doctor whose skill lay in doing nothing but making predictions – and in facilitating a 'good death'.[14] A second temptation of the scholastic legacy against which we should guard is to take the university physicians always at their own self-estimation, as the only healers who really mattered. If, as Hugh Trevor-Roper once urged, we roll back the linoleum of time and observe the teeming life that lies beneath, then we begin to detect the activity of numerous female healers – the first and largest casualty of scholasticism triumphant, as well as of contemporary chauvinism more generally.[15] A range of empirics then becomes noticeable: healers by no means necessarily unlettered.[16] Finally, we catch sight of nurses and others attending the sick: men and women whose exertions were so demeaned by university-type physicians, and who are, for that and related reasons, so poorly documented, that only lately has their medieval history begun to be written.[17]

[11] M. R. McVaugh, *Medicine before the Plague: Practitioners and their Patients in the Crown of Aragon, 1285–1345* (Cambridge, 1993), pp. 218–25; Ziegler, 'Practitioners and Saints'.

[12] See now Jacquart, *Médecine médiévale.*

[13] *Western Medical Thought* is unusual among recent synopses in devoting a chapter to regimen.

[14] F. Getz, *Medicine in the English Middle Ages* (Princeton, 1998), pp. 3–4, on the last illness of Archbishop Hubert Walter and his 'non-treatment' by Gilbertus Anglicus as reported by Ralph of Coggeshall, *Chronicon Anglicanum*, ed. J. Stevenson, RS 66 (London, 1875), pp. 156–9.

[15] Green, 'Documenting'.

[16] K. Park, 'Stones, Bones and Hernias: Surgical Specialists in Fourteenth- and Fifteenth-Century Italy', in *Medicine from the Black Death to the French Disease*, ed. R. French et al. (Cambridge, 1998), pp. 110–30.

[17] Rawcliffe, 'Hospital Nurses'.

The topic of nursing naturally brings me back to hospitals. Here anti-scholastic revisionism is still more inchoate. Attention has largely been absorbed by whether or not hospitals had doctors on their staffs. Florence carries off the prize for precocity; England trails in last, with the Savoy hospital.[18] Medicalization of this kind – medicalization in the literal sense of the arrival of *medici* – is presented as the one development that really mattered. It is also presented, for the most part, as a development *ex nihilo*, on the assumption that nothing else preceding it was really medicine. Medicalization becomes, indeed, the leitmotif of an implicit teleological narrative – of the victory of cure over care, of doctors over nurses, and (again) of treatment over regimen.

The work of Carole Rawcliffe and John Henderson, on English and Florentine hospitals respectively, subverts this teleology: so, at least, I read the fruits of their research.[19] Contrast the hospital of Santa Maria Nuova with that of St Giles, Norwich (the 'Great Hospital' as it became after the Reformation). Santa Maria Nuova had its retained corps of physicians who admitted only patients with acute but not life-threatening conditions and discharged them rapidly. St Giles helped the chronically sick and elderly to live out their days in minimum pain. The contrast could hardly be starker. The future of hospitals seems to lie on one side, the Tuscan side; their past on the other, in East Anglia. Yet this contrast, as Rawcliffe and Henderson remind us, is surprisingly superficial. More importantly, both hospitals were religious institutions, with liturgy at their heart.[20] Patients in both lay within sight of the sacrament on the altar. In both, their daily life was punctuated far more deeply by the monastic 'hours' than by the 'ward round'. Exposure to the host, even without reception;[21] regular confession[22] (without which the

[18] K. Park and J. Henderson, '"The First Hospital among Christians": The Ospedale di Santa Maria Nuova in Early Sixteenth-Century Florence', *Medical History* 35 (1991), 164–88; *The Hospital in History*, ed. L. Granshaw and R. Porter (London and New York, 1989), chs. 1–3.

[19] Rawcliffe, 'Medicine for the Soul' and *Medicine for the Soul*; J. Henderson, 'Splendide case di cura: spedali, medicina ed assistenza a Firenze nel trecento', in *Ospedali e città: L'Italia del Centro-Nord, XIII–XVI secolo*, ed. A. J. Grieco and L. Sandri (Florence, 1997), pp. 15–50. I am grateful to Dr Henderson for allowing me to read some of the typescript of his *The Renaissance Hospital* (forthcoming).

[20] Rawcliffe, *Medicine for the Soul*, ch. 4 and 'The Eighth Comfortable Work: Education and the Medieval English Hospital', in *The Church and Learning in Late Medieval Society*, ed. J. Stratford and C. Barron (Stamford, forthcoming), generously shown to me in typescript by the author. Henderson, 'Splendide case', p. 48; Saunier, '*Le pauvre malade*', ch. 3. I am also indebted to forthcoming work by Christopher Page on hospitals' collections of liturgical music.

[21] K. Thomas, *Religion and the Decline of Magic*, Penguin edn (Harmondsworth, 1973), pp. 36, 39; Rawcliffe, 'Medicine for the Soul', p. 319.

[22] Saunier, '*Le pauvre malade*', pp. 112–13; F. Kudlien, 'Beichte und Heilung', *Medizinhistorisches Journal* 13 (1978), 1–14. In the sixteenth century Alvise Luisini claimed that physicians could detect objective physical improvements in patients who had confessed one day previously. The psychological freedom from anxiety which the confession produced led directly to better health, including the remission of fever.

hospital would be contaminated by sin);[23] the proximity of relics, their power absorbed either in a single dramatic moment or more slowly and osmotically;[24] contemplation of devotional pictures with their appropriate symbolism of the sure avenue to health;[25] the prayers and Christian magic of nurses;[26] the pleasing ambience of gardens and (sometimes) water courses:[27] all these possible features of hospital life, mentioned by Rawcliffe and Henderson and a few like-minded students of medieval hospitals, erode the starkness of the contrast between England and Italy. They suggest to me a characterization of the hospital less in terms of the presence or absence of doctors and more as a 'total therapeutic environment'.

It is within this approach that I locate my focus on hospital music. I want to use that topic to push the analyses offered by Rawcliffe and Henderson further, and in two directions. One direction is medieval: it leads to the background theory of this environmental view of hospital therapy. The other is modern: conceptual in a different way. It is an attempt to break down the dualism that still seems to order our thinking about such matters as the role of the Mass in the promotion of well-being. We speak of *medicina sacramentalis* or 'medicine of the soul' as against secular medicine; we juxtapose *medicina del corpo e medicina dell'anima*, in a manner which, although apparently justified by many medieval texts, is surely too Cartesian to be without anachronism.[28] The subtext we mistakenly attribute to such binary categorization is, first, that 'sacramental medicine' ministers only to the soul

See R. Palmer, 'The Church, Leprosy and Plague in Medieval and Early Modern Europe', SCH 19 (1982), 79–99 (p. 86), citing [A.] Luisini, *Tractatus de confessione a die decubitus instituenda* (Venice, 1563), pp. 74–5. See also Ralph of Coggeshall, *Chronicon Anglicanum*, ed. Stevenson, p. 158, on the therapeutic effect of the final confession of Hubert Walter.

[23] A composition between St John's Hospital, Bruges, and its chaplain stressed that the latter must meet his obligation to confess each patient on arrival: if just one sin 'slipped through', the whole house would be imperilled: E. van der Elst, *L'Hôpital Saint-Jean de Bruges de 1188 à 1500* (Bruges, 1975), pp. 61–2, a reference I owe to Carole Rawcliffe.

[24] Rawcliffe, 'Medicine for the Soul', p. 325; Orme and Webster, *The English Hospital*, p. 56; Saunier, *'Le pauvre malade'*, pp. 114–17.

[25] R. A. Koch, 'Flower Symbolism in the Portinari Altarpiece', *Art Bulletin* 46 (1964), 76–7, a reference I owe to John Henderson. See also A. Hayum, *The Isenheim Altarpiece: God's Medicine and the Painter's Vision* (Princeton, 1989); Thomas, *Religion*, p. 29; M.-L. Windemuth, *Das Hospital als Träger der Armenfürsorge im Mittelalter*, Sudhoffs Archiv, Beiheft 36 (Stuttgart, 1995).

[26] Rawcliffe, 'Medicine for the Soul', p. 323.

[27] Rawcliffe, 'Hospital Nurses', pp. 58–9; R. Gilchrist, *Contemplation and Action: The Other Monasticism* (London and New York, 1995), p. 43.

[28] J. Agrimi and C. Crisciani, *Medicina del corpo e medicina dell'anima: note sul sapere del medico fina all'inizio del secolo XIII* (Milan, 1978); Rawcliffe, *Medicine for the Soul*, pp. 160–1. See also Agrimi and Crisciani, 'Charity and Aid', pp. 174–6. Note also the title of Risse, *Mending Bodies, Saving Souls: A History of Hospitals*. For an early, seemingly Cartesian, statement of the theme, see *Acts of Thomas* 95, trans. M. R. James, *The Apocryphal New Testament* (Oxford, 1924), p. 406.

while secular medicine assists only the body; second, that sacramental 'medicine' is not quite 'real' medicine in the familiar (that is, modern) sense – which of course doctors alone can administer. The 'psychosomaticism' of ancient and medieval thought – *corpus sanum de mente sana* as it might be – is downplayed. Rigorists in medical matters, like St Bernard, might have approved of that.[29] The Fathers gathered at the Fourth Lateran Council (1215) would have been less pleased. For them, famously, 'sickness of the body may sometimes be the result of sin', and spiritual health improves the response to secular medicine, not least because it could banish the pathogenic fear of death.[30]

II

The best evidence in medieval medical history always seems to come from the east. Hospital music-making of expressly therapeutic intent is exemplified for us most fully in the large Islamic hospitals of medieval and Ottoman times. The first surviving discussion of music in hospitals which treats Byzantium as precursor is not Hujwiri's; it is the 'epistle' on music of the 'Brethren of Purity' (*Ikhwan al-Safa'*), a fraternity that flourished in Basra in the second half of the tenth century and dedicated to the pursuit of holiness and truth, especially the truth of (ancient) Greek science.[31] Its members composed a vast encyclopaedia in the form of fifty-two epistles with a summary. That dealing with music asserts that the Greek philosophers

> also invented another melody which they used in the hospitals, at the break of day, and which had the virtue of solacing the pains due to the infirmities and ills suffered by the patient, alleviating their violence and even curing certain sicknesses and infirmities.[32]

The therapeutic power of hospital music came to seem quite uncontroversial. In the mid-eleventh century Sa'id ibn Bakhtishu', of the famous Baghdad medical family, could take it for granted in his treatise on medicine that patients' psychological problems – the quieting of their nerves – would be

[29] Bernard of Clairvaux, *The Steps of Humility*, trans. G. B. Birch (Cambridge, MA, 1942), pp. 58–60, cited by Ziegler, *Medicine and Religion*, p. 225 n. 34.

[30] Canon 22, trans. N. Tanner, *Decrees of the Ecumenical Councils*, 2 vols. (Washington, DC, 1990), I, 245–6.

[31] A. Shiloah, 'Jewish and Muslim Traditions of Music Therapy', in *Music as Medicine: The History of Music Therapy since Antiquity*, ed. P. Horden (Aldershot, 2000), pp. 69–83 (pp. 73–4, 80–1), and *Music in the World of Islam: A Socio-Cultural Study* (Aldershot, 1995), pp. 50–1; Dols, *Majnun*, pp. 170–1.

[32] 'The Epistle on Music of the Ikwan al-Safa', trans. A. Shiloah, *Documentation and Studies 3: Department of Musicology and the Chaim Rosenberg School of Jewish Studies* (Tel Aviv, 1978), pp. 16–17, repr. in Shiloah, *The Dimension of Music in Islamic and Jewish Culture*, CS393 (Aldershot, 1993), article III.

addressed in hospitals by the performance of, among other things, entertaining song.[33]

Those are generalized testimonies, prescriptive in character. There is, though, some medieval evidence of music in specific foundations. One of the designated expenditures at the Mansuri hospital in Cairo, founded by the Sultan al-Mansur in 1284, was for troupes of musicians who would entertain the patients daily. At the hospital founded at the behest of the Mamluk sultan, al-Nasir, in Aleppo in 1354, music was played in the courtyards for the benefit of the inmates.[34] For a more detailed account of such performances and their therapeutic rationale, however, we have to wait until Ottoman times and the report of the noted seventeenth-century traveller, Evliya Chelebi.[35] Musicians, he tells us, were employed at the hospital of Muhammad II (d. 1481) to amuse the sick and, especially, to cure the insane patients. At the Nuri hospital in Damascus, which Evliya visited in 1648, concerts were reportedly given thrice daily. At the Edirne hospital established by Bayezid II, three singers and seven musicians visited the hospital three times a week.[36] We should not assume from pronouncements in modern synopses, about the hostility to music of orthodox Islam, that these hospital performances can never have been religious in character.[37]

It is all reminiscent of the intense musical life of some of asylums in eighteenth- and nineteenth-century Europe.[38] We should be careful, though, not to splice scattered references in partisan accounts too tightly together and make of them a hospital tradition. Music therapy of this lavish and expensive kind may have been the prerogative of the wealthiest patients and could, overall, have been very occasional, no matter what Evliya says. Of the application of music therapy as a regular element in the physician's armoury we have no direct evidence. The oldest and largest collection of case histories from the Islamic Middle East, that compiled by students of Rhazes (al-Razi) in the early tenth century, makes no mention of the use of music.[39] Rhazes was successively director of two hospitals, in Rayy and Baghdad; and, if his casebook reflects his hospital practice at all, then the fullest evocation we have of hospital medicine would contradict several of the references just assembled.

The Islamic material is important here because it illustrates not so much a

[33] *Über die Heilung der Krankheiten der Seele und des Körpers*, ed. and trans. F. Klein-Franke (Beirut, 1977), fol. 74b (trans. p. 57, modified Savage-Smith).

[34] Dols, *Majnun*, pp. 121, 171.

[35] Shiloah, 'Jewish and Muslim Traditions of Music Therapy', p. 75.

[36] Dols, *Majnun*, pp. 171, 173.

[37] Shiloah, *Music in the World of Islam*, ch. 4; J. C. Bürgel, *The Feather of Simurgh: The 'Licit Magic' of the Arts in Medieval Islam* (New York and London, 1988), ch. 4. See also Dols, *Majnun*, p. 172.

[38] C. Kramer, 'Music as Cause and Cure of Illness in Nineteenth-Century Europe', in *Music as Medicine*, pp. 338–52 (pp. 348–9).

[39] C. Álvarez-Millán, 'Practice versus Theory: Tenth-Century Case Histories from the Islamic Middle East', in *The Year 1000*, pp. 293–306.

solid tradition as a 'horizon of expectation', a cultural possibility. Medieval Islamic scholars seized on the full range of Antiquity's theoretical legacy concerning music therapy: a collection of anecdotes attributing astonishing feats to Pythagoras and other sages, a theory of the educative ethos of particular types of music; the cosmological explanation of musical healing in terms of an 'attunement' of the individual to the 'harmony of the spheres' through the intermediary of *musica instrumentalis*. All this was taken up and elaborated into a comprehensive alignment of zodiacal signs, planets, tones, elements, and bodily humours.[40] One can see why Hujwiri, and also the Brethren of Purity,[41] should have held Greek – and presumably, by extension, Byzantine – example dear. According to Ibn Abi Usaybi'ah, the first medical men were the Greeks who invented the reed pipe and healed body and soul with their playing.[42] The debt to Galen above all, but also to Rufus of Ephesus, ensured that much attention would be given in Islam to 'psychiatry', a therapy directed at the mind because the mind affected the body.[43] In the increasingly available insane wards in hospitals, physical restraint (often of a brutish kind) was thus counterbalanced by music, fountains – and even alcohol.[44] Orthodox wariness of music and dancing was quietly overridden by this Galenic enthusiasm for the creation of a therapeutic environment.

On the basis of scattered passages in Galen and Hippocrates (the latter known largely through Galen's commentary), medieval Islamic physicians developed a conception of health which was to be crucial to the recommendation of music as medicine for centuries to come.[45] Its briefest exposition can be found in the work later known to Western medicine as the *Isagoge* [*Introduction*] of Johannitius (Hunayn ibn Ishaq; died *c.* 877), an Arabic synopsis so convenient that, in partial Latin translation, it was widely diffused across medieval Europe.[46] This text distinguishes between the 'naturals' (chiefly the four elements, qualities such as hot or moist, and the four humours), the 'contra-naturals' (disease, its causes and 'sequels'), and the 'non-naturals'. The last are the pertinent ones. They are the determinants of health. They include air and the environment, eating and drinking, exercise and baths,

[40] M. West, 'Music Therapy in Antiquity', and P. Horden, 'Commentary on Part II, with a Note on the Early Middle Ages', both in *Music as Medicine*, pp. 51–68, 103–8 (pp. 103–4); Shiloah, 'Jewish and Muslim Traditions of Music Therapy'.

[41] Shiloah, 'Jewish and Muslim Traditions of Music Therapy', p. 74.

[42] Dols, *Majnun*, p. 166.

[43] C. Burnett, '"Spiritual Medicine": Music and Healing in Islam and its Influence in Western Medicine', in *Musical Healing in Cultural Contexts*, ed. Gouk, pp. 85–91 (pp. 85–6); Dols, *Majnun*, chs. 1–3.

[44] Dols, *Majnun*, pp. 119–35, 165–73.

[45] Burnett, '"Spiritual Medicine"', pp. 89–90; W. F. Kümmel, *Musik und Medizin: Ihre Wechselbeziehungen in Theorie und Praxis von 800 bis 1800*, Freiburger Beiträge zur Wissenschafts- und Universitätsgeschichte 2 (Munich, 1977).

[46] 'Johannicius, Isagoge ad Techne Galieni', ed. G. Maurach in *Sudhoffs Archiv für Geschichte der Medizin* 62 (1978), 148–74.

sleep, coitus, and the 'passions [or 'accidents'] of the soul'.[47] Johannitius writes:

> Sundry affections of the mind produce an effect within the body, such as those which bring the natural heat from the interior of the body to the outer parts or the surface of the skin. Sometimes this happens suddenly, as with anger; sometimes gently and slowly, as with delight and joy . . . some affections disturb the natural energy both internal and external, as, for instance, with grief.[48]

Those sentences represent the conceptual gateway through which music comes into medicine – under the heading of 'delight and joy'. Music – of the appropriate ethos – can manipulate the accidents of the soul, emotions such as joy, or the workings of the imagination. It can mitigate those feelings that, through their impact on the humours, cause disease, and strengthen those that prevent it. The *Isagoge* is the fount of a whole tradition in Islamic medical writing of discussing 'soul medicine', psychosomatic therapy as we might call it, in terms of the regulation of this particular non-natural.[49]

III

The accidents of the soul as an ingredient in health formed, then, an idea with a future. That future in Islamic medicine is not to the point here. The future of its translated, Latin, version will be. Before I come to it, however, I want to consider whether the non-naturals in their full Islamic glory were essential to the therapeutic role in medieval hospitals which I envisage for religious music. Was the Islamic 'medicalization' of the emotions an essential pre-condition? Or could a vulgarized form of late Antique Galenism serve almost as well? For answer I turn back to early Byzantium. This is partly to enquire further into what might have prompted Hujwiri's misconception about Byzantine therapy, but mainly to look more generally at the beginnings of another hospital tradition and the role of medicine and music within it.

The first major philanthropic foundation in Byzantium was that of St Basil, called the Basileias by later church historians.[50] This 'new city', as it was

[47] For the non-naturals, see G. Olson, *Literature as Recreation in the Later Middle Ages* (Ithaca and London, 1982), pp. 40–4; L. García-Ballester, 'On the Origin of the "Six Non-Natural Things" in Galen', in *Galen und das Hellenistische Erbe*, ed. J. Kollesch and D. Nickel, Sudhoffs Archiv, Beiheft 32 (1993), pp. 105–15; P. Gil-Sotres, 'Modelo téorico y observación clínica: las pasiones del alma en la psicología medica medieval', in *Comprendre et maîtriser la nature au Moyen Age: mélanges d'histoire des sciences offerts à Guy Beaujouan* (Geneva, 1994), pp. 181–204; H. Mikkeli, *Hygiene in the Early Modern Medical Tradition* (Helsinki, 1999).

[48] *Sourcebook of Medieval Science*, pp. 708–9.

[49] Burnett, '"Spiritual Medicine"', pp. 88–9.

[50] Sozomen, *Historia ecclesiastica* VI.xxxiv.9; p. 291. For what follows see the summary accounts of P. Rousseau, *Basil of Caesarea* (Berkeley, Los Angeles and Oxford, 1994),

lauded in the funeral oration pronounced by Gregory of Nazianzus, was a philanthropic 'multiplex' outside Basil's episcopal seat at Caesarea.[51] Gregory describes it as a centre in which disease is studied philosophically (*philosopheitai*); he makes it out to be a school of charity, an academy of compassion. The objects of its compassion were above all lepers, limbless (as they often were) victims of 'social death', expelled from all the forms and arenas of association that characterized the ancient *polis*: family, household, fraternity, assembly, bathhouse, public place, city space generally. They existed in name only since their wasted bodies could no longer individuate them. Only music, in Gregory's interesting recollection, could express their identity. They were – to the extent that the disease's ravages had left them any voice at all – 'masters of pitiful songs'.[52] Basil also lodged the transient poor, almost as unwelcome in the *polis* as were lepers, along with those (presumably) local people whose infirmity necessitated care. In a letter to the governor of Caesarea, in which Basil defended his subversion of the social priorities of the city, he anticipates those who would refuse to equate the history of medicine with the history of doctors. He does not sharply differentiate nursing from medicine: he writes, in that letter, not of doctors (*iatroi*) but of those who are doctoring (*iatrouontai*).[53] But if his physicians were amateurs (in the strict sense) from the monastery, that does not entitle us to envisage them as crass empirics with merely a few herbal panaceas in their arsenal. They had Basil's personal example to guide them into a more theoretical approach.

According to Gregory, Basil's own ill health as well as his philanthropy originally turned him towards medicine. Like Gregory, he had studied the care of the sick and medical treatment: the 'deep structure' of the discipline – 'not as far as it relates to what is visible . . . but as far as it is based on principle [*dogmatikon*] and is philosophical'.[54] We cannot know how much actual Galen Basil had read. But he presumably absorbed at least the rudiments of Hippocratic–Galenic thinking about the psychosomatic aspect

pp. 139–44; Temkin, *Hippocrates*, pp. 162–4; D. Constantelos, *Byzantine Philanthropy and Social Welfare*, 2nd edn (New Rochelle, NY, 1991), pp. 75–6, 119–20; T. Miller, *The Birth of the Hospital in the Byzantine Empire*, 2nd edn (Baltimore and London, 1997), pp. 85–8; P. van Minnen, 'Medical Care in Late Antiquity', in *Ancient Medicine in its Socio-Cultural Context*, ed. P. J. van der Eijk, H. F. J. Horstmanshoff and P. H. Schrijvers, 2 vols., The Wellcome Institute Series in the History of Medicine, Clio Medica 27–8 (Amsterdam and Atlanta, 1995), I, 153–69 (pp. 157–9). The political circumstances (and the precursors) of Basil's initiative have been re-examined by Peter Brown in his Menahem Stern Lectures (2000), 'Poverty and Leadership in the Later Roman Empire', the text of which he kindly allowed me to read in advance of its delivery.

[51] Gregory of Nazianzus, *Oratio* xliii.63; *PG* 36, 577C.

[52] *PG* 36, 580B, with Temkin, *Hippocrates*, p. 162.

[53] Basil, *Epistulae* 94, in *Saint Basile: Lettres*, ed. Y. Courtonne, 3 vols. (Paris, 1957–66), I, 206.

[54] Gregory of Nazianzus, *Oratio* xliii.23 (*PG* 36, 528B), with Temkin *Hippocrates*, ch. 13.

of health, the potentially pathogenic and the beneficial aspects of the 'accidents of the soul'. In the treatise *On the Nature of Man* (another text with a future) by Basil's near contemporary, Nemesius, bishop of Emesa in Syria, a Christianized and Aristotelian Galenism allows a large conceptual space for the physiology of the emotions and for a 'two-way' traffic between soul and body in matters of daily regimen.[55] People become ill, Basil himself wrote, when diverted from their natural state. For they are deprived of health either because of poor regimen (principally but not exclusively food and drink) or because of something morbific. In the same way the soul is made ill – diverted from its natural state – by sin. The medicine of the body is a paradigm for the therapy of the soul. It is a model conceded to us by God.[56] But that does not make the medicine of the soul a mere metaphor. It actually falls within the province of the ideal physician. Such a figure will be ambidextrous: he will not confine his art to healing the body but will seek also the cure of diseases of the soul.[57] Medicine in the relatively narrow sense of dietary prescription, medication and surgery is certainly, for Basil, a model that helps us understand a greater medicine. Yet the imperative that one should place only limited trust in physicians does not entail that medicine is to be conceived as narrowly somatic in scope. This is borne out if we turn to the more conventionally religious aspects of Basil's philanthropic initiative. Basil is, of course, a major figure in the history of Orthodox liturgy as well as in the history of philanthropy. The two aspects of his achievement are, however, seldom if ever considered in tandem or seen as in any way connected.

Presumably there were priests to attend the needy inmates of the Basileias and officiate in its chapel – priests drawn, if nowhere else, from the numbers of those 'doctoring' monks.[58] Like John Chrysostom while patriarch of Constantinople a few decades later, Basil would have founded a hospital with 'pious presbyters' as well as medical attendants.[59] Within his 'new city', the church would have provided a focus to the philanthropic complex comparable to that of a cathedral in a *polis*. In it would have been heard the 'pitiful songs' which were all that the leprous patients had to offer. What effects could have been attributed to the chants of its divine liturgy? Medical analogies are easy to find in Basil's output, but the 'psychotherapeutic' effects of psalmody are also described in his homilies on the Psalms and in his

[55] Nemesius, *De natura hominis*, 17–20, ed. M. Morani, Teubner edn (Leipzig, 1987), pp. 75–82; M. Morani, *La tradizione manoscritta del* De natura hominis *di Nemesio* (Milan, 1981); medieval Latin translation in *Nemesius d'Emèse* De natura hominis, ed. G. Verbeke and J. R. Moncho, Corpus Latinum commentariorum in Aristotelem Graecorum, Suppl. 1 (Leiden, 1975).

[56] Basil, *Quod deus non est auctor malorum* 6 (*PG* 31, 344A), with Temkin, *Hippocrates*, pp. 172–3.

[57] Basil, *Epistulae* clxxxix.1; ed. Courtonne, II, 132.

[58] Rousseau, *Basil*, p. 142.

[59] Temkin, *Hippocrates*, p. 164.

correspondence.[60] 'A Psalm is a tranquillity of soul . . . it settles one's tumultuous and seething thoughts. It mollifies the soul's wrath [or even 'passion of the soul': *tes psyches to thumoumenon*] and chastens its recalcitrance'; 'the consolation of hymns favours the soul with a state of happiness and freedom from care', and so on: sentiments that can be given either a theological or a medical gloss – or both simultaneously.[61] Basil knows all the anecdotes bequeathed by antiquity about the power of music – a power also shown, and to exemplary effect, by David:

> The passions born of illiberality and baseness of spirit are naturally occasioned by this sort of music. But we must pursue that other kind, which is better and leads to the better, and which, as they say, was used by David, that author of sacred songs, to soothe the king in his madness.[62]

For the fullest exposition in late Antiquity of the therapeutic benefits of liturgy, however, we have to look, not (for once) eastward but to the west. One of the now more obscure names in the patrology, Niceta, bishop of Remesiana (modern Bela Palanka, east of Niš, in the former Yugoslavia), who died after 414, was well-known in his time, to Paulinus of Nola and to Jerome among others. He 'theologizes' the power of David's singing over the demon in Saul in a way that will resonate throughout the Middle Ages and be repeated in the *Malleus Maleficarum*:

> He subdued the evil spirit which worked in Saul – not because such was the power of his cithara, but because a figure of the cross of Christ was mystically projected by the wood and the stretching of strings.[63]

Yet his other evocations of the possible effects of psalmody seem to blur any distinction between the literal or somatic and the celestial (or analogical) sense of therapy:

[60] For context, see P. Weitmann, *Sukzession und Gegenwart: zu theoretischen Äußerungen über bildende Künste und Musik von Basileios bis Hrabanus Maurus* (Wiesbaden, 1997), pp. 14–15; R. Taft, *The Liturgy of the Hours in East and West: The Origins of the Divine Office and its Meaning for Today* (Collegeville, MN, 1986), ch. 2; J. Quasten, *Music and Worship in Pagan and Christian Antiquity* (Washington, DC, 1983), ch. 4.

[61] Basil, *Homilia in psalmum I* 2 (*PG* 29, 212–13), trans. J. McKinnon, *Music in Early Christian Literature* (Cambridge, 1987), no. 131, p. 65; *Epistulae* ii.2, ed. Courtonne, I, 8, trans. McKinnon, no. 138, p. 68.

[62] Basil, *Ad adulescentes* 7 (*PG* 31, 581), trans. McKinnon, no. 140, p. 69. I Samuel 16. 16, 23.

[63] Niceta, *De psalmodiae bono* (*de utilitate hymnorum*) 4, ed. C. Turner, 'Niceta of Remesiana II', *Journal of Theological Studies* 24 (1922), 225–52 (p. 235); trans. McKinnon, no. 304, p. 135. P. Murray Jones, 'Music Therapy in the Later Middle Ages: The Case of Hugo van der Goes', in *Music as Medicine*, pp. 120–44 (p. 127), quoting J. Sprenger and H. Institoris, *Malleus maleficarum*, trans. M. Summers (London, 1928), p. 41.

> A psalm consoles the sad, restrains the joyful, tempers the angry [in true Aristotelian-Galenic fashion], refreshes the poor . . . To absolutely all who will take it, the psalm offers an appropriate medicine . . . effective in the cure of disease by reason of its strength . . .[64]

I think we should again be chary of dismissing the medicine there as merely metaphorical.

IV

A fully-fledged conception of the non-naturals, such as was developed in Islam, may not, then, have been necessary for the appreciation of hospital music as a type of therapy. Music, even if it took the rudimentary form only of liturgical chant in a small hospital chapel, could, through its effects on the soul, be medicinal for the body. Such, at least, was the perception. This is as true, I suspect, of the earliest hospitals in Europe as it is of the first Byzantine ones. From the very start they were institutions of psychosomatic religious healing.[65] According to the hagiographer of Caesarius of Arles, this sixth-century Frankish bishop

> had a very great concern for the sick and came to their assistance. He granted them a spacious house, in which they could listen undisturbed to the holy office [being sung] in the basilica. He set up beds and bedding, provided for expenses, and supplied a person to take care of them and heal them.[66]

No great disjunction there between medicine and religion. It may be no coincidence that the preceding paragraph in Caesarius's *Vita* should picture the bishop attempting to prevent the laity from gossiping in church by ordering them 'to learn psalms and hymns by heart and to sing sequences and antiphons in a loud and rhythmic voice'. The subject of liturgical musical participation as an educative measure led the writer by a natural association to the subject of sickness and the liturgical arrangements of Caesarius's hospital.

Centuries later, the theoretical stimulus given to learned medicine in Europe by the diffusion of Latin translations of the Arabic undoubtedly gave the 'passions of the soul' a currency greater than that enjoyed by any related notion

[64] Niceta, *De psalmodiae bono* 5, ed. Turner, pp. 235–6, trans. McKinnon, nos. 305–6, pp. 135–6.

[65] T. Sternberg, *Orientalium more secutus: Räume und Institutionen der Caritas des 5. bis 7. Jahrhunderts in Gallien*, Jahrbuch für Antike und Christentum, Ergänzungsband 16 (Münster, 1991), pp. 174–7.

[66] *Vita Caesarii* i.20, and, for what follows, i.19, trans. W. E. Klingshirn, *Caesarius of Arles: Life, Testament, Letters*, Translated Texts for Historians 19 (Liverpool, 1994), p. 18. On liturgy in Merovingian Gaul see Y. Hen, *Culture and Religion in Merovingian Gaul, AD 481–751* (Leiden, 1995), chs. 2–5.

in Caesarius's time. Still, it was not as wide a currency as it might have been. The culture of musical therapy nurtured by Islamic scholar-physicians was not transmitted in all its fullness to the West. No European hospital that I know of employed visiting musicians. No European hospital until the early modern period, and then only that of Santo Spirito in Rome, used non-liturgical music of any kind as a regular diversion for its patients.[67] Sometimes, in monasteries, secular music was indeed permitted as an aid to therapy, but it was unlikely to have been heard in the infirmary. Take for example the thirteenth-century Customary of St Augustine's Abbey, Canterbury:

> In the infirmary, there should be no disturbing clamour at any time, but nor in that same place should there be any music of any musical instrument played openly in general hearing. But, for reasons of greater need, if it be judged very useful for improving someone's condition – as when it happens that any brother be so weak and ill that he greatly needs the sound and harmony of a musical instrument to raise his spirits – that person may be led into the chapel by the *Infirmarius*, or carried there in some manner, so that, the door being closed, a stringed instrument may be sweetly played before him by any brother, or by any reliable and discreet servant, without blame. But great care should always be taken lest music or melody of this kind be heard at any time in the hall of the infirmary or – perish the thought – in the chambers of the brothers.[68]

Of course, if music in the infirmary was prohibited in this way, it had presumably sometimes been played there. One piece of evidence that supplies a possible context for its medicinal use in English monasteries is a passage in the register of Adam of Orleton, bishop of Hereford. This reveals that in 1318 the canons of Wigmore Abbey were diverted with wanton songs (*cantilenis inhonestis*) while being bled. To protect other patients from the pollution of blood, such prophylactic phlebotomy was, however, less likely to have taken place in the main infirmary than in a separate room, or even in a detached 'seyney hall'.[69]

[67] Kümmel, *Musik und Medizin*, pp. 260–1; P. de Angelis, *Musica e musicisti nell'Arcispedale di Santo Spirito in Saxia dal Quattrocento all'Ottocento* (Rome, 1950), ch. 6.

[68] *Customary of the Benedictine Monasteries of St. Augustine, Canterbury, and St. Peter, Westminster*, ed. E. M. Thompson, 2 vols., Henry Bradshaw Society 23 and 28 (London, 1902–4), I, 329–30; trans. C. Page, 'Music and Medicine in the Thirteenth Century', in *Music as Medicine*, pp. 109–19 (pp. 110–11).

[69] *Registrum Ade de Orleton*, ed. A. T. Bannister, Canterbury and York Series 5 (London, 1908), p. 102, cited in Page, 'Music and Medicine', p. 118. On monastic infirmary regimen see B. Harvey, *Living and Dying in England 1100–1540: The Monastic Experience* (Oxford, 1993), pp. 91–9, and (also on Westminster Abbey) 'Before and After the Black Death: A Monastic Infirmary in Fourteenth-Century England', in *Death, Sickness and Health in Medieval Society and Culture*, ed. S. J. Ridyard, *Sewanee Medieval Studies* 10 (2000), 5–31; and (most comprehensively, despite its subtitle), C. Rawcliffe, '"On the Threshold of Eternity": Care for the Sick in East Anglian Monasteries', in the forthcoming Festschrift for Norman Scarfe, ed. C. Harper-Bill and C. Rawcliffe, of which the author kindly sent me a typescript.

One possible reason for this comparatively 'low-key' approach to musical therapy may have been that much of the relevant literature in Arabic which could have encouraged such therapy among the learned was simply not translated. Neither the musicological discourses on therapy that correlated astrology, music and humours, nor the treatises on 'soul medicine' found their way into Latin.[70] But commentaries on the *Isagoge* and the like served as partial substitutes. Regimen had a place in European medicine after *c.* 1200 that it simply could not have gained earlier.[71] In the promotion of a health-giving cheerfulness, the benefits of 'wine, women and song' (alongside, incidentally, a 'good read')[72] became widely recognized.

The consequences of that for the European hospital were several. First, nursing was in effect medicalized. I do not mean that nurses became equivalent to physicians; no aspirant doctor would have conceded so much. Rather, since medicine and doctoring were not, despite appearances, coterminous, nursing could be accorded a status within medical theory. The nurses who ensured that their patients enjoyed a refreshing night's rest and (ideally) the peace and quiet of hospital surroundings, or who tended a fragrant herb garden in the hospital precinct, or who removed the source of noxious smells, were all performing tasks that were, in theory, just as much medicine as was phlebotomy, or medication with complex and exotic drugs, or subtle and penetrating diagnosis.[73] The same applied on a more exalted and occasional level. When Christine de Pisan urged the merits of charitable work upon ladies and extolled the benefits of a royal visit she too was thinking medically. The good princess, she wrote, should tour the hospital in her finery with a magnificent retinue because this would raise the spirits of the poor inmates.[74] That was sound medical theory. In the 'non-natural' scheme of things, the most therapeutic emotion was cheerfulness.

A second relevant consequence of this notion of 'emotional hygiene' was that the distinction between secular and sacred became blurred. The context in which an Aristotelian moderation of the non-naturals appears in the medical *consilia* (physicians' letters of advice) of the later Middle Ages is nearly always secular.[75] But occasionally the patient requesting the advice is a religious and then the recommendations are modified. One sick Franciscan was for example advised by Bartholomaeus da Montagnana to avoid strong emotions such as anxiety or those inspired by reading stories of martyrdoms. Yet, in another *consilium*, Bartholomaeus urges the study of moral or

[70] Burnett, '"Spiritual Medicine"', pp. 87–90.

[71] García-Ballester, '*Artifex factivus sanitatis*'; P. Gil-Sotres, 'The Regimens of Health', in *Western Medical Thought*, pp. 291–318.

[72] Olson, *Literature as Recreation*, ch. 2.

[73] Rawcliffe, 'Hospital Nurses', pp. 49–50.

[74] Christine de Pisan, *The Treasure of the City of Ladies*, trans. S. Lawson (London, 1985), p. 53.

[75] J. Agrimi and C. Crisciani, *Les 'consilia' médicaux*, Typologie des sources du Moyen Age 69 (Turnhout, 1994).

theological narratives, *along with the singing of psalms*, as among the exercises 'that bring delight'.[76]

The non-naturals themselves as it were migrated easily from medical to religious discourses. John Mirfeld (d. 1407), who lived for forty years in rooms in St Bartholomew's Hospital, London, composed a *Breviarium* of excerpts from medical texts for those (such as hospital attendants presumably) without a suitable library.[77] It includes a number of Christian charms (perhaps to be said by nurses) to assist women, which may be a reflection of St Bartholomew's reputation as a harbour for unwed mothers. It also inevitably includes a discussion of the non-naturals, as indispensable to basic hospital know-how. Towards the end of his life Mirfeld prepared a comparable anthology of religious texts, the *Florarium*. In that later work he reproduced the passages on the *regimen sanitatis* that had originally appeared in the *Breviarium*.[78] As a model of self-discipline, a therapeutic or preventive regime would obviously serve in either a medical or a pastoral context. But was the other reason for repeating the regimen that, in quite general terms, it belonged as much to religion as to medicine? It is significant that, according to an inventory of 1448, the London hospital of St Mary Elsing, Cripplegate, included a copy of the *Florarium* in its remarkable library.[79]

'In theory, if less often in practice, the precisely regulated environment of the medieval hospital lent itself especially well to the implementation of a system which integrated earthly and spiritual medicine in a carefully balanced way.'[80] Liturgical music was a part of that integrated system. Of course there had long been votive masses of therapeutic intent, such as the mass in honour of St Sigismund for the relief of fever; but the saint, not the mass, is supposed to be the source of healing.[81] Any mass, however, votive or not, whether sung simply in a hospital chapel, or elaborately in some grander church, could potentially have beneficial effects on the accidents of the soul through the positive emotions that it inspired in its singers or auditors.

Now historians have tended to make undocumented assertions about how beneficial it would have been for patients to have heard sung liturgy regularly. The 'gret criynge and joly chauntynge' which the Reformers castigated in the thrice-daily masses heard in the hospital of St Giles, Norwich, were likely to have been differently perceived in the Middle

[76] Olsen, *Literature as Recreation*, pp. 61–2.

[77] Getz, *Medicine*, pp. 49–50.

[78] P. Horton-Smith Hartley and H. R. Aldridge, *Johannes de Mirfeld of St Bartholomew's, Smithfield: His Life and Works* (Cambridge, 1936), p. 154.

[79] *Londinium Redivivum*, ed. J. P. Malcolm, 4 vols. (London, 1803–7), I, 29, cited by Rawcliffe, 'Eighth Comfortable Work', n. 76.

[80] Rawcliffe, 'Hospital Nurses', p. 54.

[81] F. S. Paxton, 'Liturgy and Healing in an Early Medieval Saint's Cult: The Mass *in honore Sancti Sigismundi* for the Cure of Fevers', *Traditio* 49 (1994), 23–43; A. Angenendt, 'Missa specialis: zugleich ein Beitrag zur Entstehung der Privatmessen', *Frühmittelalterliche Studien* 17 (1983), 153–221.

Ages.[82] 'The soothing and often melodious routine [of the hours] . . . may itself have proved extremely therapeutic.'[83] Is it possible to confirm this intuition? When, around 1500, a local priest left money for masses to be sung every week in the hospital of the Holy Cross, Orléans, 'for the sustenance of the bodies and souls of the poor', what could he have had in mind?[84] His bequest was unusual by that time in that the first-named beneficiary of the mass was the inmate, not the donor. And the living inmate, not the dead one. The priest seems to have envisaged something more than an abbreviation of future purgatory. In hospitals where the services were sung (an important qualification) how might the liturgical music of plainchant or polyphony have affected body and soul?

There is a tradition of theoretical writing which is bread and butter to medieval musicologists but 'caviare to the general' as far as medical historiography is concerned. I should like to end by simply drawing attention to it and urging its integration into our analysis of how a medieval hospital liturgy might, in ideal circumstances, have worked – worked therapy if not wonders.

The anecdotes of ancient feats of musical correction, moral improvement and healing, replayed throughout the European Middle Ages in copies of, and commentaries on, Boethius's *De Musica*, and endorsed by the theory of the non-naturals, ensured that the medicinal power of music became a topos of medieval discussion.[85]

For example, Gerald of Wales, in famous passage in the *Topographia Hiberniae*:

> The sweet harmony of music not only gives pleasure but renders important services. It greatly cheers depressed spirits, smoothes furrowed brows . . . Moreover, music soothes disease and pain. The sounds which strike the ear . . . either heal our ailments or enable us to bear them more readily . . . there are no sufferings which music will not mitigate, and many which it cures.[86]

Or take the *Summa musice*, a manual for teaching boys to sing from plainchant notation, written around 1200 by two authors, one of them probably a *decanus* in Würzburg Cathedral:[87]

82 Rawcliffe, *Medicine for the Soul*, pp. 123–4.

83 Rawcliffe, 'Medicine for the Soul', p. 317.

84 Saunier, '*Le pauvre malade*', p. 104.

85 Horden, 'Commentary on Part II', pp. 103–4; C. Page, *The Owl and the Nightingale: Musical Life and Ideas in France 1100–1300* (London, 1989), pp. 29, 139. For context see T. J. McGee, *The Sound of Medieval Song: Ornamentation and Vocal Style According to the Treatises* (Oxford, 1998), and, for the tradition in medieval musicological treatises, L. Zanoncelli, *Sulla estetica di Johannes Tinctoris* (Bologna, 1979), pp. 117–26.

86 *Giraldus Cambrensis Opera*, ed. J. F. Dimock and J. S. Brewer, RS 21, 8 vols. (London, 1861–91), V, 155–6.

87 *The 'Summa musice': A Thirteenth-Century Manual for Singers*, ed. and trans. C. Page (Cambridge, 1991), p. 12.

> Music has medicinal properties and performs miraculous things. Music cures diseases, especially those which arise from melancholia and sadness. Through music one can be prevented from falling into the loneliness of pain and despair.... Music calms the irascible, gladdens the sorrowful, dissipates anxious thoughts and destroys them. What is greater still, music terrifies evil spirits and banishes them, just as David the string player . . . expelled the demon from King Saul when he was possessed by a devil.[88]

Or consider this, from the *Treatise on the Two-fold Practice of Church Music in Divine Services* by Egidius Carlerius (d. 1472), dean of the cathedral chapter of Cambrai, later a theologian in the Collège de Navarre, Paris, and (in all likelihood) friend of the composer Guillaume du Fay:

> Now let us turn our pen to the question as to how harmonious music may be most acceptable to God, and let us reveal how praiseworthy and useful it is in church . . . The first of [music's special claims] is that it is a reflection of heavenly joys . . . the second special claim is that music tempers mental passions [standard anecdotes from Boethius follow] . . . The third special claim is that music calms physical passions. For the first book of Boethius's *De Musica*, referred to earlier, mentions that when some Pythagoreans suffered sleepless nights because of the worries that plagued them, a soft and peaceful slumber crept over them with certain melodies . . . euphonious music has sometimes even cured severe illnesses, and no wonder! . . . The fourth special claim is that music drives away evil spirits. For they cannot endure music in praise of God . . . Let us therefore praise harmonious music that rouses the sleeping and gives hearing to the deaf.[89]

We thus do not have to rely on informed intuition in attributing a potentially therapeutic effect to liturgical music in hospitals. Of course the ancient topoi from which the above quotations descended were by no means all necessarily appreciated in Lanfranc's hospital at Canterbury, with which I began, or indeed in any given hospital among the other, later ones which I have mentioned. That, quite generally, medieval 'hospitals, clinics, and health spas sounded with rhythm and melody'[90] seems unlikely. All I would conjecture is the topoi provided hospital life with a general background of possibility: they brought music therapy within donors', priests', and patients' 'horizon of expectation'. To be sure, the liturgical musical round can numb with boredom. That was recognized in the Middle Ages as it can be today.[91] But chant, whether in New Age or Middle Age guise, can also be

88 *'Summa musice'*, ed. Page, pp. 55–6 (trans.), 145–6 (text). For the later medieval debate on the power of music over demons see Page, *The Owl and the Nightingale*, pp. 158–60; Jones, 'Music Therapy in the Later Middle Ages', pp. 123–4.

89 *On the Dignity and Effects of Music: Two Fifteenth-Century Treatises*, ed. and trans. R. Strohm and J. D. Cullington, Institute of Advanced Musical Studies, King's College London, Study Texts 2 (London, 1996), pp. 26–32 (trans.), 42–7 (text).

90 M. P. Cosman, 'Machaut's Medical Musical World', *Annals of the New York Academy of Sciences* 314 (1978), 1–36 (p. 1).

91 Page, *The Owl and the Nightingale*, p. 158.

hailed as therapeutic. The hope that amelioration, or even cure, might come through hearing it could contribute to an atmosphere of confidence and trust. And such an atmosphere is crucial to successful medicine of any kind, in any age. Osler would have understood. 'Faith in *St Johns Hopkins*, as we used to call him, an atmosphere of optimism, and cheerful nurses, worked just the same sort of cures as did Aesculapius at Epidaurus . . . The Christian Church began with a mission to the whole man – body as well as soul – and the apostolic ministry of health has never been wholly abandoned.'[92]

[92] W. Osler, 'The Faith that Heals', *British Medical Journal* (18 June 1910), I, 1470–2 (p. 1471).

Medicine and Heresy

Peter Biller

My theme is medicine and the Cathar and Waldensian heretical movements. That Cathar and Waldensian preachers in southern France in the early to mid thirteenth century practised medicine has long been known by scholars. Occasionally it has attracted comment.[1] Looking at Cathars, the French Catholic Jean Guiraud invoked the magico-mystical prestige of medicine in the countryside, and talked of heretics' cunning in exploiting this in order to convert people to Catharism.[2] The Marxist Gottfried Koch saw medical practitioners as part of a literate stratum in the middling bourgeoisie which led the Cathar movement.[3] In the sixteenth and seventeenth centuries Waldensian historians preserved the memory of the medical practice of medieval Waldensian Brothers,[4] while the standard Waldensian history of the late twentieth century continued to envisage the Waldensians as holy men who were engaged simultaneously in spiritual and physical healing. This was now confined to one area and period (early thirteenth century Quercy), and one inquisition record reference to touch was generalised as the Brothers' method: the laying on of hands.[5] Two articles on medicine and heresy appeared in the same year, 1982, both of them based extensively on inquisition records, each of them concentrating on one heretical movement. One was a note on Cathar doctors by Walter Wakefield, the genial patriarch of American heresiologists and a scholar

[1] H. C. Lea, *A History of the Inquisition of the Middle Ages*, 3 vols. (New York, 1887–8), II, 32; A. Borst, *Die Katharer*, Schriften der Monumenta Germaniae Historica 12 (Stuttgart, 1953), p. 125 and n. 19; J. Duvernoy, *La religion des Cathares* (Toulouse, 1976), p. 200, and *L'histoire des Cathares* (Toulouse, 1979), p. 259; Wickersheimer, *Dictionnaire biographique*, I, 43 (Arnaud Bos, Arnaud Fabre), 44 (Arnaud Sicre), 49 (Arnaude), 228 (Guillaume Bernardi Dairos); Jacquart, *Milieu médical*, p. 125 n. 1. See nn. 2–6 and 11 below.

[2] J. Guiraud, *Histoire de l'inquisition au moyen âge*, 2 vols. (Paris, 1935–8), I, 351–3; see also II, 87–9.

[3] G. Koch, *Frauenfrage und Ketzertum im Mittelalter: Die Frauenfrage im Rahmen des Katharismus und des Waldensertums und ihre sozialen Wurzeln (12.–14. Jahrhundert)*, Forschungen zur mittelalterlichen Geschichte 9 (Berlin, 1962), p. 73.

[4] Quoted and discussed in Biller, *'Curate infirmos'*, pp. 56–7.

[5] A. Molnar, *Storia dei Valdesi 1: Dalle origine all'adesione alla Riforma* (Turin, 1974), p. 113, which is based on and generalizes J.[= Giovanni] Gonnet and A. Molnar, *Les Vaudois au moyen âge* (Turin, 1974), p. 159.

steeped in the depositions of Languedoc, and the other an article by me on Waldensian doctors.[6]

I am returning now to this theme to see what can be gained by doing what these 1982 articles did not do: systematically comparing the two movements, while also asking questions about the medical milieu and gender. In the following I look first at the sources, secondly at the civilian medical world in its relations with these heretical movements, and finally at the movements themselves. Both of the groups I discuss were divided into two strata, one of 'perfect' or full heretics, men and women who had professed according to a certain rite, and who lived the life of a religious and preached to others, the other of 'imperfect' or not-full heretics, men and women who lived in the world while receiving the preaching and sharing the faith of the 'perfect' heretics.[7] 'Perfect' and 'imperfect' were terms used by inquisitors to label strata whose relation had analogies with the relation between Catholic clergy and religious on the one hand and laity on the other. For the 'perfect' heretics of one group I use the words they used, 'Brothers' and 'Sisters', and also the term the Church used, 'Waldensians' (more strictly 'Waldenses' from *Valdenses*), while for the 'perfect' heretics of the other group I also alternate between their own words, 'Good Men', 'Good Women', and the Church's term, 'Cathars'.

My principal sources are seven manuscripts and one printed text, which from the point of view of their fruitfulness and their problems fall into three groups. In the first group there is a manuscript, surviving in a seventeenth-century copy, consisting of material relating to 742 no-longer-extant sentences delivered by the inquisitor Peter Sellan in 1241–2 on persons implicated with Waldensians and Cathars.[8] What survives in each case is a brief extract drawn from the fuller record of question and answer in an interrogation, confined to things which made a person guilty and drawn up with a view to the sentencing of the guilty person and the imposition on her or him of appropriate penance. The extract, therefore, excludes dates and names and material regarded by the inquisitor as irrelevant to such sentencing. In the same group falls a text which was printed in the seventeenth century, the *Liber sententiarum* of Bernard Gui, which contains 930 sentences on 638 heresy suspects delivered between 1307 and 1323, and also summaries of suspects' interrogations, drawn up prior to sentencing, which are comparable to Peter Sellan's extracts.[9]

6 W. L. Wakefield, 'Heretics as Physicians in the Thirteenth Century', *Speculum* 57 (1982), 328–31; Biller, '*Curate infirmos*'. See also P. Biller, 'Cathars and Material Women', in *Medieval Theology and the Natural Body*, ed. P. Biller and A. J. Minnis, YSMT 1 (York, 1997), pp. 61–107 (pp. 104–105). See n. 11 below on further study of medicine and heresy.

7 Useful definitions, based on mid-thirteenth-century discussions, can be found in Bernard Gui, *Practica inquisitionis* IV.iii.2; ed. C. Douais (Paris, 1886), p. 218.

8 Doat 21.

9 Gui, *Liber sententiarum*.

The second group is of five manuscripts, surviving in seventeenth-century copies, which contain depositions in front of inquisitors, mainly in Toulouse, between 1237 and the mid-1280s.[10] Here inquisitors have not weeded irrelevant detail, but the seventeenth-century copyists seem to have excluded depositions in which a person denied involvement with heresy and was not challenged.

The third group consists of one manuscript, referred to henceforth as 'Toulouse 609'.[11] This is a copy made in 1260 of originals from 1245–6, and it contains the depositions from this period of over 5000 people, arranged by parishes. Negative depositions have not been weeded. Thus, for example, the manuscript preserves depositions of three men from Gardouch, one described as *medicus* and two as *raseire*, whose denials of implication in heresy seem to have been accepted by the inquisitor.[12] In this way reconstruction of the ambient non-heretical medical world is sometimes enabled by Toulouse 609, whereas it is usually obstructed in the other records.

There are other distortions and problems. Fragmentary survival from earlier inquisitions skews our geography of Catharism, illuminating some tiny villages while usually leaving the great city of Toulouse in darkness. The inquisitor Peter Sellan was more consistently interested in the cost of medical services than other inquisitors: hence our varying knowledge of cost reflects first of all variations in inquisitors' inquisitiveness.

More elusive is the root of a larger contrast between the extracts from interrogations of Waldensian followers on the one hand by Peter Sellan, which are saturated with medical practice, and on the other hand by Bernard Gui, in which medical practice is absent. One Waldensian is described as a barber, and he has his basin, but no trace of his doing a barber's job enters the extracts.[13] Had the role of medical practice within the Waldensian ideal withered away? Or was Gui simply not interested? Perhaps there had been a development in inquisitors' thought, which had by now come to hold that the giving and receiving of conventional medical services was a peripheral matter, which did not touch upon faith? If this was the case, Waldensian medical practice could have continued to flourish, while leaving no traces in the records.

The inquisitorial records of Languedoc are so rich that their areas of silence can be forgotten, and the extraordinary dominance of inquisitors'

10 Doat 22–6.

11 Toulouse 609. This manuscript is the principal source of M. Pegg's *The Corruption of Angels: Heresy, Two Friar-Inquisitors, and the World of the Lauragais*, forthcoming from Princeton University Press, which also discusses medical practice. I wrote the current paper before seeing the manuscript of this book, which Mark Pegg kindly made available to me.

12 Toulouse 609, fol. 112r: Willelmus medicus; fols. 112v–113r: W. raseire; fol. 113v: Arnaldus raseire.

13 Gui, *Liber sententiarum*, p. 344: 'vocabatur Stephanus Bordeti, et erat barbitonsor'; p. 359: 'Stephanum, et videbatur esse barbitonsor quia secum portabat bassinum.'

interests in their shaping can go without sufficient challenge. Let us ponder two analogies, the first bearing upon the apparent decline of Waldensian medical practice. There is a contrast between Cathars and Waldensians eating food, as this action appears in the depositions. There is much about Cathars eating, and virtually nothing about Waldensians. Why? Because Cathar hostility to certain sorts of food attracted inquisitors' interest on the one hand, while on the other hand there was nothing out of the ordinary in Waldensians' attitudes to particular foods. Hence silence in the records: one which does not mean that the Waldensians did not eat! The second bears upon civilian non-heretical medical practice. Let us mention the glaringly obvious contrast. There is description of heretical belief and practice which is quite extraordinary in its extensiveness, colour and detail, whereas for obvious reasons Catholic lay practice and belief is only glimpsed incidentally. Yet in reality lay Catholicism was the mass-phenomenon. Although the parallel is not exact, there is something of a lesson here for the civilian non-heretical medicine which we also glimpse incidentally in the extant inquisition records. It is an obvious one: its past reality was much bigger.

Where medical cases are attested they usually have no control, because they are only testified once. Are there problems of nomenclature? *Medicus* seems clear enough, and for barbers the terms *barbitonsor* and *rasor*, which are used interchangeably in Toulouse 609, as is also the vernacular *raseire*. Fairly frequent incidental references to a barber blood-letting confirm the medical role of the numerous barbers encountered in the depositions. How do we read the female *medica* and female vernacular barber, *raseiritz*?[14] One way is suggested by John Mundy's comment on a Toulouse woman, *Geralda, medica*, who was implicated with the Cathars and sentenced in 1237: 'wives usually took their husband's names or designations'.[15] In the sentence Geralda is followed immediately by three women married to men whose jobs are given – but the women are identified as wives, not with the female noun of their husband's job: 'invenimus etiam Geraldam Medicam, Lauram uxorem quondam Raymundi Pelliparii, Aicelinam de Roaxio, et Bernardam uxorem quondam Guillelmi Vitalis Campsoris diffamatas et infectas'.[16] In inquisition records those women I have found, who were the wives of men designated *medicus* or *raseire*, were not called *medica* or *raseiritz*.[17] Dissenting reluctantly

[14] At Montesquieu there was 'Audiardis raseiriz': Toulouse 609, fol. 107r.

[15] J. H. Mundy, *The Repression of Catharism at Toulouse: The Royal Diploma of 1279*, PIMS, Studies and Texts 74 (Toronto, 1985), p. 89.

[16] Doat 21, fols. 150v–151r.

[17] For example, Roquevidal had two medics, neither of whose wives had the name *medica*: 'Raymunda Terrena, uxore [*sic*] Guillelmi Medici de Rocavidal' (Doat 25, fol. 98r); 'Bernarda Massarona, uxor quondam Gauberti Medici de Rocavidal' (Doat 25, fol. 111r). Auriac had two barbers, Faure *raseire* or *rasor* and his son *Ramundus rasor*, father and son, and Faure's wife was not designated *raseiritz*: 'Willelma, uxor den Faure raseire' (Toulouse 609, fol. 94v).

from John Mundy, who knows these records better than any living scholar, I read these terms as meaning female practitioners.

This still leaves the problem identified by Monica Green, women who engage in medical care without being given a job-title,[18] and there is in the case of the Valdenses the use of the male noun, *Valdenses*, to cover both sexes. What of *hospitalarius* and *hospitalaria*? John Mundy suggests that one should regard *hospitalarius/-a* as meaning a hospital worker, or someone running a hospital.[19] I am going to use these men and women as part of the picture – but with reserve, for a question-mark hovers over the precise functions and therefore relevance of the 'hospitals' we find in the little communities of Languedoc.

The sources usually available to the compilers of biographical registers of medieval medical practitioners skew towards themselves – that is to say, towards those practitioners who appeared in law-suits, left wills and received formally accounted sums of money. What is left is elite, urban and male. Inquisition records are also undeniably skewed, towards the question of involvement or non-involvement with heretics, but they are not skewed in *those* ways towards the upper echelons of the profession.[20] I am preparing a longer study of the medical world which they reveal, but in describing here the medical milieu in which the heretics lived and worked, I confine myself to a few salient points.[21]

Combing the inquisition records allows one to name nearly thirty communities, mainly rural, and to list in each case one or several in the categories *medici*, barbers, leper-houses, hospitals and hospital workers. At Auriac we can see two barbers, and one widow with no title who is, nevertheless, glimpsed making a potion from a herb to minister to a leg ailment. Baziège has a *rasor* and one female hospital-worker.[22] Montgaillard has a female hospital-worker.[23] Renneville has a *medicus*.[24] Laurac has three barbers, a leper-house and a hospital.[25] Montesquieu has a leper-house and a female

[18] Green, 'Documenting'.

[19] Personal communication.

[20] While the French biographical registers noticed the most prominent heretical preachers who were also medical practitioners (see n. 1 above), the majority of medics mentioned in the inquisition registers who were not preachers escaped them.

[21] Toulouse 609 has been used for this purpose, but not the Doat manuscripts, by John Mundy in his 'Village, Town and Society in the Region of Toulouse', in *Pathways to Medieval Peasants*, ed. J. A. Raftis, PIMS, Papers in Medieval Studies 2 (Toronto, 1981), pp. 141–90 (pp. 160–2 and 180–2, nn. 50–5). Mundy's account is characteristically sharp and witty, but it bypasses many references to medical practitioners.

[22] 'Bernarda, hospitaleira' (Toulouse 609, fol. 59r); 'W. Jordarn [*sic*], rasor' (fol. 60v); 'Petrus, hospitaleirs' (fol. 61v).

[23] 'Na de Petiz, hospitalaria' (Toulouse 609, fol. 47r).

[24] 'Ramundus . . .medicus' (Toulouse 609, fol. 53r).

[25] 'Raimundus Marti de Calhau, barbitonsor' (Toulouse 609, fols. 71v, 74v); 'Iohannes Bertholomeu, barbisasor / Bartholomaeus, raseire' (fols. 74v, 129v); 'Willelmus d'Armanhac, rasor' (fol. 192r); 'domus leprosorum' (fols. 74v, 75v); 'hospitale' (fol. 198r).

barber.[26] Fanjeaux has a medic who seems to have been to medical school, *Magister Arnaldus phisicus*,[27] a barber, a hospital and a hospital-worker who was a Cathar Good Man.[28]

Mas-Saintes-Puelles can be taken as an example. Walter Wakefield reckoned that in the thirteenth century this community will have been probably not much smaller than it was in 1968, when its population was 682.[29] Toulouse 609 signals four people who practised in Mas. One, Garnier, was referred to both as *medicus* and *phisicus*, and he is glimpsed in his medical practice travelling from Mas to Avignonet, to treat a sick noble-man, with whom he stayed overnight. He was an active adherent of Cathars, engaging in the rite of adoration and hearing their sermons around 1233, and his sentence of excommunication survives.[30] Another practitioner was a woman called Alissen, referred to as *medica*. She did not support the Cathars.[31] Another woman was one of the persons of highest estate in the community, the Lady (*Domina*) Richa. She did not bear any professional title, but was on at least two occasions a practitioner. Around 1235 she let blood (*flebotomavit*) for two female Cathars, and did the same for four female Cathars around 1238. Lady Richa was a passionate devotee of the Cathars, who included her son, and her imposing Hall was used for important Cathar assemblies.[32] Finally, there was a *divinatrix* called Alisson.[33] The *divinatrix* outlined her

[26] 'Domum leprosorum de Monte Esquivo' (Toulouse 609, fol. 100v); 'Audiardiz raseiritz' (fol. 107r).

[27] Toulouse 609, fol. 151v.

[28] 'Fuxus barbitonsor' or 'rasor', otherwise 'W. de Fuxo', or 'Fois' appears Toulouse 609, fols. 151v–162v, *passim*; 'hospitale' (fol. 158v); fol. 158r: 'Willelmo hospitalario heretico'.

[29] W. Wakefield, 'Heretics and Inquisitors: The Case of Le Mas-Saintes-Puelles', *Catholic Historical Review* 69 (1983), 209–26 (p. 210).

[30] Toulouse 609, fols. 5v, 6v, 13r, 23v; Wakefield, 'Heretics and Inquisitors', 222; *Documents pour servir à l'histoire de l'inquisition dans le Languedoc*, ed. C. Douais, 2 vols. (Paris, 1900), I, 74–5.

[31] Toulouse 609, fol. 11r, deposing on July 1 1245.

[32] Toulouse 609, fol. 21r: 'Narricha. [= Domina Richa]..in domo Willelmi de Canast. Bru vidit duas hereticas et ipse [*sic*] testis flebotomavit ibi dictas hereticas'; fol. 21v: 'vidit in domo Ermengarde Boerie Lunars et sociam suam, hereticas, et duas alias hereticas, et ipsa testis flebotomavit ibi dictas hereticas'. See also Wakefield, 'Heretics and Inquisitors', 216, 218, 219 and n. 39.

[33] Toulouse 609, fol. 6v, deposing July 3 1245: 'Alisson, divinatrix, dixit quod pluries mandavit infirmis quod mitterent sibi zonam vel camisiam vel peplam vel sotulares, et quando habebat ipsa dictas zonas vel camisias vel sotulares coniurabat Christi stallum [? christallum], et postea dicebat, "Faciatis tale emplastrum" vel "tale de herbis"; et hoc totum dicebat ut posset habere denarios. Item, dixit quod multociens iescit plumbum infirmis, ut haberet denarios, et nullam virtutem credebat in plumbo. Item dixit quod Na Garesada de Vilario coniuravit multociens plumbum, et dedit intelligere gentibus quod cum plumbo coniurato liberabantur ab infirmitatibus.' In his 'Village, Town and City', p. 161, Mundy takes the *divinatrix* Alisson and the *medica* Alissen to be the same person. Difference in spelling of a name happens throughout the register and is of no use in settling this matter. Sharing a name seems to be the only argument, and this

sick clients, to whom she offered divination, plasters and herbs. Alisson presented herself as a cynic. She had no belief in the efficacy of her divination, she claimed to the inquisitors, she just did it for the money. Nor did she have the slightest belief in the Cathars.

This example is bristling with interest for the 'medical market' historian. Four in a population of five hundred or so is quite dense, while the proportions are also interesting. Two of the four have titles, and one of these is a woman. One part-time practitioner is female, as also one unconventional practitioner, and the majority of practitioners are female. Although I cannot give examples of other communities where women predominate, the proportion of women involved is higher than in conventional biographical registers and tends to confirm Monica Green's hypotheses about concealment. Qualitatively, in Mas-Saintes-Puelles, non-rational medicine becomes even more marginal through its practitioner's claim not to believe in it. This is confirmed when we look elsewhere: it is difficult to find more than a tiny handful of non-rational practitioners in the registers.[34]

This is only one tiny example from our broader but very patchy picture of the ambient medical world and its relations with the Cathars. The picture is *pointilliste,* that is to say, it has the colour-spots of details but it is difficult to see the broader brush strokes of consistent patterns. The Good Men and Women lived, worked and travelled in this 'medical milieu', and their contacts were many and various.

What of affiliation? Those with the title *medicus* or *medica* range from Catholicism to the full Cathar commitment of the *medicus* William, at St Paul–Cap-de-Joux, who received the Cathar *consolamentum* before dying in 1227.[35] The *medicus* at St Martin Lalande, Jean Traver, who refused to treat a Cathar with a broken arm may have done this through fear. He may also have been a Catholic who disliked Cathars. *Both fear* and Catholicism may have been at

is weak, for the communities contained many individuals who shared the same name, and this applies to practitioners as well. Two of Gardouch's three practitioners were called William, but they were different people: one was a *medicus,* the other a *raseire.* Why should Mas not have two Alissons? *Medicus* and *medica* were respectable appellations, *divinatrix* was not. Why should one Alisson appear respectable before the inquisitor, and then on another occasion the opposite? Why should *one* person make two appearances, in both of which there was denial of implication in heresy?

[34] Two diviners were attested in Sorèze, Raimundus *de Puteo* (Doat 25, fols. 122v–123v, and Doat 26, fol. 25r–v), and Arnaldus Baussani (Doat 25, fol. 283v). It was alleged that Raimundus did auguries specially for believers in Cathars (Doat 26, fol. 25v). See the long description of a consultation in *Le registre d'inquisition de Jacques Fournier, évêque de Pamiers (1318–1325): Manuscrit no. Vat. Latin 4030 de la Bibliothèque Vaticane,* ed. J. Duvernoy, 3 vols., Bibliothèque Méridionale, s. 2, 41 (Toulouse, 1965), II, 39–41. See the conversation in *Le registre d'inquisition de Jacques Fournier,* III, 210, which marginalizes this sort of thing. Worrying about birds and auguries is dealt with sarcastically (and prejudicially): 'tale factimationes curare est vetularum'.

[35] Toulouse 609, fol. 75v.

work.[36] There seems no consistent pattern of commitment to Cathar faith at different levels of *medici*. Thus two *medici* with the title *magister* in Carcassonne were heavily implicated in Catharism.[37] But the *phisicus magister* at Fanjeaux, a Cathar centre, was not involved.[38]

Many barbers seem to have been implicated, but barbers are numerically predominant in the lists I have compiled, and some were not implicated. The two at Gardouch denied involvement, though the claim of one of them to have 'heard' that his mother was a Cathar reminds us of the often no longer separable layers of lies and truth in these testimonies. And the more detail we get, the more complex is the affiliation which we glimpse. The barber Peter Fornier at Fanjeaux came from a family of Cathar adherents, and wanted to receive the Cathar *consolamentum* as he lay dying. But the Cathars argued with him about money he still owed them, from his father's legacy, which had not been executed. The squabble ended with the dying barber using abusive words when telling the Cathars to go away.[39] Sadly, the barber's precise words are not preserved, but their tenor can readily be imagined.

A woman called Arnaude was ill and lying in bed in the hospital in Cordes, and this was the setting and occasion for another woman talking, raising theological points, and converting her to Catharism,[40] while a woman was hereticated on her deathbed in the hospital in Mirepoix.[41] Peter Brunel, *hospitalarius* of the hospital at Montgiscard, claimed to be Catholic, as did Na de Petiz, *hospitalaria* at Montgaillard, and Bernarde and Peter, *hospitaleira*

[36] Toulouse 609, fol. 35r: 'Poncius Johannis . . . ballivus . . . duxit duas hereticas ad domum isius testis. Et tunc Ar. Johannis, filius dicti testis, erat infirmus, et Johannes Traver, medicus, tenebat dictum infirmum in cura. Et una de illis hereticabus habebat bracchium fractum. Et tunc dictus Willelmus Fabri rogavit dictum medicum quod teneret eam in cura sua; quod dictus medicus facere noluit. Et tam cito dictus W. Fabri recessit cum dictis hereticabus.' This is again attested in fol. 40r. The women were captured the next day and burnt.

[37] 'Pontius de Villa Sicca medicus de Carcassonna', 'magister' (Doat 26, fols. 181v and 239r); 'magister Guillelmus de Aquis Vivis medicus de Carcassonna' (fol. 189v).

[38] See above and n. 27.

[39] Toulouse 609, fol. 159v: 'intravit domum P. Fornier, barbitonsoris, et volebat succendere quandam candelam. Et vidit ibi Ramundum Rigaut et socium suum, hereticos, et vidit ibi cum eis ipsum P. Fornier, qui iacebat infirmus infirmitate qua decessit, et Arnaldum Tornier et Stephanum Piquer et Ramundam, concubinam ipsius P. Fornier. Et tunc dictus infirmus rogabat dictos hereticos quod hereticarent ipsum. Et ipsi dicebant quod non facerent quousque redderent eis illud quod pater suus et mater sua dedit eis in morte. Et dictus P. Fornier dixit dictis hereticis quod ipse habebat xx et sex sextarios vini denarios, et daret eis de illo vino et de blac quousque tenerent se pro pagatis de patre suo et de matre sua et de ipso, et quod reciperent ipsum. Sed noluerunt facere, quia non erat consuetudo in secta hereticorum. Et tunc dictus infirmus fecit eos expelli de domo, et dixit eis multa convicia et obprobria.'

[40] Doat 25, fols. 55v–61v.

[41] Toulouse 609, fols. 191r–192r.

and *hospitaleirs* at Baziège,[42] while Naufressa, *hospitalaria* at Montauban and Veziada, *hospitalaria* at Montcuq, were followers of the Waldensians.[43] But Durantia, another *hospitalaria* at Montauban, listened to Cathar preaching on at least one occasion,[44] and William, *hospitalarius* at Fanjeaux, was a Cathar Good Man.[45] In the case of some leper-houses what we hear is the activity of the Good Men, but no more. This applies to Verdun, in whose leper-house a Cathar was seen around 1220–1,[46] and St Paul–Cap-de-Joux, where Cathars hereticated the dying leper Calvet in the leper-house around 1229. At St Paul Willelma, who looked after a leper, denied belief in the Cathars.[47] The rector of the *domus leprosorum* at Laurac was a believer in the Cathars,[48] as were the leper inmates Aumenz and William Rigaut, and Cathar Good Women were seen in the leper-house's gardens. A woman dying there received both the Church's eucharist and the Cathar *consolamentum*.[49]

From this complexity and variety we can elicit, however, a few more general themes. Let the first hang upon the example of a practitioner in Laurac, the barber Raimon Marti. One of his acts of bloodletting is mentioned. Like many barbers, Raimon heard Cathar sermons, and like a smaller number, he was asked about individual articles of Cathar belief. Raimon said that God had not made this world and bodies in it. The host is not the body of God. Dead bodies will not be resurrected. Marriage is damnable, and so on.[50] Here, then, we have an explicit individual example of an extraordinary tension between metier and belief. It will also have been present in the hearts and minds and practice of other civilian medical practitioners who adhered to Cathar belief. They believed that human bodies were the evil material creations of the evil God, and at the same time they used their skills to help to cure and repair and prolong the life of these evil material bodies. What was produced by this tension is not now precisely recoverable.

The clients of these civilian medical practitioners included the Cathars themselves, and a notable area of practice was bloodletting. Our first line of explanation must be the fact that phlebotomy was one of the principal

42 Toulouse 609, fols. 47r, 59r, 61v, 65v.

43 Doat 21, fols. 224v and 264v–265r.

44 Doat 21, fol. 265v.

45 See n. 28 above.

46 Toulouse 609, fol. 251v.

47 Toulouse 609, fol. 75v.

48 Doat 26, fol. 22r.

49 Toulouse 609, fol. 75v.

50 Toulouse 609, fol. 74v: 'Ramundus Marti de Calhau, consanguineus Bertrandi Martini Episcopi hereticorum, . . . vidit plures hereticos in pluribus locis et pluries adoravit et rasit eos et flebotomavit [perhaps 'flebotomaret'] . . . audivit hereticos dicentes quod deus non fecerat visibilia et quod baptismus aque nichil valet et quod hostia sacrata non est corpus Christi et quod non est salus in matrimonio et quod mortui non resurgent; et ipse testis credidit omnibus predictis erroribus et sunt xviii anni.'

remedies of medieval medicine. However, its profile in the sources seems unusually high. The Raimon Marti we have just mentioned often did this for the Cathar Good Men. Three occasions of bloodletting are attested for an individual Good Man, Peter Sans, in the early fourteenth century.[51] Earlier, between 1229 and 1236, W⟨illelmus⟩ *raseire* bled Cathar Good Men at least three times. In 1229 or 1231 he went to Montségur and bled the very important Good Man Guilabert de Castres and his fellow Cathars, in 1233 he went to a little cave near Mirepoix where seven or eight Cathars were living and bled three of them, and in 1236 on another visit to Montségur he bled the Cathar Bonet and 'many others' in the place.[52] We also have two instances, already mentioned, of female Cathars having blood-letting.[53] If further explanation is needed, comparison with Catholic religious may be useful. Joseph Ziegler has recently described discussions around 1300 about phlebotomy as a remedy for religious celibates who were anxious to avoid sexual desire and sin.[54] Sexual sin was an even darker matter for a Cathar, even more desperately to be avoided, and there may well be a medical echo of this in their marked recourse to blood-letting.

There are two curious points in the testimony of the barber who let blood for Cathars in Montségur. The first case he described was in an important and formal setting, the house of the Cathar bishop, Guilabert, and the bloodletting was done with Cathar religious ceremony. 'When he began to blood-let, he would say, "Bless", and the heretics [= Cathars] would reply, "May God bless you"; and he adored [= Cathar ritual of *melioramentum*] the heretics, as has been said above [= according to the previously described ritual]. And they gave him the witness [food] to eat, but he did not eat with the said heretics at the same table.' The odd mixture of perfect and imperfect tenses in the verbs may arise from the witness (a) giving evidence about *one* past visit (and therefore using the perfect tense), and (b) describing how such blood-lettings were wont to take place (and therefore using the imperfect). We are dimly glimpsing, I suggest, blood-letting having a special role and a ceremonial form among the Cathars. The other curious point is that Cathars asked W⟨illelmus⟩ *raseire* to sharpen for them on a grindstone two forceps and a razor, and they paid him a large sum, seven and a half shillings, to do

[51] Gui, *Liber sententiarum*, pp. 119, 139.

[52] Doat 22, fols. 183v–186v: 'venerunt ad domum dicti Guilaberti et ipse testis tunc minuit dictum Guilabertum et socios eius hæreticos, et quando ipse testis incipiebat minuere dicebat, "Benedicite", et hæretici respondebant, "Deus vos benedicat". Et ipse tesis adoravit dictos hæreticos sicut dictum est, et dederunt eidem testj ad comedendum set ipse testis non comedit cum dictis hæreticis ad unam mensam . . . hæretici . . . rogauerunt eum quod præpararet eis ad molam duas forprpeels [last letters unclear, but it appears later as 'forcipes'] et unum rasor [*sic*] . . . minuit dictum Bonedum hæreticum et plures alios de Monte Securo . . . apud Cauanacum iuxta Mirapiscem ubi stabant septem vel octo hæretici in quadam cauaneta et ibi ipse testis minuit tres de prædictis hæreticis.'

[53] See above and n. 32.

[54] Ziegler, *Medicine and Religion*, pp. 265–6.

this and bring the instruments to them in Montségur. Unfortunately we are not told why.

In his *Lives of the Brethren*, written 1259–60, the Dominican historian Gerard de Frachet reminisced about a medical practitioner called Peter of Aubenas.[55] Peter thought for a long time about becoming a Waldensian, only deciding to become a Dominican after being shown a dream in which jolly smiling Dominicans contrasted with grim and lugubrious Waldensians. Though this man eventually turned towards orthodox friars, his story is a reminder. Medical practitioners constituted one group from which the ranks of Cathar Good Men and Women and Waldensian Brothers and Sisters could be recruited. Medical practitioners could cross from a civilian world into the (in one sense) religious Orders which these heretical preachers constituted.

With this failed would-be Waldensian I turn to this world, the Cathar and Waldensians themselves as medical practitioners, beginning with numbers. I have counted eighty-two cases of Waldensian medical treatment, and thirty-six Cathar. In the case of Waldensian medical practitioners we only get one named individual, a Peter *de Vallibus*. It would be grossly mistaken, however, to think only of this one named Waldensian. *Valdenses* in the plural acted to cure people – *curabant* and *medicabant* – and people went for help to plural Waldensians, *ad Valdenses*. The optical illusion arises because we know about these Waldensian practitioners only through Peter Sellan's sentences, which usually omit most details, including names. Only the use of the female rather than male accusative of *quidam*, *quamdam Valdensem*, a certain Waldensian, survives to tell us that at least once a Waldensian Sister is (probably) the medical practitioner.[56]

We get to know about Cathar practitioners principally via the second and third groups of records I described above, depositions which are much more detailed, and consequently we get to know the names of more practitioners, seven or eight in all (see the end of this paragraph). There is still some optical illusion about numbers, for Cathar Good Men and Good Women travelled and worked in pairs, and it was usually the senior partner who got the attention of inquisitors and later historians; he or she was named, while the junior was often left unnamed. Arnaut Faure is one of the famous Cathar doctors, for example, and he worked with his brother Pons. If the cases are

[55] 'Frater Petrus de Albenacio, qui in Provincia fuit prior et lector . . . Cum ipse . . . in civitate Ianuensi in phisica practicaret . . .': Gerard de Frachet, *Vitae Fratrum ordinis praedicatorum* iv.13, ed. B. M. Reichert, Monumenta Ordinis Fratrum Praedicatorum Historica 1 (Louvain, 1896), pp. 183–4. Peter died around 1245. See on him J. Quetif and J. Echard, *Scriptores ordinis praedicatorum*, 2 vols. (Paris, 1719–21), I, 117–18. On Gerard, see T. Kaeppeli and E. Panella, *Scriptores Ordinis Praedicatorum medii aevi*, 4 vols. (Rome, 1970–93), 2, 35–8.

[56] P. Biller, 'The Preaching of the Waldensian Sisters', *Heresis* 30 (1999), 137–68 (p. 157); 'probably', because the phrase runs 'quamdam . . . medicum'; I suggest that gender prejudice makes 'medicum' more likely to be the error than 'quamdam'.

examined carefully it is clear that Pons was also a doctor, and one who shared his more famous brother's high reputation as a doctor.[57]

Further, the usual archival veil is cast over women. There are two cases of a Cathar Good Woman acting as medical practitioners, but neither has the title *medica* attached to her. The Good Woman Arnauda of Lamothe stayed in the house of Lady Assaut for a week or a fortnight, tending and 'medicating' Lady Assaut's ill daughter, and the use of the plural, *medicabant*, indicates that her fellow Good Woman, her unnamed *socia*, was also acting medically.[58] The designation of another Good Woman indicates that her metier was that of a barber – 'Willelma raseiridz' – but she is not seen in action: she is number eight in my 'seven or eight practitioners'.[59] Note the proportions among the named Cathars, two women and six men, and note also that one can find women among the unnamed Cathar medical practitioners. At Moissac 'P⟨eter⟩ Stephani consulted a heretic [female] many times about illness'.[60] At this level as well, the minority among medical practitioners which is formed by women continues to be proportionately larger than the minority in biographical registers.

When due allowance has been made for distortion in the sources, eighty-two cases with one named practitioner and thirty-six cases with seven or eight named practitioners may seem much of a muchness. If they give this impression, we need to think again. The Waldensians were a tiny minority among those seen as heretics in southern France in this period, only attested in some strength in Montauban and a few other communities in Quercy. The majority of all evidence about these Waldensians lies in the 280 extracts from sentences passed by Peter Sella on those involved with them in that region, and it is these that attest Waldensian medical practice. Let us put this another way. This is the largest cache of evidence about Waldensians in southern France, and over a quarter of the 280 sentences in this cache includes Waldensians practising medically. For Waldensians of this area and time, medicine was one of the main things they did.

The Cathars had an 'astonishing number' of doctors, according to previous historians of Cathars.[61] And they quote the statement by one deponent recorded in Toulouse 609, that the Cathars were *obtimi medici*, the best of

[57] See the use of plural verbs for the actions of these two: 'ut curarent', 'habebant in cura', 'medicabant', Toulouse 609, fols. 131r, 131v, 132v; see below and n. 62 on the reputation both had as 'obtimi medici'.

[58] Doat 23, fol. 72r–v: 'Dixit quod, cum Arpais filia dictæ Dominæ Assaut de Manso Daurin infirmaretur apud Mansum Dauri, Arnauda de Lamota et socia eius hæretica venerunt ibi ad domum dictae Dominæ Assaut, et ibi steterunt per octo dies, vel per quindecim dies, et serviebant predictæ Arpaii infirmæ, et medicabant dictam infirmam prædictæ hæreticæ.'

[59] Toulouse 609, fol. 95r.

[60] Doat 21, fols. 297v–298r: 'P. Stephani pro infirmitate consuluit hæreticam multotiens, et visitauit hæreticas.'

[61] The phrase is from Arno Borst (cited in n. 1 above): 'Ärtzte treffen wir unter den Katharern . . . erstaunlich oft.'

doctors. But more reflection is needed. The Cathars formed the vast majority of those seen as heretics in southern France. The Cathar (rough) equivalents of Catholic clergy, monks and nuns, the Good Men and Women, must have been getting on for a thousand in their hey-day around 1200. We know the order of magnitude from a happy event of in 1206, when around 600 of them attended a *consolamentum*, and from a tragic event in 1210, when a fraction of their number, 140, was executed at Minerve. So far I have been emphasizing the fragmentariness of southern French inquisition records, and their lacunae and distortions, but we need also to look at these records in a broader way. Compared to very slight evidence about the Waldensians, there is a vast amount about the Cathars. In the largest of the manuscripts I am using, Toulouse 609, the depositions amount to nearly half a million words. They name several hundred Cathar Good Men and Women, and detail thousands of their actions. It is an extraordinarily small fraction of this and the other inquisition records which is represented by thirty-six cases and seven named practitioners!

Descriptions of the most famous Cathar doctor, William Bernard d'Airoux, can put his description as *medicus* first, before *hereticus*: 'William the doctor the Cathar'.[62] This contains a hint of the most likely explanation of the Cathar *medici*. There was nothing special about them or their appearance among the Cathars. Medics just *happened to be* among the educated strata from which Cathar Good Men were recruited. This is why the Cathars also included notaries and jurists. What of the further special point, the Cathars as 'very good' doctors? One of the Faure brothers possessed a book of medicine, *liber medicine*,[63] both were *medici* and both Cathar Good Men, and they were recruited from a family in which there was perhaps a tradition of medical practice. The statement that Cathars were *obtimi medici*, 'the best of doctors', made by a deponent in Toulouse 609, has been misused by previous historians, including me. The deponent only meant that *these two* brothers, Arnaud and Pons Faure, were very good doctors.[64] The statement is not nor was it ever meant to be a general statement about Cathar doctors in general.

Geography is one clue to the nature of past Cathar medical practice. In the few places where such well-known practitioners as the Faure brothers or William Bernard of Airoux lived for a few years, some people went to them for medical help. What about the majority of the communities where there were Cathar Good Men and Women? Our evidence is mainly confined to the Cathar Good Men and Women themselves. See, for example, the extract from the confession of 'A⟨rnaldus⟩ medicus' of Montauban, who 'bound the leg of

62 For example, Toulouse 609, fol. 67r, and n. 72 below.

63 Toulouse 609, fol. 94r: 'fama est apud Auriacum . . . quod Ber. de Planis de Auriaco habuit quendam librum medicine ex deposito ab Arnaldo Faure heretico''

64 Toulouse 609, fol. 132v: 'P. Pis . . . vidit Arnaldum Faure et Poncium Faure, haereticos, in quodam nemore prope Caramanh; et portavit eis quendam puerum ipsius testis, qui erat infirmus, quia Poncius de Sancto Germerio dixerat ipsi testi quod obtimi medici erant.'

a certain heretic, and together with his master had twenty shillings from this . . . and gave them an ointment, and got two shillings for this . . . [he produced?] medicine for the work of the heretics . . . gave one of them a consultation about his illness'.[65] Dealing with the Cathars seems to have formed a significant part of Arnold's medical practice. It seems that when the Cathar Good Men wanted bone-setting or cure of an illness, they themselves usually consulted civilian medics. This is presumably because the vast majority of Cathars were not medical practitioners – although, as we shall see later, one aspect of their religious practice did require some medical knowledge.

When we turn to Waldensians we find a contrast. We have one sentence on a woman who visited ill Waldensians,[66] but never a sentence on a civilian practitioner medicating a Waldensian: the effect of Waldensians themselves practising. They had no need. If medicine was one of the main things Waldensians did and intrinsic, therefore, to what they were, with Cathar medical practitioners we have something very different. Their presence was an aspect of Cathar recruitment among quite well educated people, and their medical activity was not integral to the religious activity of a Cathar Good Man or Woman.[67]

I am now going to suspend comparison, and look more closely at these groups individually, beginning with the Waldensians, with whom I shall deal summarily, for a fuller account referring the reader to my earlier article on them. In the usual absence of comparative evidence about civilian medical practice in Quercy at this time, it is difficult to tell what was distinctive to the Waldensian religious, and what was simply normal medical practice. The eighty-two cases concerned physical ailments, sometimes specified (two cases of eye ailments, one concerning a hand, one a shin, and possibly one concerning a wound). Waldensian historians have taken *tetigit*, 'he touched', of one Waldensian *medicus* tending an ill person, to indicate a holy man laying on hands, but there is nothing to indicate that this was not conventional medical 'touching', of the pulse for example.[68] Everywhere there is medical vocabulary about consultation, getting a *consilium*, the Waldensians as *medici*, and about the remedies they employed, such as the application of a plaster, ointment for eyes, a poultice on a shin, and the giving of a herb for an illness.

Among those consulting the Waldensians there were those who believed in them, but also some who believed in Cathars and also Catholics. Although

[65] Doat 21, fols. 256v–257r: 'A. Medicus . . . ligavit tibiam cuiusdam hæreticis [*sic*] fractam et habuit inde viginti solidos cum magistro suo . . . Item . . . dedit eis unguentum et accepit ab hæreticis duos solidos . . . Item Medicinam ad opus hæreticorum. . . . Item dedit uni consilium de infirmitate sua.'

[66] Doat 21, fol. 281r.

[67] On the fundamental contrast between Cathar and Waldensian medical practice, see the perceptive comment by Duvernoy, *Religion des Cathares*, p. 200.

[68] See Biller, '*Curate infirmos*', pp. 62–3 n. 28.

individuals consulted on behalf of themselves, many were family affairs, one person consulting on behalf of another in the family, a man on behalf of his wife or brother, or, very frequently (sixteen cases), a woman summoning or consulting on behalf of a child or husband. One case shows consultation involving three generations in one family, almost suggesting Waldensians as family doctors. In the sentences the gender of the ill people treated runs almost but not quite even, thirty-eight females to forty-four males. I suspect that there are some occasions of male nouns being used to cover both sexes, *pro filio* for example, carelessly replacing *pro filia*, and that this is slightly skewing something which in reality was near to 50:50. Families of all estates seem to have been among the clients. In at least a third of the cases it is made explicit that one or several Waldensians visited the house in which the sick person lay to attend to her or him medically. Sometimes they stayed to prolong the medical attention (in one case for three days), and sometimes they prolonged the medical attention by frequently repeated visits (in one case over a period of two months).

There is no trace of Waldensian doctors trying to use medical consultation as an opportunity to convert people, or preach to them or involve them religiously. On one occasion we see a Waldensian staying on after someone had died, to keep vigil overnight and talk to those who were around, but we know nothing of what he said, and there is no reason to suspect anything unusual.[69] The Waldensian doctors are praised for their efforts and assiduity in trying to heal people physically, and their clients' statements of their love for them, especially where these were followers, are striking. In only one area can we be sure of a contrast. In the case of a civilian doctor of Montauban, Arnold, and his medical dealings with the Cathars, what we see immediately is cash. He charged two shillings for an ointment, and sharing with his master twenty-two shillings for binding the broken leg of a Cathar Good Man.[70] The Waldensian doctors of Montauban refused money. 'She gave them wine since they would not accept money', said one former patient, while another who gave food said that 'if they had been willing to receive she would have given them more'.

So, there is one point here in our fragmentary picture of the medical market-place in Quercy in the early thirteenth century – civilian doctors charging money, and the concurrent and presumably competitive medical practice of mendicant religious Brothers and Sisters who would only take small amounts of payment in kind. The broader point is the religious importance of poverty in this mendicant movement, as in the early Franciscans, and the proposition which I argued in 1982. Despite the fact that they had been condemned in 1184, the Waldensians still lived pretty freely on early thirteenth-century Quercy – some of those interrogated by inquisitors

[69] Doat 21, fol. 247r: 'mortuo viro suo quidam Valdensis vigilavit ibi de nocte et praedicavit astantibus'.

[70] See n. 65 above.

could claim persuasively that they did not know that Waldensians were condemned by the Church – and their medical activities make it pretty clear what they had done with Christ's injunction to the apostles in Matthew 10, 'preach and heal the sick'. They had taken the latter to be as important as preaching, and they had interpreted it plainly as physical healing. An early orthodox Waldensian hospital at Elne, projected as a fifty-bed building for the distressed, the poor, the sick, abandoned children, and poor women in childbirth had been another expression of this. I have already suggested that later silence in inquisitorial records may be rooted in later inquisitorial lack of interest. This possibility does not exclude others. There may well have been some real dwindling of both open preaching and physical healing of the sick as a consequence of the curtailing of activities made necessary by persecution and the Waldensian Brothers and Sisters having to go underground and develop a secret organization.

I turn now to the Cathar medical practitioners. Ailments, medical consultations and medication are described in broadly similar terms. 'Bertrand Audeberti saw a heretic and consulted him about the health of his body, and on his advice he cauterised himself.'[71] 'Guillelmus Bernardus d'Airoux, *medicus*, who was a heretic . . . tended the said ill man and medicated him, and made for him a plaster and other necessary things . . . and when he had stayed for a few days he left.'[72] Unlike the Waldensians Cathar doctors on occasion took money, although most of the time we do not hear about this. Like the Waldensians they did sometimes stay in a house, attempting a cure for a night or two or a week, but unlike the Waldensians there is no special comment from deponents on their assiduity. Unlike the evidence about the Waldensians, the evidence about Cathars occasionally shows possible friction, the taking over of a case from a civilian doctor and an argument,[73] or making medical aid depend on conversion.[74]

If the conscientiousness of Waldensian medical care and their refusal to take money provoked comment from deponents, this is what we would expect, since curing was an expression of their form of religious life. And if there was no such generalizing comment from deponents about Cathar

[71] Doat 21, fol. 206r: 'Bertrandus Audeberti vidit hæreticum et consuluit eum de salute corporis, et cauteriauit se de eius consilio.'

[72] Doat 23, fol. 199v: 'Guillelmus Bernardus Dairos medicus qui erat hæreticus . . . serviebat dicto infirmo et medicabat ipsum, et faciebat ei *emplaustz* et alia necessaria . . . et cum stetissent per aliquot dies recesserunt inde.'

[73] Toulouse 609, fol. 245r–v.

[74] Toulouse 609, fol. 246r: 'Guillermus Deumer . . . cum ipse esset vulneratus gravi vulnere et omnes medici relinquerent ipsum, dictum fuit ei quod, apud Baucium erat quidam medicus qui curaret ipsum, si posset ipsum habere. Et tunc ipse testis fecit se portari apud Baucium Et invenit ibi illum medicum. Et erat hereticus, sed non recolit de nomine eius. Et dictus hereticus tenuit ipsum testem in cura sua per mensem. Et pluries rogavit ipsum testem quod faceret se hereticum; quod ipse testis facere noluit. Et propter hic dictus hereticus noluit ipsum testem habere in cura sua, et dimisit eum.'

doctors, then this is also what we should expect, since with the Cathars medical practice was occasional and an accident of recruitment. There is still a medico-religious theme in Cathar medical practice, but it is a very different one. It is the theme already adumbrated with Raimon Marti of Laurac, namely the possible areas of tension between the fundamental beliefs of a Cathar Good Man or Woman and their efforts with sick human bodies.

Let me introduce this topic with examples of Cathar attitudes to material bodies, from birth to death. First, believing in the evil nature of procreation, Cathar Good Women as well as Men preached that a pregnant woman had the devil in her belly and if she died in this condition she was damned.[75]

Secondly, touching people. Cathars went to great lengths to avoid touching the bodies of the other sex; the examples which survive are all gender-skewed, indicating the danger for male Cathars of touching female flesh.[76]

Thirdly, dying bodies. After receiving the Cathar *consolamentum* a very ill Cathar believer would be assured of salvation when he or she was dead – that is to say, when his or her spirit escaped the evil envelope of its body and fled off to the heaven of the Good God where there would be, of course, no resurrection of bodies. Dying soon would help, in that one would avoid any chance of a defilement which would ruin this happy outcome, and this explains why one male Cathar believer got terribly angry with his wife for secretly breast-feeding their very ill baby after it had received the *consolamentum*, for this milk was among the prohibited defiling foods.[77]

Fourthly, dead bodies. One deponent who was given the dead bodies of Cathar Good Men threw some into a pit, the others into the river Tarn – thereby showing an utter lack of special regard for dead bodies which was strictly in accord with Cathar theology.

Now this last example provides a warning about what we may hope to find about Cathar medical practice and human bodies. Things were not so simple, not always so logically Catharist. Some dead bodies of Cathars were thrown away, but we also find different treatment, in an ascending scale. One level is a hole in the ground being dug in a forest for a dead Cathar body; one level above this is dead Cathar bodies being interred in places referred to as 'cemeteries', and many levels above this is the ashes and bones of Cathars who had been burnt to death being venerated by Cathar followers as relics. One hypothesis is to regard these as first, following Cathar logic, then Cathar logic slightly modified, then further modified by the pressure of convention and tradition, and then finally thoroughly taken over and imbued with traditional Catholicism.[78] Whether this grid works or not, these examples remind us that the Cathar Good Women and Men lived in a real world and

[75] Biller, 'Cathars and Material Women', pp. 99–101.
[76] Biller, 'Cathars and Material Women', pp. 103–5.
[77] Biller, 'Cathars and Material Women', p. 102.
[78] See my 'Cathar Peace-Making', forthcoming in *Christianity and Community in the West: Essays for John Bossy*, ed. S. Ditchfield, St Andrew's Studies in Reformation History.

(in a non-pejorative sense) compromised with it and were coloured by it. We shall rarely encounter absolutely clear examples of tension between Cathar theology and human medicine, and we are usually left with no more than question-marks.

I begin with childbirth. We have one clear example of Catholic midwives reacting with horror when assisting a woman in childbirth, whose Cathar belief they deduced from her cries, but we have no direct examples of the thoughts and actions of the many women of Cathar belief who acted as midwives while believing in the evil nature of what was taking place.[79] With medical care of the living who suffered from ailments from which they could recover, we have no sign that medical care, once undertaken, was not followed through as effectively as possible. There are slight signs of oddity, however, when Cathar doctors were considering undertaking care. Here we have a female deponent, Geraldine, wife of William Faure. She had a medical problem on her face, she said, and she went to see the Good Man William Bernard of Airoux at Saix. But the Good Man, she said, was unwilling to undertake her care; she was refused.[80] This example brings to mind one peculiar pattern among clients. Bearing in mind that Waldensian clients came fairly near to an even sex-ratio, we find, when we turn to Cathar clients, an odd sex-ratio. The cases involved treated thirty-one males and only five females, and this should be coupled with the fact that William Bernard d'Airoux refused treatment to one or two women.[81] Rather hesitantly I suggest that because of the physical touch necessarily entailed in much conventional medical treatment, the doctors who were also Cathar Good Men may have been reluctant to provide medical treatment for women. Seventy or so years after William Bernard a regular penance for accidental brushing contact with a female body seems to have been general among Cathar Good Men.

Finally, dying. One of the most frequent phrases in depositions is 'ill with the illness from which he or she died'. Repeated hundreds of times in the depositions, it introduces a Cathar's visit to administer the *consolamentum*. A Cathar Good Man called Raimond Sans, not otherwise known as a doctor,

[79] See Biller, 'Cathars and Material Women', pp. 100–1 and n. 162.

[80] Toulouse 609, fol. 57v: 'Geralda uxor Willelmi Fabri . . . dixit quod ⟨cum⟩ haberet quandam infirmitate in facie ivit ad Sac ad W. Ber. D'Airos hereticum – sed nesciebat ipsum esse hereticum. Et dictus hereticus noluit recipere ipsam testem in cura sua.'

[81] The second case: 'Domina Geralda . . . dixit quod cum ipsa testis patetetur quadam vice tersanam, misit Begonem de Rocovilla, militem sororium ipsius testis, ad W. B. D'Airos hereticum medicum, et ipse testis [*sic*] adduxit eum ipsi testi ad Montem Guiscardum, et fuit dictus hereticus in domo ipsius testis et viri sui Estolt per unam diem et noctem; et quia erat circa mensem Augusti noluit ipsam testem recipere in custodia neque facere ei aliquam curam'; Toulouse 609, fol. 66r–v. See Toulouse 609, fol. 67r, for the testimony of the knight Sichard de Gavaret, who saw the two Cathars in Estolt's house and claimed they were medicating her. This is either discrepant or refers to another occasion. See Biller, 'Cathars and Material Women', pp. 104–5.

takes the pulse of a very ill man, to see if he is dying. He pronounces that the man is going to live, and goes away.[82] Although Cathar Good Men were usually not doctors, they did need a narrowly focussed range of expertise here, namely assessing whether a person was going to survive or was going to die, and gauging the approach of death. Further, some evidence suggests that more positive steps could be taken to shorten life after the reception of the *consolamentum*.[83] One witness questioned by the famous Jacques Fournier said that he had heard that if after reception of the *consolamentum* Cathars were bled until all the blood had left their bodies, they were doing a good deed, and thus could die quickly and quickly come to the glory of the Father.[84] One example survives in a very late Cathar adherent, a woman called Cerdana or Esclarmonde, who perhaps should be counted as a medical practitioner. In 1309 she helped a Cathar Good Woman after several failed attempts to kill herself or be killed, supplying her with a potion of wild cucumber juice which did the job.[85]

Scholars used to argue about this dramatic and terrible material, Catholic polemicists generalizing it and Cathar apologists seeing it as a myth, and it is now generally accepted that it was characteristic only of (a) a restricted element in (b) very late Catharism. No attention has been paid to investigating the more moderate and restrained, but still distinct attitude, of which this was an out-growth. During the illness from which her son-in-law died, Alazayt visited him, as did also an unknown man, and Alazayt was instructed to say 'if asked who this man was, who had been there, to reply that he was a medic'. This confirmed Alazayt in her suspicion that he was a Cathar, 'because this man had done nothing to the ill man of the sort that a doctor would do, and she believes that he had come to the ill man to do what the Cathars do to ill people'.[86] What do we find when we go back to the 1220s and 1230s? Where Cathar doctors came to the bedsides of the dying, there is no hint of any attempt to cure. We see the well-known Cathar doctor William Bernard of Airoux often hereticating the dying, but never attempting to medicate them. In Soreze, after visiting one dying man, he said that 'it had gone well with him', meaning that the man had received the *consolamentum*,

[82] 'Bertrandus Quiders . . . cum ipse testis infirmaretur graviter in domo sua apud Avinionem . . . Ramundus Sans, hereticis, tetigit pulsum ipsi testi et dixit quod valeret vivus': Toulouse 609, fols. 139v–140r.

[83] For a brief sane discussion of the *endura*, see A. Murray, *Suicide in the Middle Ages*, vol. 1, *The Violent against Themselves* (Oxford, 1999), pp. 189–91.

[84] *Le Registre d'inquisition de Jacques Fournier*, III, 247–8.

[85] Gui, *Liber sententiarum*, pp. 70, 76, 94. See a contemporary herbal, *The Herbal of Rufinus*, ed. L. Thorndike (Chicago, 1945), p. 117, where the fatal power of wild cucumbers is illustrated by the account of the execution in Bologna of a *vetula* who had administered it.

[86] Gui, *Liber sententiarum*, p. 114: 'si aliquis peteret ab eo quis erat ille homo qui fuerat ibi, responderet quod medicus erat, . . . credidit quod ille homo esset hereticus . . . quia ille homo nihil fecerat infirmo quod pertineret ad medicum . . . quod ille homo veniret ad infirmum ad faciendum illud quod heretici faciunt infirmis'.

while the dead man's sister, Ermessende, hit her cheeks to stop herself crying until the heretics had got a long distance away.[87] Nothing *proves* my point, but there is a chill note to this story, which accords well with what common sense would suggest follows from the extraordinary contrast between Cathar and Catholic Christian attitudes to the body. This is that *when* the logic of Catharism was followed, there was a distinct curtailment of the medical aspiration to cure and to preserve life.

[87] Doat 25, fols. 253v–254r: 'quæsivit de statu dicti infirmi, et respondit ei dictus Guillelmus. B. hæreticus quod bene contigerat ei, et bene fecerat factum suum, et per hoc ipse testis perpendit et intellexit quod hæreticaverunt eum. Deinde dictus Adam Barta duxit eos ad domum suam, prout dixit, et dictus Raymundus Petri et ipse testis accesserunt ad domum prædicti infirmi ubi, cum iam obisset, Ermessendis soror eius percussebat genas suas cum palmis, non audens clamare donec hæretici supradicti longe se absentassent.'

The *Incubus* in Scholastic Debate: Medicine, Theology and Popular Belief[1]

Maaike van der Lugt

Medieval physicians not infrequently offered naturalistic explanations for mysterious and supposedly supernatural events. Certainly – and it is important to stress this – they were far from denying the possibility of divine or demonic intervention in earthly affairs. From the second half of the thirteenth century on, medical practitioners even routinely collaborated in canonization processes to authenticate miracles.[2] But in their role as expert witnesses, medieval physicians were guided by the assumption that supernatural causation should only be posited after a medical explanation had been ruled out.[3]

[1] When writing this article I benefited from a grant from the Niels Stensen Stichting at Amsterdam. I wish to express my gratitude to the foundation for its support. The article develops a chapter of my doctoral dissertation 'Le ver, le démon et la vierge: Les théories de la génération extraordinaire (v. 1000 – v. 1350). Une étude sur les rapports entre théologie, philosophie naturelle et médecine' (Universiteit Utrecht/ EHESS, 1998) (publication forthcoming). To avoid misunderstanding I should make it clear that the first version of this chapter was researched and written months before, and completely independently of an article in Dutch on the same subject: Eerden (van der), 'Incubus', esp. pp. 117–26. Van der Eerden does not study the *incubus* theory in scholastic medicine but concentrates on its earlier development. On the *incubus* in the ancient world see also W. H. Roscher, '*Ephialtes*, eine pathologisch-mythologische Abhandlung über die Alpträume und Alpdämonen des klassischen Altertums', *Abhandlungen der philologisch-historischen Classe der königlich Sächsischen Gesellschaft der Wissenschaften* 20–2 (Leipzig, 1903). Roscher collects a lot of references to ancient mythology and medicine, but he presents his subject in a very muddled way; see also C. Lecouteux, 'Mara – Ephialtes – Incubus. Le cauchemar chez les peuples germaniques', *Études germaniques* 42 (1987), 1–24, especially for the terminology of the nightmare in vernacular tongues. Unfortunately, Lecouteux's failure to distinguish between the different *incubus* traditions renders his analysis rather unreliable. The same is true for an article by M. Blöcker-Walter, 'Imago fidelis-Incubus. Die Umdeutung eines Traumbildes im Mittelalter', in *Variorum munera florum: Latinität als prägende Kraft mittelalterliche Kultur. Festschrift für Hans F. Haefele zu seinem sechzigsten Geburtstag*, ed. A. Reinle, L. Schmugge and P. Stotz (Sigmaringen, 1985), pp. 205–10; see also E. Jones, *On the Nightmare* (London, 1949) for a psychoanalytical interpretation of the *incubus*.

[2] See Ziegler, 'Practitioners and Saints'.

[3] For instance, to distinguish between apoplectic seizures and miraculous resurrection, Pietro d'Abano, a contemporary of Bernard of Gordon, applies the rule that the patient must have lain dead for at least three days: Pietro d'Abano, *Conciliator*, diff. 182, propter 3, fol. 239vab.

They were inclined to limit the role of supernatural forces as far as possible, a tendency which could easily bring them into conflict with church authorities and more generally with all who were prepared to allow the supernatural much larger scope.[4]

In his *Lilium medicinae*, written around 1305, Bernard of Gordon, a famous professor of medicine at the university of Montpellier, offered a typical and interesting example of medieval medicine's naturalistic approach. In the part on diseases of the head, Bernard included a curious disease called *incubus*, which he described as follows:

> *incubus* is an apparition (*phantasma*) that presses on the body and weighs it down during sleep, disturbing both movement and speech. *Incubus* is the name of a demon and that is why some people think that when the *incubus* is directly above the human body – especially when a person lies on his back – he presses the body down by his corrupting influence, to such an extent that the patient thinks he is going to suffocate. When this happens to babies, they often do suffocate, because they cannot bear so great a corruption. Such is the opinion of the theologians. But the common people (*vulgares*) believe that the *incubus* is an old woman (*vetula*) who tramples on and presses down the body. This is nonsense. The physicians (*medici*) have a better opinion.[5]

Bernard of Gordon then mentions the medical aetiology of *incubus*. According to physicians, the suffocating feeling, which moved up from the feet to the breast, and either stopped the patient from moving and crying out, or made him moan and scream in fear, could arise from both internal and external causes. As external causes, Bernard of Gordon mentioned a sudden cooling off of the head, or a full stomach; as internal causes, corrupted humours blocking the circulation of spirits in the vital organs – the heart and the brain.[6] He prescribed different cures for each cause, and he especially

[4] Even when physicians accepted a miracle, they could be misunderstood. Despite his explicit affirmation of the miraculous nature of the resurrection of Lazarus, Pietro d'Abano was accused after his death of having denied this miracle. Cf. Marangon, *Pensiero ereticale*, pp. 87–8.

[5] 'Incubus est phantasma in somnis, corpus comprimens et aggrauans, motum et loquelam perturbans. Incubus nomen est daemonis et ideo volunt aliqui quod quando ille incubus directe est supra corpus humanum et potissime quando iacet dormitque resupinus ratione corruptae influentiae, aggrauat corpus, ita quod videtur patienti quod suffocetur. Et si adueniat pueris lactantibus, frequenter suffocantur, quia tantam corruptionem sustinere non possunt, et est opinio theologorum. Vulgares autem dicunt quod est aliqua vetula calcans et comprimens corpora, et hoc nihil est. Medici autem melius opinantur': Bernard of Gordon, *Lilium medicinae* ii.24 (Lyons, 1550), pp. 220–1.

[6] 'Incubus autem prouenit ex causa intrinseca et ex causa extrinseca. Si extrinseca, vt quando dormit, venit subito frigiditas, caput comprimens et oppilans, aut quando aliquis dormit supra nimiam repletionem cibi et potus. Causa intrinseca est vapor corruptus, ab humoribus resolutus, oppilans et grauans cerebrum et cor, ita quod spiritus non possint plenarie se diffundere ad totum corpus et ita quia primo deficiunt in extremis, ideo videtur patienti quod illud phantasma incipiat ascendere

recommended a friend sitting by the patient's bedside and waking him up whenever an *incubus* crisis occured. The friend then had to rub the patient's feet, hands and head, spray water in his face, make him vomit and administer different kind of drugs.[7] We see that Bernard of Gordon distinguished three interpretations of the term *incubus,* which corresponded to three different explanations of the same experience: a suffocating sensation during sleep accompanied by the impression that something or someone presses heavily upon one. Both theologians and the common people considered that these symptoms, which could be so severe in babies as to cause cot death, were induced by a being attacking the dreamer. However, while theologians held that this assailant was a demon called an *incubus,* popular opinion had it that the *incubus* was an old woman. For their part medieval physicians put forward a strikingly different interpretation of nocturnal suffocation. They attributed this affliction – which modern medicine identifies as a respiratory anomaly – to purely natural causes, and they suggested that the nocturnal attacker was nothing but a bad dream, a figment of the imagination. Bernard of Gordon adhered to this medical point of view, and rejected the theological and especially the popular explanations of *incubus.*[8]

However straightforward Bernard of Gordon's discussion of the *incubus* may at first seem, the closer we look at the beliefs he so confidently refuted the more puzzling his account becomes. Anyone familiar with medieval and early modern demonology is bound to have heard of demons called *incubi.* These *incubi* were known for sleeping with women, especially witches. The cold sperm of the devil described in witchcraft trials has almost become a commonplace. However, these *incubi* only partly resembled the demons described by Bernard of Gordon, whose activity, although harmful, was not sexual at all. They choked adults and caused cot deaths. Consequently, the medical opinion about the *incubus* as described by Bernard of Gordon cannot simply be understood as an attempt to rationalize and explain away the well-known medieval belief in the existence of demons who slept with women. And the distinction made by Bernard of Gordon, between a theological and a popular opinion about the identity of the *incubus,* also needs further attention.

a pedibus et deinde paulatine occupat totum corpus, secundum quod vapores plus aggrauant et ideo loquitur mugiendo, petens auxilium si posset loqui, et est totus perterritus, propter farcinae aggrauationem, id est, fumum corruptum oppilantem et obnubilantem spiritum, qui fumus aliquando prouenit ex sanguine, aliquando a cholera grossa, aliquando a phlegmate, aliquando a melancholia.'

7 'In primis iste cui consueuit euenire, habeat socium dilectum, qui statim cum audit ipsum sic vociferantem, et quasi lamentantem, quod excitet eum et quod fricet pedes et manus et caput multum fortiter et aspergat faciem eius cum aqua ros et quod procuret vomitum et quod det sibi dianthos cum musco aut diambram [. . .]'

8 Bernard of Gordon's rationalization of *incubus* is not an isolated case in his work. In another chapter of the *Lilium* (ii.15, p. 192), he does not hesitate to interpret supposed cases of religious ecstasy as a disease of the head called *congelatio,* which immobilizes the patient and renders him insensitive to external stimuli.

In order fully to understand the significance of Bernard's account of the *incubus,* we need to trace the history of the medical tradition and the authorities upon which he built. For, as Bernard himself acknowledged, he was far from being the first to envisage the *incubus* as a dream and sleeping disorder. Moreover, as may already be clear, terminology is not always a useful guide in discussions about the *incubus.* The same word could vary in meaning according to author and context, while the same concept could be referred to by different terms. We must start with a more thorough analysis of the cluster of concepts and traditions associated with the term *incubus.* We have already seen that the most familiar meaning of the word was that of a sexual demon. This went back to Augustine's *City of God* and to Isidore of Seville's *Etymologies.* According to Augustine (354–430), *incubus* was the popular name (*vulgo vocant*) for the sylvan figures and fauns of pagan Greco-Roman mythology: half-gods who had a reputation for seducing and harassing women. Augustine further likened *incubi* to *Dusii,* who were mysterious divinities of the indigenous people of Gaul and for whom we have no other independent source. In Augustine's Christian eyes, of course, *incubi* were demons, not gods. His discussion of sexual demons was part of a debate on the exegesis of an obscure passage in Genesis about the origin of the giants present on earth before the Flood (Genesis 6. 1–4). Augustine dismissed a Jewish interpretation, accepted by some Christian fathers, according to which these giants sprang from the union between fallen angels and women. Nevertheless, because of the weight of witnesses' accounts of the intervention of such demons he did not reject outright the possibility of intercourse between demons and women.[9]

Isidore of Seville (*c.* 560–636) built on Augustine's definition of the sexual *incubus,* adding several elements from other pagan and Christian sources. In his hands the *incubus* acquired the company not only of sylvan figures and fauns but also of Pan, another mythological divinity with erotic connotations. In addition there were the more mysterious *inui* who were so called 'from their having sex indiscriminately with animals' (*ab ineundo passim cum animalibus*). For their definition and association with fauns, Pan and *incubi,* Isidore relied on Servius Grammaticus's commentary on Virgil.[10] Isidore assimilated all these demonized pagan gods to the biblical *pilosi* ('hairy ones')

[9] 'Et quoniam creberrima fama est multique se expertos vel ab eis, qui experti essent, de quorum fide dubitandum non est, audisse confirmant, Silvanos et Faunos, quos vulgo incubos vocant, inprobos saepe exstitisse mulieribus, et earum appetisse ac peregisse concubitum; et quosdam daemones, quos Dusios Galli nuncupant, adsidue hanc immunditiam et temptare et efficere, plures talesque adseverant, ut hoc negare, impudentiae videatur.' Augustine, *De civitate Dei* XV.xxiii.1; IV, 142. See also his *Quaestionum in heptateuchum libri VII* i.3, ed. I. Fraipont, CCSL 33 (Turnhout, 1958), pp. 2–3.

[10] *Servii Grammatici qui feruntur in Vergilii carmina commentarii,* vi.775, ed. G. Thilo and H. Hagen, 3 vols. (Leipzig, 1881–1902), II, 109. Servius uses the term *incubo* instead of *incubus;* the two terms are used interchangeably by Isidore.

mentioned in Isaiah's prophecy about the destruction of Babylon (13. 21–2: 'but wild beasts shall rest there [. . .] and the hairy ones[11] shall dance'), taking his cue from a commentary on Isaiah by Jerome to which I shall return shortly. Isidore also introduced a very influential etymology of the term *incubus.* According to him, this word came from the verb *incumbendo,* a term he in turn glossed by *stuprando,* to rape.[12]

From the twelfth century on, scholastic theologians took up again the patristic discussion about *incubi* and their capacity for sexual intercourse and procreation. Encouragement came not only from a general preoccupation with theological problems that involved speculation about the functioning of the body and its links to the soul,[13] but also from new narratives about demonic procreation, such as the legend of Merlin, son of the devil. The theological debate developed around two central problems: the question of the human nature of the devil's offspring, and the question of the ability of demons who lacked a body of flesh and blood to have sex and procreate. Exploring the intricacies of these discussions would take too long here,[14] and for the present purpose we need only to note that by the 1250s a compromise had been reached. According to this, demons could sleep with women by temporarily taking on an artificial body made from air or a human corpse. They were unable to procreate, but they could impregnate women with the sperm of men, with whom they had first slept in the shape of a woman. Thanks to the use of human seed, the children resulting from these diabolical unions were purely human. The theory of artificial insemination with stolen sperm was accepted by all later medieval theologians and it gradually found its way into encyclopaedias, manuals of penance and influential tracts on demonology and witchcraft such as Johannes Nider's *Formicarius* and the *Malleus Maleficarum.*

We have seen that neither Augustine nor Isidore explicitly linked the intervention of sexual demons to the night or to sleep, that Isidore presented intercourse between demons and women as involuntary on the part of the women, and that this was much less clear in Augustine. In medieval narratives about sexual intercourse between demons and women, we find

[11] Modern English translations of the Bible render 'satyr' here; however, the Latin vulgate version by Jerome that was used by medieval authors reads *pilosus.*

[12] 'Pilosi, qui Graece Panitae, Latine incubi appellantur, sive Inui ab ineundo passim cum animalibus. Unde et incubi dicuntur ab incumbendo, hoc est stuprando. Saepe enim inprobi existunt etiam mulieribus, et earum peragunt concubitum: quos daemones Galli Dusios vocant, quia adsidue hanc peragunt inmunditiam. Quem autem vulgo incubonem vocant, hunc Romani faunum ficarium dicunt': Isidore of Seville, *Etymologiae* viii.11, ed. W. M. Lindsay, 2 vols. (Oxford, 1911), I, 103.

[13] Cf. C. Walker-Bynum, 'The Female Body and Religious Practice in the Later Middle Ages', in eadem, *Fragmentation and Redemption: Essays on Gender and the Human Body in Medieval Religion* (New York, 1991), pp. 181–238 (p. 226).

[14] For a detailed study of these debates see van der Lugt, 'Le ver, le démon et la vierge' and 'La personne manquée: Démons, cadavres et *opera vitae* du début du douzième siècle à saint Thomas', *Micrologus* 7 (1999), 205–21.

two possibilities. The *incubus* either seduces a woman when she is awake, or he rapes her when she is asleep. Thus two twelfth-century versions of the story of Merlin – the original Latin text of Geoffrey of Monmouth and a French adaptation by Robert of Boron – adopt the first and the second alternative respectively.[15] In the thirteenth century, Caesar of Heisterbach and Thomas of Cantimpré report examples of both, taking their information from written accounts, hearsay or confession.[16] By the fifteenth century the idea of women voluntarily engaging in or even seeking intercourse with the devil had become predominant, as part of a complex of misogynist ideas associated with witchcraft.

There are of course evident similarities between the belief in sexual *incubi* and the beliefs described by Bernard of Gordon. But they are by no means identical. On the one hand we have seen that women who had intercourse with demons were not always described as passive sleeping victims of sexual harassment. On the other hand, the important fact remains that there was no reference to anything sexual in Bernard of Gordon's discussion of the *incubus*, while certain elements in his description, like the killing of children, were absent from the accounts of sexual demons. Bernard of Gordon did not present the *incubus* as a gendered disease. But sexual *incubi* in the large majority of cases had it in for women, even though medieval theologians recognized the existence of demons who assumed the shape of a woman to sleep with or seduce men. However, these *succubi*, like the fairies of medieval folklore with whom they were identified by the theologians, were always portrayed as beautiful young girls, not as malicious old women. If we are to understand Bernard of Gordon's discussion of the *incubus*, we have to look further.

Apart from sexual demons there was another although far rarer meaning for the term *incubus* in medieval literature. Ultimately this alternative interpretation goes back to the *Vita sancti Pauli* of St Jerome and to his commentary on Isaiah to which I have already alluded. In the *Vita sancti Pauli*, the term *incubus* was used to refer to one of St Paul's companions in the desert, a hybrid – half man, half goat – who claimed to be a mortal being and who was hoping for salvation.[17] While Jerome associated the *incubus* with satyrs and fauns, he did not attribute to the *incubus* the traditional character-

[15] Geoffrey of Monmouth, *Historia regum Britanniae* 107, ed. N. Wright (Cambridge, 1985), p. 72; analysis of pseudo-Robert of Boron's *Merlin* in F. Dubost, *Aspects fantastiques de la littérature narrative médiévale (XIIème–XIIIème siècle): L'Autre, l'Ailleurs, l'Autrefois* (Geneva, 1991), pp. 711–30.

[16] Caesar, *Dialogus* iii.6–8 (I, 116–21); Thomas of Cantimpré, *Bonum universale de apibus* II.lvii.13–5 (Douai, 1605), pp. 547–8. Thomas of Cantimpré opens his series of examples with the remark that 'Incubos daemones oppressise feminas quasdam, alias Venereis confabulationibus ad concubitum illexisse, in confessione pluries audivimus.'

[17] 'Mortalis ego sum et unus ex accolis eremi quos vario delusa errore Gentilitas Faunos Satyrosque et Incubos vocans colit': Jerome, *Vita sancti Pauli primi eremitae* 8, in *PL* 23, 23.

istics of these mythological creatures. The desert monster had no indecent intentions when approaching Paul; Paul's *incubus* was mortal, whereas Christians tended to see satyrs and other pagan gods as demons. Jerome mentioned *incubi* again in his commentary on the prophecy of the destruction of Babylon in the book of Isaiah, where he put forward as a gloss for *pilosus*, *incubo;* not *incubus* – the two terms were used interchangeably, although medieval authors preferred the latter. The precise nature of the *incubus* was more ambiguous here than in the *Vita sancti Pauli*, because Jerome on the one hand associated *incubi* with wild men of the woods (*homines silvestres*) but on the other hand cited the idea that they were demons.[18]

Whatever his nature – monster, wild man or demon – Jerome's *incubus* was clearly no better a match for the theological and popular beliefs described by Bernard of Gordon than the sexual *incubus*. Bernard is not our only medieval source for a belief in demons or other evil beings who attacked people in their sleep and tried to suffocate them, though in non-medical contexts these non-sexual stranglers were rarely referred to by the term *incubus*. We encounter them under a wide variety of names of different origin. The most common of these terms were *larva* and *lemur*, words from Classical Latin which seem to suggest that the nightly oppressors were ghosts; *lamia*, *masca* and *stria*, words that refer to witchcraft; a group of terms from the German vernacular root *Mahr* (giving rise to both 'nightmare' and *cauchemar*). And last but not least was *ephialtes*, from a Greek verb meaning 'to jump onto someone or something' and which was thus a close relative of the Latin *incubus*, from the verb 'to lie on something or someone'.[19]

The origin of the belief in nocturnal stranglers is difficult to trace. We find it sporadically in Antiquity, mainly in medical refutations of the belief. In medieval sources it was quite common, especially from the twelfth century on. There is a famous example in Guibert de Nogent's *Autobiography*, where the author tells us about a demon who tried to suffocate Guibert's mother at night during his father's captivity. He lay down on top of her, *incubuit:* Guibert did not use a noun to describe the aggressor. The demon was finally driven away by the intervention of the Virgin Mary.[20] For his part, Peter the Venerable recounted in his *De miraculis* the terrifying experience of a novice, who claimed to have been nearly suffocated at night by a demon in the shape of an enormous bear.[21] At the beginning of the thirteenth century Gervase of Tilbury mentioned non-erotic nocturnal stranglers in a chapter of his *Otia imperialia* entitled 'of *lamiae* and nocturnal *larvae*'. The activities of these

[18] 'pilosi [. . .] vel incubones, vel satyros, vel silvestres quosdam homines, quos nonulli fatuos ficarios vocant, aut daemonum genera intelligunt': Jerome, *Commentariorum in Esaiam libri I–IX* 5, ad 13. 21–2, ed. M. Adriaen, CCSL 73 (Turnhout, 1963), pp. 165–6. Isidore of Seville uses the term *fauni* instead of *fatui*, cf. n. 12 above.

[19] For these terms see Lecouteux, 'Mara – Ephialtes – Incubus'.

[20] Guibert de Nogent, *De vita sua* i.13, ed. E.-R. Labande (Paris, 1981), p. 90.

[21] Peter the Venerable, *De miraculis* i.18, ed. D. Bouthillier, CCCM 83 (Turnhout, 1988), pp. 55–6.

creatures were multifarious, explained Gervase. Not only did they harass dreamers but they also ate food in the house, lit lamps, tampered with human bones, drank human blood and snatched babies from their cots. After recounting several stories about the *lamiae*'s actions, Gervase cited at the end of the same chapter the passage from Augustine about sexual demons. Gervase used the words *larvae* and *lamiae* as umbrella terms for all sorts of evil creatures of the night, but throughout his discussion he left their nature – demons or evil men and women – ambiguous.[22]

While a modern reader might be tempted to interpret the experience of Guibert de Nogent's mother as a rape fantasy and as a sign of sexual frustration, it is medieval intellectual categories whose understanding is our main concern and we must remember that Guibert does not refer to anything explicitly sexual. Moreover, even though some medieval authors, like Gervase of Tilbury, assimilated sexual and non-sexual nocturnal demons, others explicitly distinguished between them. In the 1230s, William of Auvergne, bishop of Paris and well known for his interest in popular traditions, reserved the term *ephialtes* for the non-sexual demon, while using *incubus* for the sexual one, and he carefully kept his discussions of them separate. Like Gervase of Tilbury, William of Auvergne also mentioned *lamiae*, but he used this term to refer specifically to the belief in evil women who stole, lacerated and roasted small children. William regarded the idea that these *lamiae* or *stryges* were real women as a popular superstition. But instead of rejecting the belief outright, he christianized it by saying that *lamiae* were in fact demons who assumed the shape of old women and who did from time to time kill children, in order to punish parents who loved their offspring more than they loved God.[23] In this way William of Auvergne tried to bring some order into all sorts of beliefs on nocturnal visitors about which he had read or heard, and did his best to integrate them into a Christian framework.

Gervase of Tilbury and especially William of Auvergne bring us a lot closer to understanding Bernard of Gordon. William's description of popular and christianized beliefs in nocturnal stranglers, some of whom specifically aimed

[22] Gervase of Tilbury, *Otia imperialia* iii.86, in *Des Gervasius von Tilbury* Otia imperialia *in einer Auswahl neu herausgegeben und mit Anmerkungen begleitet*, ed. F. Liebrecht (Hanover, 1856), pp. 39–40. See also iii.85.

[23] '[. . .] de aliis malignis spiritibus, quas vulgus stryges et lamias vocant, et apparent de nocte in domibus in quibus parvuli nutriuntur, eosque de cunabulis raptos laniare vel igne assare videntur. Apparent autem in specie vetularum, videlicet quae nec vere vetulae sunt, nec vere pueros devorare possibile est eis. [. . .] Interdum autem permittitur eis parvulos occidere in poenum parentum, propter hoc quia parentes eosque interdum diligunt parvulos suos, ut Deum non diligant': William of Auvergne, *De universo*, II.iii.24, in *Opera omnia*, I, 1066. 'De nocturno vero daemone, quem ephialtem multi vocant [. . .] possibile est hanc potestatem malignis spiritibus, ut consimiles oppressiones dormientibus de nocte faciant et quandoque etiam suffocant' (p. 1069). William of Auvergne also mentions suffocating demons in *De universo* I.i.46, p. 656.

to hurt children, corresponds quite closely to the popular belief and the *opinio theologorum* described by Bernard. The only significant difference lies in the terms they use (see the diagram, below). Now that we have identified the beliefs Bernard of Gordon referred to in his discussion on *incubus*, we can turn to the development of medical theories about nocturnal suffocation.

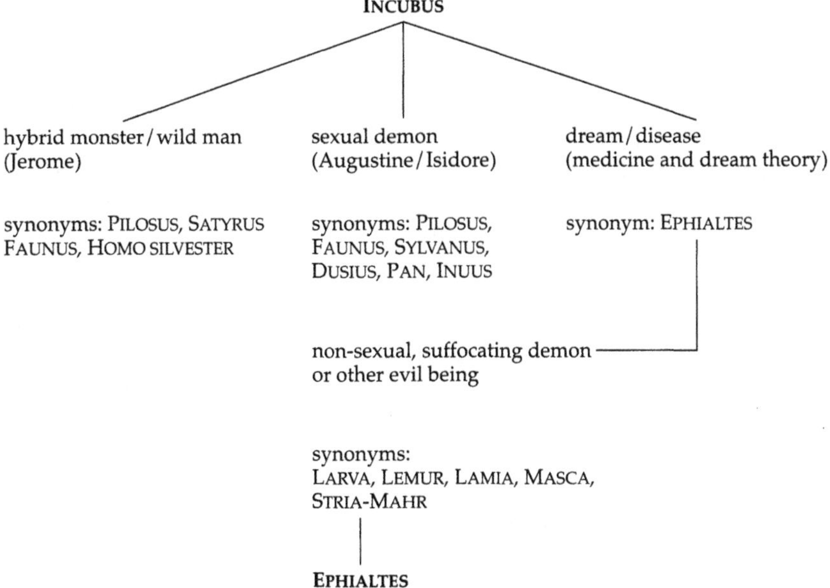

Family of terms and concepts associated with the term *incubus*

Classical Sources of the Medical *Incubus*

The concept of the *incubus* as a disease, the main symptoms of which are a sense of strangulation and of being unable to move or speak, goes back to ancient medicine and more precisely to the Methodist school. Without spelling out the details of the development and ramifications of the *incubus*-theory in Antiquity, it will be helpful to identify the intellectual foundations of the medieval debate.[24]

In Greek medicine, the disease was generally called *ephialtes*. This term was copied into some early Latin translations of Greek medical works, which explains its presence in medieval sources. In Latin disease classification the *incubus* first appeared in Caelius Aurelianus's fifth-century treatise on chronic disease, a Latin adaptation of a lost Greek work of Soranus from the beginning of the second century. Caelius Aurelianus's treatise seems to

[24] Fuller discussion of *incubus* and *ephialtes* in ancient medicine in Roscher, 'Ephialtes', pp. 18–29 and Eerden (van der) ,'Incubus', pp. 117–21.

have been practically unknown during the Middle Ages.[25] However, the *incubus* also appeared in several early medieval translations of Greek medical texts. One was the third book of Paul of Aegina's encyclopaedia, which was probably translated in the ninth century. Another, and much more important, was the fourth-century medical encyclopaedia of Oribasius. This was translated twice during the sixth century and circulated quite widely during the early Middle Ages, until it was gradually eclipsed, from the twelfth century on, by the corpus of Galenic medical works translated by Constantine the African.[26] One of these Latin versions gives both the Greek and Latin terms (*ad ephialtu, quod nos incybum dicimus*). Apart from its presence in ancient medical works and translations, the notion of the oppressive, suffocating dream had, by the beginning of the fifth century, also been incorporated in a non-medical text that was to become extremely influential: Macrobius's commentary on the *Somnium Scipionis*. Macrobius did not use the term *incubus*, however, but rather its Greek counterpart, *ephialtes*.

In the eleventh century the Salernitan physician Gariopontus inserted the *incubus* into his medical encyclopaedia, the *Passionarius*, a work that owed its success in the Middle Ages largely to its attribution to Galen.[27] The *incubus* did not appear in the *Pantegni* and the *Viaticum*, the new Constantinian translations which dominated medical debate about disease until the middle of the thirteenth century. Among the medical works translated from the Arabic by Gerard of Cremona and his team during the last quarter of the

25 Caelius Aurelianus, *Tardarum passionum* i.3, in *On Acute Diseases and On Chronic Diseases*, ed. I. E. Drabkin (Chicago, 1950), pp. 474–7; see also pp. xii–xiii. The work survives only in an early printed edition. A manuscript referred to in two ninth-century catalogues of the library in Lorsch is no longer extant. Three leaves of the manuscript used by the Renaissance editor of the text were discovered in 1921 and 1922; they may have been part of the Lorsch manuscript. An extant manuscript from Lorsch erroneously attributes a fragment from the *Physica Plinii* to Caelius Aurelianus. The title may nevertheless be an indication of a joint circulation of the *Physica Plinii* and Caelius Aurelianus's works. Cf. U. Stoll, G. Keil and A. Ohlmeyer, *Das Lorscher Arzneibuch: Übersetzung der Handschrift Msc. Med. 1 der Staatsbibliothek Bamberg* (Stuttgart, 1989), p. 70. Caelius's description of *incubus* may have circulated as well in an abridged version of his works, the so-called *Medicinales Responsiones*, parts of which survive in ninth-century northern French and Reichenau manuscripts. Lorsch also possessed three books of the *Responsiones*. Cf. V. Rose, *Anecdota Graeca et Graecolatina* (Berlin, 1870), II, 169–73; G. Baader, 'Die Anfänge medizinischen Ausbildung im Abendland bis 1100', in *La scuola nell'Occidente latino dell'alto medioevo*, 2 vols., Settimane di Studio del Centro Italiano di Studi sull'Alto Medioevo, 19 (Spoleto, 1972), II, 669–718 (pp. 697–8).

26 Oribasius, *Synopsis* viii.4, ed. A. Molinier in *Oeuvres d'Oribase*, ed. U. C. Bussemaker and C. Daremberg (Paris, 1873–6), VI, 205–6. For the circulation of the text in the early Middle Ages, Eerden (van der), 'Incubus', p. 121. The translation of Paul of Aegina's third book containing the chapter on *incubus* had a much weaker circulation. For manuscripts see Paulus Aeginata, *De arte medendi*, ed. J. L. Heiberg (Leipzig, 1912), pp. iii–xiii; text p. 36 no. 60.

27 Gariopontus, *Passionarius* v.17 (Basel, 1536), pp. 303–6.

twelfth century, however, both Avicenna's *Canon* and Rhazes' *Liber ad Almansorem* mentioned the disease. Avicenna and Rhazes were not widely used until the second half of the thirteenth century, but from that time on they constituted the principal works of reference on the matter.[28]

I shall confine myself for the moment to the medical sources – Macrobius's dream treatise needs separate treatment. All these medical texts put forward roughly the same description of the symptoms of the *incubus*. The patient suffering from an *incubus* almost suffocated during sleep and he dreamt that something heavy was pressing him down and strangling him. According to Caelius Aurelianus the dreamer sometimes imagined that his aggressor urged him to satisfy sexual needs.[29] However, the more widely read sources did not mention this erotic aspect at all; the characteristic trait of the disease remained the feeling of suffocation.

The opposition between the medical *incubus* and the belief that nocturnal suffocation was caused by a real being attacking the dreamer was already visible in ancient medicine. According to Caelius Aurelianus, Soranus showed that the *incubus* was neither a god, a half-god or a Cupid, and Oribasius explicitly rejected the demonic explanation of nocturnal suffocation.[30]

The aetiology of *incubus* put forward by the physicians differed from author to author, but all agreed that the causes were purely natural. Oribasius, for instance, asserted that the disorder was due to a superabundance of black bile in the head, which blocked sensation. He recommended a treatment which combined bloodletting to purge the body of bad humours, medication on the basis of black hellebore, and a simple diet of little food and lots of liquid.[31] Gariopontus attributed nocturnal suffocation to an excess of blood and bad humours, as well as to too much or too little food, or too much drink. Sleeping on one's back worsened the condition. Those suffering from *incubus* should first of all balance their diet. To stop a heavy attack, Gariopontus recommended more draconian remedies: pulling the patient's hair, or throwing cold water in his face.[32] The accounts of Avicenna and Rhazes were rather brief and differed little from earlier Greek and Latin

[28] Avicenna, *Canon* III.i.5.5, fols. 191vb–192ra; Rhazes, *Liber ad Almansorem* x.12, in *Opera parva* (Lyons, 1511), fol. 148v. The work of Serapion, also translated by Gerard of Cremona, does not mention the *incubus*.

[29] 'Quidam denique ita inanibus adficiuntur visis, ut et se videre credant irruentem sibi et usum turpissimae libidinis persuadentem': Caelius Aurelianus, *Tardarum passionum* i.3, p. 474.

[30] '[. . .] nam quod neque deus, neque semideus, neque cupido sit, libris Causarum quos Aetiologumenos Soranus appellavit, plenissime explicavit': Caelius Aurelianus, *Tardarum passionum* i.3, p. 474. Oribasius, *Synopsis* viii.4; VI, 205–6. (trad. Aa): 'Ad ephialtu, quod nos incybum dicimus. Incybus non est demon, sed quedam aegritudo fortis'; (trad. La): 'Non est qui vocatur inquibus [*sic*] demon malus, sed est quaedam aegritudo fortes [*sic*].'

[31] Oribasius, *Synopsis* viii.4; VI, 205–6.

[32] Gariopontus, *Passionarius* v.17, pp. 303–6.

descriptions. Rhazes suggested that the disease was caused by an excess of blood, and he prescribed abstinence from wine and sweet foodstuffs which stimulated the production of blood.[33] Avicenna attributed the feeling of suffocation to a cooling off of the brain and the rising of noxious vapours that blocked the circulation of spirits.[34]

Almost all the physicians mentioned here classed the *incubus* among the diseases of the head, like epilepsy, apoplexy or mania.[35] They thought that nocturnal suffocation was not very dangerous in itself, unless it became chronic or started occurring in the daytime. In certain such cases *incubus* could forebode more serious diseases of the head and even lead to death.[36]

Before examining the reception of these theories by medieval physicians and the development of debate about *incubus* in medieval medicine, we must turn back to Macrobius's commentary on the *Somnium Scipionis*. Until the middle of the thirteenth century learned debate about *incubus* was dominated by this treatise, and during this earlier period it was commentators on Macrobius rather than physicians who offered the more interesting and comprehensive discussions of the suffocating dream.

Incubus and *Ephialtes* in the Macrobian Classification of Dreams

In his commentary on the *Somnium Scipionis,* Macrobius divided dreams into five categories, which ranged from purely physiological dreams that signified nothing to prophetic dreams. The *ephialtes* (we have already seen that Macrobius did not use the term *incubus*) belonged to an intermediary category called *visum* or *phantasma,* a type of dream without signification which occurred in a state between waking and deep sleep:

> In this drowsy condition the dreamer thinks he is still fully awake and imagines he sees spectres rushing at him or wandering vaguely about, differing from natural creatures in size and shape, and hosts of diverse things, either delightful or disturbing. To this class belongs the *ephialtes,* which according to popular belief rushes upon people in sleep and presses them with a weight which they can feel.[37]

[33] Rhazes, *Liber ad Almansorem* ix.12, fol. 148v.

[34] Avicenna, *Canon* III.i.5.5, fols. 191vb–192ra.

[35] Paul of Aegina, who associates the *incubus* with stomach ache, is an exception.

[36] See for example Oribasius, *Synopsis* viii.4; VI, 205–6: (trad. Aa) 'Patitur enim suffocationem et gravis sine voce efficitur et frequenter nocte hoc patitur; quae passio si diu perseveraberit et frequenter majores supervenire significat passiones, id est aut apoplexia aut mania aut epilempsia. Nam in capite sensu oppresso humore melancholico hec passio generatur, et ideo cito in supradictas vertitur passiones. Quaecumque enim ephilemptici in die vigilando patiuntur, hoc ephialtici patiuntur dormientes.' Caelius Aurelianus, *Tardarum passionum* i.3, p. 474: 'Cum enim vehementer impresserit praefocatio, quosdam interficit.'

[37] 'Phantasma vero, hoc est visum, cum inter vigiliam et adultam quietem in quadam, ut aiunt, prima somni nebula adhuc se vigilare aestimans, qui dormire vix coepit,

While not explicitly refuting the popular explanation of nocturnal suffocation, Macrobius clearly thought that the aggressor existed only in the imagination of the sleeping person.

Although copying and glossing of the *Commentary on the Dream of Scipio* went back to the early Middle Ages, Macrobius's classification of dreams did not attract widespread attention until the twelfth century, when one of the most important commentators was William of Conches.[38] William and his followers developed a theory of dreams which emphasized their physical causes.[39] We have seen that for Macrobius the *ephialtes* was simply a dream linked to a particular state of consciousness, between waking and deep sleep, without any particular danger. Macrobius insisted on the psychological aspects and even though he suggested that the dream was purely natural, he did not identify any physical causes. The medieval glossators, however, gave a medical twist to the *ephialtes*. They described *ephialtes* as a pathological condition, which could even lead to death.

According to William of Conches, the suffocating sensation was caused by the obstruction of vital organs, the brain or the heart, which gave rise to a general feeling of heaviness. When someone slept on his back, the anterior ventricle (*cellula*) of the brain pressed on the posterior ones. When he slept on his left side, the liver, gallbladder and stomach pressed down on his heart.[40]

aspicere videtur irruentes in se vel passim vagantes formas a natura seu magnitudine seu specie discrepantes, variasque tempestates rerum vel laetas vel turbulentas. In hoc genere est ephialtes, quem publica persuasio quiescentes opinatur invadere, et pondere suo pressos ac sentientes gravare': Macrobius, *Commentarii in somnium Scipionis* I.iii.7, ed. J. Willis (Leipzig, 1963), p. 10; *Commentary on the Dream of Scipio*, trans. W. H. Stahl (New York, 1952), p. 89. On Macrobius's dream theory see S. F. Kruger, *Dreaming in the Middle Ages* (Cambridge, 1992), pp. 21–32.

38 Cf. A. M. Peden, 'Macrobius and Mediaeval Dream Literature', *Medium Aevum* 54 (1985), 59–73 (pp. 61–2). See also Peden's unpublished study of Macrobian glosses before the twelfth century written under her maiden name: A. M. White, 'Glosses Composed before the Twelfth Century in Manuscripts of Macrobius's Commentary on Cicero's *Somnium Scipionis*' (unpublished D.Phil. thesis, University of Oxford, 1981). I owe the second reference to Irene Caiazzo, who has edited an anonymous twelfth-century commentary in an unpublished doctoral dissertation; see also her recent article 'Le glosse a Macrobio del codice Vaticano lat. 3874: un testimone delle *formae nativae* nel secolo XII', *AHDLMA* 64 (1997), 213–34.

39 On the naturalization of dreams, see Peden, 'Macrobius'; M. Fattori, 'Sogni et temperamenti', in *I sogni nel medioevo. Seminario internazionale, Roma 2–4 ott. 1983*, ed. T. Gregory (Rome, 1985), pp. 87–109; Kruger, *Dreaming*, pp. 70–3, and Ricklin, *Traum*.

40 'Est enim epialtes [*sic*] in hoc genere: id est suprapremens. [. . .] Ephialtes autem ex modo iacendi oritur. Cum enim homo iacet supinus, cerebrum de duabus cellulis anterioribus in posteriorem descendit cellulam et ideo capite sic gravato totum etiam corpus adeo gravatur, quod videtur aliquod grave sibi superincumbere [. . .]. Item cum quis supra sinistrum latus iacet, fel et epar et stomachus opprimunt cor, quod est fons et principium motus in corpore, unde sic ipso adgravato reliqua etiam membra aggravantur et contingit etiam inde multociens mors subitanea': William of Conches, *Glosae super Macrobium* ad I.iii.7, in Munich, Bayerische Staatsbibliothek,

Other glossators copied William of Conches' explanation of the *ephialtes*, and added supplementary causes in the same vein: the suffocation of the heart by blood or vapours, the disturbance of the brain by vapours, or more generally an excess of blood in the body.[41]

Interestingly, the causes mentioned by the glossators only partially corresponded to those put forward by Oribasius, the main medical authority on the subject at that period, or to those cited by less well known authors such as Paul of Aegina or Caelius Aurelianus. They also did not agree with the causes mentioned by the Salernitan physician Gariopontus, the only contemporary physician known to have discussed nocturnal suffocation. We cannot entirely exclude the possibility that the glossators built on specific, but not yet identified, medical discussions of *incubus.* But it seems more likely that they forged their own psychosomatic dream theory out of more general psychological, physiological and anatomical principles found in the Salernitan medical corpus.[42]

The Macrobian classification of dreams also left traces outside the commentaries. It was copied by John of Salisbury in his *Policraticus* (after 1164?). Beyond the circles of Chartres it was also copied by the anonymous Cistercian author (often identified as Alcher of Clairvaux) of the very influential *Liber de spiritu et anima*, a compilation on psychology, which passed for a work by Augustine. John of Salisbury did not develop the causes of *ephialtes*, but he mocked the realistic interpretation of nocturnal suffocation.[43] The author of the *Liber de spiritu et anima* followed the glossators in attributing the phenomenon to a vapour rising to the brain from the stomach or the heart.[44]

Like Macrobius, William of Conches, John of Salisbury and the author of

MS CLM 14557, fols. 110v–111r (transcribed in Ricklin, *Traum*, p. 456). Ricklin transcribes five manuscripts of William's commentary, which, for our passage, differ in phrasing but not substantially in meaning.

41 Cf. Peden, 'Macrobius', p. 64.

42 Peden, 'Macrobius', p. 64. Eerden (van der), 'Incubus', pp. 122–3, thinks that William of Conches copies the *ephialtes* theory from a medical source, because of its discrepancy with the Augustinian concept of the sexual *incubus* which William also accepts in the *Philosophia mundi* and the *Dragmaticon.* However, it is not impossible that William developed the *ephialtes* theory himself. The doctrinal positions of medieval authors are strongly conditioned by the context in which they treat a particular problem, which can easily lead to contradictions. Moreover, it must be borne in mind that William uses different terms, *ephialtes* for the oppressive dream, *incubus* for the sexual demon.

43 John of Salisbury, *Policraticus, sive de nugis curialium et vestigiis philosophorum libri VIII* ii.15, ed. C. Webb, 2 vols. (London, 1909), I, 89, and *Frivolities of Courtiers and Footprints of Philosophers,* trans. J. B. Pike (Minneapolis and London, 1938), p. 76. See Peden, 'Macrobius', p. 65.

44 'In hoc genere [of *phantasma*] est ephialtes, quem publica persuasio quiescentes opinatur invadere, et pondere suo pressos ac sentientes gravare. Quod non est aliud nisi quaedam fumositas a stomacho vel a corde ad cerebrum ascendens, et ibi vim animalem comprimens': *Liber de spiritu et anima* 25, in *PL* 40, 798.

the *Liber de spiritu et anima* referred to the bad dream only under its Greek name, *ephialtes*. The term *incubus* did appear, however, as a synonym for *ephialtes* in one late eleventh-century gloss on Macrobius[45] and in a treatise on the origin and interpretation of dreams written about 1165 in Constantinople: the *Liber thesauri occulti* of Pascalis Romanus.[46] In 1212 or 1213, Ralph of Longchamp also used the term *incubus* in his commentary on Alan of Lille's *Anticlaudianus*.[47] Pascalis Romanus had made wide use of William of Conches' theory of the psychology and physiology of dreams, and he listed the same types of causes as William of Conches and the glossators: sleeping on the back or on the left side, suffocation of the heart by blood, disturbance of the brain.[48] However – and here he ran counter to William and the glossators – Pascalis added that *incubus* was not necessarily a sign or symptom of some internal dysfunction of the body. According to him, the phenomenon could also be provoked 'accidentally' in people in good health, by external *stimuli* such as bed-linen pressing on the dreamer's throat. With this last idea, Pascalis moved back to Macrobius's original non-pathological description. Like Macrobius, Pascalis Romanus also cited and rejected the popular explanation of the disease (*vulgaris opinio*), according to which the *incubus* was not a dream but a little animal looking like a satyr that suffocated dreamers at night-time.[49]

[45] 'Effialtes, id est incubi [*sic*], id est inde aliquis dormiens sentiens opprimitur': Biblioteca Apostolica Vaticana, MS Vat. lat. 1546, fol. 11r (cited by White, 'Glosses', II, 267).

[46] 'In quo genere est ephialtes, id est supersiliens qui lemur vel incubus dicitur [. . .]': Pascalis Romanus, *Liber thesauri occulti* 10, in S. Collin-Roset, 'Le *Liber thesauri occulti* de Pascalis Romanus: Un traité d'interprétation des songes du XIIe siècle', *AHDLMA* 30 (1963), 111–98, esp. pp. 157–8. See the reassessment of Pascalis by Ricklin, *Traum*, pp. 247–69.

[47] Ralph of Longchamp, *In Anticlaudianum Alani commentum* i.54, ed. J. Sulowksi (Wrocław, 1972), p. 57. On the author and the part on dreams see also Ricklin, *Traum*, pp. 378–407.

[48] Pascalis never cites William of Conches explicitly, but the correspondences between Pascalis's and William's general dream theory and discussion of the *ephialtes* are very strong, cf. Collin-Rosset, 'Le *Liber thesauri occulti*', p. 128. Ricklin, *Traum*, pp. 259–62, also accepts William's influence on Pascalis, but he is puzzled by the fact that, while William attributes the suffocation of the heart to the pressure on organs, Pascalis evokes the compression of humours and blood around the heart. However, this last cause was mentioned by at least one anonymous glossator, and it would thus seem that Pascalis also used one of these anonymous commentaries.

[49] 'De incubo autem habet vulgaris opinio quod sit animal parvum ad similitudinem satiri, et sic comprimit dormientes noctu et pene suffocando extingit. Sed secundum rei veritatem quidam sanguis est in corpore humano, qui non discurrit per venas neque per aliquos certos meatus, sed est in corde vel circa cor. Hic itaque sanguis quando aliquis dormit, iacens super latus sinistrum vel etiam resupinus, quedam habundantia humorum ad eandem partem decurrit corque suffocat; itaque est proximum sinistro lateri quod non potest aperiri vel claudi. Nam cor, quia sedes est semper spiritus, est in motu naturaliter nec vult impediri. Cum autem cor ita suffocatum est a sanguine et humoribus, quod non potest se libere aperire et

Little is known about Ralph of Longchamp, apart from links to the medical circles of Montpellier. These seem firmly established, although Ralph does not seem to have been a physician himself.[50] As for the symptoms, causes and treatment of *incubus/ephialtes*, Ralph cited Galen, though in fact he was just paraphrasing Gariopontus's *Passionarius*, which passed, it will be recalled, for a work by Galen. In his discussion of dreams Ralph also cited Aristotle's recently translated *Liber de somno et vigilia* and an anonymous commentator on this work who has recently been identified as David of Dinant.[51] Though he was one of the earliest authors to cite the *Liber de somno et vigilia*, his discussion on dreams was based on the Macrobian classification, and the impact of the new Aristotle remained very slight.

From the beginning of the thirteenth century on, we find the Macrobian dream classification in a wide variety of sources, particularly in handbooks on psychology and encyclopaedias. For the most part these works simply copied the account of the pseudo-Augustinian *Liber de spiritu et anima*.[52] Paradoxically, as the Macrobian dream theory started to reach a larger public, Macrobius's authority gradually began to weaken in more technical literature, in favour of Aristotle.[53] Even if the concept of the medical *incubus* survived in late medieval dream theory, most often under its Greek name *ephialtes*, it gave rise to few interesting developments.

One of the exceptions were the Latin and vernacular commentaries on Dante's *Purgatorio*. In the eleventh *canto*, verses 26 and 27, Dante had described the souls of the proud, praying and weighed down by their sins, 'like that of which one sometimes dreams' (*simile a quel che tal volta si sogna*).[54] Dante's commentators developed this oblique reference to the medical *incubus* by identifying its physical causes. Around 1333–4 the so-called *ottimo commentatore* cited corrupt humours; Francesco da Buti in the 1380s

claudere nec esse in suo motu naturali, gravantur humores in dormiente, ut putet se totam domum vel aliquam molem sustinere. [. . .] Aliquando vero fiunt fantasmata ex cerebri pertubatione. Cum enim iacet resupinus, memorialis pars cerebri opprimitur ab intellectuali et intellectualis a fantastica. [. . .] Fit preterea fantasma et accidentaliter nichil predictorum significans, quando cuilibet iacenti stragula, vel aliquod cooperimentum vel etiam sua ipsius vel alterius manus sive bracchium gulam lento modo compresserit et viam spiritus vel sanguinis impedierit. Quod qui aliquociens patitur per noctes, si mox evigiliaverit inveneritque pannum vel aliquid super gutur suum, hoc sciat fuisse causam illius fantasmatis, sin autem in fundamentis nature sanguinis sui, vel cerebri sede patitur, ut predictum est': Pascalis Romanus, *Liber thesauri occulti* 10, pp. 158–9.

50 Cf. Ralph of Longchamp, *In Anticlaudianum*, pp. xlix–l.

51 Cf. Ricklin, *Traum*, p. 395.

52 For examples see Kruger, *Dreaming*, pp. 62–3, 98 and 116–19.

53 See Peden, 'Macrobius', pp. 65–7.

54 Dante Alighieri, *Purgatorio* xi.26–7. We may add that Dante mentioned in *Inferno* xxxi.83–111 a giant named *Fialt*, one of two brothers already named by Virgil, and placed him among the giants chained in hell for having tried to rebel against the upper god. Cf. *Enciclopedia dantesca*, 2nd edn, 6 vols. (Rome, 1984), II, 848–9. Dante's *Fialt* is unrelated to the *incubus* concept.

attributed the heavy feeling to the congestion of blood around the heart,[55] and Benvenuto of Imola, a Bolognese master of grammar active during the second half of the fourteenth century, noted in his Latin commentary that Dante referred to

> a kind of natural disease (*morbus naturalis*) that can happen to someone at night when he dreams. And it seems to him, as I have heard from experts, that he has the whole world on top of him, and he feels that he is suffocating under such a weight. The physicians call this disorder *incubus*.[56]

While twelfth-century commentators of Macrobius developed their own explanations of *ephialtes* out of general medical theory, dream theorists in the fourteenth century recognized the expert knowledge of the physicians and confidently had recourse to medical opinion. By this time, the focus of the debate about the medical *incubus* had shifted from dream theory to scholastic medicine.[57]

The *Incubus* in Scholastic Medicine

The chronology of the medical debate about the *incubus* differs perceptibly from that in dream treatises. In the West, the first medieval physician to have left a discussion on *incubus* seems to have been the Salernitan physician Gariopontus. After this, learned medicine seems to have neglected the subject

[55] 'E dice, che cosiì [. . .] soto il peso andavano simile a quello, che alcuna volta li uomini per corrotti omori sognano avere sopr' a sè': *L'ottimo commento*, ad *Purgatorio* xi.26–27, ed. A. Torri, 3 vols. (Pisa, 1828), II, 183; 'imperò che l'omo sogna spesse volte avere grande peso addosso, et àe grande angoscia, massimamente quando l'omo dorme rivolto, che 'l sangue corre al cuore et grava il cuore, sicchè para a l'omo avere tutto 'l mondo addosso': Francesco da Buti, *Commento sopra la Divina Comedia di Dante Allighieri*, ad *ibidem*, ed. C. Giannini, 3 vols. (Pisa, 1858–62), II, 255.

[56] '"simile a quel che tal volta si sogna". Ad cuius intelligentiam est notandum quod est quoddam genus morbi naturalis accidens homini in nocte in somnio, quia videtur ei, ut audio ab expertis, quod habeat totum mundum super se, et videtur suffocari sub nimio pondere; et vocatur a phisicis incubus': Benvenuto Rambaldi da Imola, *Comentum super Dantis Aldighierii Comoediam*, ad *Purgatorio* xi.26–7, ed. G. Warren Vernon and J. P. Lacaita, 5 vols. (Florence, 1887), III, 303–4.

[57] Certain dream treatises of the later Middle Ages use the term *incubus* independently of the Macrobian classification. In the 1330s, William of Aragon in his *De prognosticatione somniorum libellus* follows the theory, widely established since the twelfth century, according to which the content of dreams depends on the temperament of the dreamer. The *incubus* appears in the class of the melancholic's frightening dreams. William mentions the *incubus* only in passing, without painting its portrait. The notion of the medical *incubus* is lost here; the term designates not a dream category but a type of image appearing during certain bad dreams. R. A. Pack, '*De Prognosticatione sompniorum* libellus Guillelmo de Aragonia adscriptus', *AHDLMA* 33 (1966), 237–97, esp. p. 260. For the link between dreams and the theory of humours see Fattori, 'Sogni e temperamenti'.

for over two centuries. The lack of editions of Salernitan medical works imposes prudence here. However, neither the texts edited by De Renzi nor the *Prose Salernitan questions* – which together give a fairly good indication of the subjects covered by Salernitan medicine – mention *incubus,* while they do contain references to related diseases of the head like epilepsy.[58] This apparent lack of interest for *incubus* in medical debate in the twelfth and the first half of the thirteenth century can probably be explained by the absence of the disorder from the two central medical texts on pathology of that period, the *Pantegni* and the *Viaticum.*

Despite the silence of learned medical works, there is nevertheless indirect evidence suggesting that the medical *incubus* had not disappeared from medical learning. Gervase of Tilbury and William of Auvergne both remarked that their own demonological interpretation of nocturnal suffocation differed from the opinion of the physicians. William described physicians as very competent in that area and he even allowed for the possibility that some cases of nocturnal suffocation were due to a compression of the heart blocking the free circulation of spirits in the body.[59] He did not tell his reader how to distinguish the pathological from the demonic version but he obviously privileged the latter explanation himself. Unfortunately, Gervase of Tilbury's and William of Auvergne's accounts of the causes and treatment of the natural form of nocturnal suffocation are not precise enough to allow us to identify their sources. It is difficult to tell whether they derived their knowledge from discussions with contemporary physicians, from traditional

[58] Of the works edited (very imperfectly) by S. De Renzi, *Collectio salernitana,* 3 vols. (Naples, 1854) only a dictionary of plants, stones, animals and pharmaceutics called *Alphita* (III, 295) contains a definition of *Incubus* ('nomen est morbi et nomen demonis et inde subincubus [var. succubus]'). This definition probably derives from Oribasius. However, the *Alphita* cites Avicenna, Aristotle and Rhazes and thus dates from the end of the thirteenth century at the very earliest, unless, of course, these references are all later additions. A study of the manuscript tradition would be needed to rule out this possibility. See also *Alphita: A Medico-Botanical Glossary from the Bodleian Manuscript, Selden B. 35,* ed. J. L. G. Mowat, Anecdota Oxoniensia: Texts, Documents and Extracts chiefly from Manuscripts in the Bodleian and other Oxford Libraries, Medieval and Modern Series 1, part 2 (Oxford, 1887), p. 86: 'Incubus nomen est morbi, et nomen demonis, et inde succubus id quod sicuta.'

[59] 'Lamias quas vulgo mascas aut in gallica lingua strias nominant, physici dicunt nocturnas esse imaginationes, quae ex grossitie humorum animas dormientium turbant et pondus faciunt': Gervase of Tilbury, *Otia imperialia* iii.86, p. 39. 'De nocturno vero daemone, quem ephialtem multi vocant, scire oportet quia multi ex peritioribus medicorum ephialtem daemonem esse negant et oppressionem illam quam eos incubens daemon facere videtur, hominibus ex compressione cordis esse dicunt, qua nervus per quem sensibilis et motivus spiritus a corde ad membra alia digreditur et permeat atque diffunditur, ibi stringitur, ut spiritus illos retineat et ad membra transire prohibeat. [. . .] Veritas autem haec est quia etsi hoc modo fieri possit et plerumque fiat huiusmodi compressio vel oppressio, nihilominus tamen possibile est hanc potestatem malignis spiritibus, ut consimiles oppressiones dormientibus de nocte faciant et quandoque etiam suffocant [. . .]': William of Auvergne, *De universo* II.iii.24, in *Opera omnia* I, 1069.

medical sources (or even, in the case of William of Auvergne, from Avicenna's newly introduced *Canon*[60]), or merely from dream books. Further proof of the presence of *incubus* in twelfth-century medical learning and practice is found in a collection of the miracles of Thomas Becket written by Benedict, abbot of Peterborough (1177–93). One of these miracles involves an English knight who had suffered from chronic nocturnal suffocation for more than thirty years. The knight was finally liberated from a demon thanks to the saint's intervention, but not after having been treated in vain by physicians who claimed that he suffered from *ephialtes*.[61]

Nevertheless, the medical *incubus* did not become a commonplace of medical debate until the end of the thirteenth century, after the assimilation of the new Arabic sources, Rhazes and Avicenna, and with the full development of scholastic medicine in the universities. In the 1280s and 1290s, William of Saliceto and Arnau de Vilanova, two eminent physicians active respectively at Bologna and Montpellier, both described the *incubus*. Bernard of Gordon followed around 1305, and the subject was also discussed by later scholastic physicians and commentators on Rhazes and Avicenna, such as Gentile da Foligno (d. 1348), Gerard of Solo (works *c.* 1350), John of Tornamira (1329–96), Jacques Despars (*c.* 1380–1458), Antonio Guaineri (first half of the fifteenth century), Giovanni Arcolano (d. 1458) and Cristoforo Barzizza (fl. 1450) .

Following their Arabic sources, these physicians all classed the *incubus* among the diseases of the head. They also repeated the idea that the disease could degenerate into more serious disorders of the same genre. As for the aetiology of *incubus*, medieval practitioners generally copied Avicenna, who attributed the disease to a cooling off of the brain and the rising of vapours that blocked the circulation of spirits, but they also mentioned causes that had appeared already in Oribasius and Gariopontus, like difficult digestion (mentioned, as we have seen, by Bernard of Gordon) and sleeping on one's back.[62] On the other hand, we do not find the idea, that sleeping on the left side

[60] William of Auvergne is among the first authors to cite the *Canon*, cf. D. Jacquart and F. Micheau, *La médecine arabe et l'occident médiéval* (Paris, 1990), p. 157.

[61] Benedict of Peterborough, *Miracula*, in *Materials for the History of Thomas Becket, Archbishop of Canterbury*, ed. J. C. Roberts and J. B. Sheppard, 7 vols., RS 67 (London, 1875–85), II, 44–5. I owe this example to Eerden (van der), 'Incubus', p. 125. Incidentally, this story illustrates the complementary roles of medicine and religion in medieval society: a religious cure is resorted to after the failure of medical treatment, a pattern that is not without analogies in the modern Western world.

[62] See for instance the list of causes in Gerard of Solo's commentary on Rhazes (chapter 12): 'Cause incubi sunt tres, scilicet primitiva et illa est duplex, una frigiditas cito ascendens usque ad posteriorem partem cerebri comprimens ipsum [. . .] alia causa primitiva est somnus diurnus immediate factus super repletionem magnam cibi et potus [. . .] Causa accidentalis principalis est materia grossa a qua elevantur fumi viam cerebri opilantes. Causa coniuncta sunt alii fumi et vapores causantes epilepsiam ratione quorum prohibetur transitio spiritum ad membra inferiora': Gerard of Solo, *Practica super nono Almansoris* (Venice, 1502), fol. 31r (*c.* 1350). Gentile da Foligno, *Super Canonem Avicennae* ad III.i.5.5 (Padua, 1477,

is just as dangerous, which had been upheld by twelfth-century commentators on Macrobius – an indication that these dream theories were either unknown to scholastic physicians, or considered unprofessional and obsolete. Some physicians, like William of Saliceto and Gentile da Foligno only described the symptoms, causes and remedies of *incubus*, while others contrasted their own opinion with alternative explanations.[63] Arnau de Vilanova (*c.* 1240–1311) opened his discussion of the *incubus* with the remark that he was reporting medical opinion, thus implicitly recognizing the existence of other explanations of the phenomenon, even though he did not describe them.[64] The first detailed description of these alternatives I have found is in Bernard of Gordon's *Lilium*. Bernard's discussion was to be very influential. In the 1350s and 1360s, his refutation of popular belief and the theological theory was copied, without significant variations, by at least two other leading medical professors from Montpellier, Gerard of Solo and John of Tornamira.[65] The *Lilium* itself remained one of the most important medical authorities until the beginning of the early modern period, and it also reached a larger public of educated laymen, thanks to translations into several vernaculars.[66]

But as we move into the fifteenth century some interesting changes take place in the way some physicians portray the beliefs they want to rationalize and explain away. In his *De egritudinibus capitis*, Antonio Guaineri, student of the great Jacopo da Forlì (who does not seem to have written about *incubus*) and also author of an important treatise on women's diseases, dropped the distinction between theological theory and common opinion. Both the idea that nocturnal suffocation is caused by a demon and that it is caused by a *vetula* were characterized here as popular beliefs. Interestingly, Guaineri also

unnumbered) mentions the idea that the *incubus* happens especially to those sleeping on their backs.

63 William of Saliceto, *Summa conservationis et curationis* 16 (Venice, 1490, unnumbered). Gentile da Foligno, *Super Canonem Avicennae*, ad III.i.5.5.

64 'Incubus in latino et ephialtes in graeco, passio est ab accidente denominata, quoniam patiens aliquid opprimens decumbere vel superiacere, sibi dormiendo existimat. Ideo determinatur a medicis esse cerebri morbus, quoniam sensibiliter impetit omnes motus, qui virtute a cerebro derivata perficiuntur [. . .]': Arnau de Vilanova, *De parte operativa*, in *Opera omnia* (Basel, 1585), 289–90.

65 '[. . .] Dico quod tres sunt opiniones de hac. Una theologorum qui dicunt quod causa huius passionis sunt demones qui sunt existentes in aere supra corpus humanum principaliter respiciunt cor et quia cor non potest sustinere aspectum illius mali spiritus et ideo non potest moveri et quia fumi vadunt ad caput, ideo non possunt loqui nec sentire. Alii dicunt quod est vetula vel merula que vadit vel scandit ad aliud seculum; et illa ponit se supra hominem et calcat et comprimit et illud nihil est. Alia est causa medicorum [. . .]': Gerard of Solo, *Practica super nono Almansoris* 12, fol. 31r. '[. . .] Incubus est nomen diaboli dicunt theologi, qui comprimit corpora de nocte dormiendo. Laici dicunt quod est vetula comprimens gentes de nocte. Sed nos medici scimus et dicimus aliter': John of Tornamira, *Clarificatorium super nono Almansoris cum textu ipsius Rasis* 12 (Lyons, 1490), fol. 23r; this was written in 1365.

66 Cf. L. E. Demaitre, *Doctor Bernard de Gordon: Professor and Practitioner*, Studies and Texts 51 (Toronto, 1980), pp. 185–90 (inventory of manuscripts, translations and early editions).

mentioned the vernacular terminology for these old women. The common people in his region (*nostri vulgares*) called them not only *striae* – a common word for witch – but also *zobiane*, a term which seems to be much more local. Guaineri added that it was believed that *zobiane* not only killed babies but also changed themselves into cats. Like Bernard of Gordon, he belittled these popular beliefs. The common people only clung to them, he said, because they were unable to understand the real causes of nocturnal suffocation and, in particular, cot death.[67]

Other physicians maintained the opposition between theological and popular belief, but they changed the definition of the theory of the theologians. Instead of associating the medical *incubus* with the notion of suffocating demons, they brought into their discussions references to the Augustinian sexual *incubus*. An example can be found in the commentary on Avicenna's *Canon* by Jacques Despars, written between 1432 and 1453. Despars, who taught medicine at the university of Paris, described the symptoms and causes of the *incubus* in the traditional manner. The patient suffering from *incubus* (*habens incubum*) had the impression that an old woman or an animal was pressing on him and suffocating him, so that he could neither cry out nor move, even though he desperately tried to do so. The disorder was due to noxious vapours that rise to the brain and block the pores. Despars insisted that the aggressor existed only in the imagination, by describing this *incubus* as an empty vision (*visio vana*) or a false apparition (*apparitio falsa*), and he derided the opinion of 'certain simpletons and idiots who believe that they have really been trampled down by an old woman or by an animal that the common people call *calcamara*'.[68]

[67] '[. . .] quod uulgares demonem homines suffocantem putant, ob hoc ergo passio hec "incubus" appellatur, quod est nomen demonis. Alii vetulas quasdam incantantes que se in formas varias ut inquiunt mutare possunt, hoc facere putant et eas strias seu zobianas nostri vulgares appellant, que ut dicunt gatorum formam sepius accipiunt. Hec crudelitas [*sic*] ob hoc ortum habuit, quia passio hec lactantes sepe deprehendit quos tunc suffocat, cuius causas uulgares ignorantes uetulas illas zobianas illud fecisse putant': Antonio Guaineri, *De egritudinibus capitis* 6 (Pavia, 1488), fol. 17rab.

[68] '[. . .] habens incubum [. . .] sentit vel sentire putat, ut verius loquamur, phantasme grave, id est falsam aliquam apparitionem seu visionem vanam, rei ponderose super se cadent et eum oppriment. [. . .] Apparet enim patienti hunc morbum quod aliqua vetula vel aliqua bestia sibi superiaceat et suffocet ipsum. Solet autem vulgo calcamara vocari. [. . .] Anhelitus huius patienti adeo angustatur quod ei videtur quod suffocetur. [. . .] Vox eius intersecatur sic quod neque loqui nec clamare potest quamvis id desiderit ut ei succurratur et excutiatur id quod ipsum opprimit. [. . .] impeditur motus eius voluntarius sic quod nec se volvere [. . .] nec erigere potest licet summe id optet ut a se excutiat opprimens phantasma. Et dum expergefit refert hec in somno sibi contigisse vel visa fuisse vel imaginative sibi occurisse. Et quidam simplicium vel idiotarum credunt veraciter se fuisse calcatos vetula aut bestia quam calcamaram vocant. [. . .] Ille qui patitur incubum forte suffocatur ex oppillatione suorum pororum id est meatuum vel ipsius cerebri a grossis vaporibus ut in apoplexia vel anhelitus eius a grossis humoribus et vaporibus quibus oppilantur anhelitus vie vel orificium arterie vocalis': Despars, ad III.i.5.5.

After refuting the popular belief, Despars moved on to the opinion of the theologians. Bernard of Gordon had attributed to them the idea of a non-sexual oppressing demon. Despars did not follow his illustrious predecessor on this point, but rather copied the entries *incubus* and *pilosus* from John Balbi of Genoa's extremely well known and influential encyclopaedic dictionary, the *Catholicon* (1286), which in turn had copied Thomas Aquinas.[69] In doing so he introduced the notion of the sexual *incubus* into the medical debate.

One contemporary of Despars, Giovanni Arcolano, a professor of medicine at the universities of Bologna, Padua and Ferrara, went even further. In his commentary on the ninth book of Rhazes' *Liber ad Almansorem*, Arcolano explained first that the disease was called *incubus* because it made the sleeping person feel 'as if a heavy fantasy lies down on him and sleeps with him', a hybrid definition that combined both the sense of oppression and of sexual intercourse. All along, Arcolano oscillated between the definition of the suffocating and the sexual demon. He evoked the idea that certain demons weighed down people in their sleep to do them harm but he also summarized the doctrine of demonic generation. Citing Augustine and Thomas Aquinas, Arcolano mentioned the theory of temporarily assumed material bodies, of stolen seed, and the biblical example of the giants in Genesis.[70]

While presenting the traditional medical causes and remedies of the *incubus*, Arcolano conceded that the demonological explanation of the disease was not wholly unfounded, saying that it 'may sometimes be true' (*forte aliquando est verum*) that demons slept with human beings and that 'it cannot

[69] 'Grammatici vero nomina exponentes et quidam theologi per incubi nomen demonem intelligunt. Unde scribitur in *Catholicone*: "Incubi pilosi quidam demones sunt et dicuntur idem incubones." Et ibidem scribitur sub nomine pilosus quod "incubi vel incubones dicuntur ab incubendo id est stuprando. Sepe enim improbi existunt mulieribus et earum peragunt concubitum quos demones galli dusios nominant quod assidue hanc peragunt immundiciam. Sed quem vulgus incubonem vocat hunc romani faunum ficarium dicunt hunc alii satirum vocant." Sed si demon sit malignus spiritus non habens carnem neque ossa mirabile videtur quod sit pilosus vel mulierum stuprator nisi corpus assumet': Despars, ad III.i.5.5.

[70] 'Incubus ab incubando dictus, eo scilicet quod appareat phantasma grave incubare homini in somniis ac si cum eo cubaret. [. . .] Propter quod sciendum de intentione Augustini 15 *De Civitate Dei* et sancti Thomae in prima parte suae [*sic*] *Theologie* quod reperiuntur daemones qui dicuntur incubi et succubi, immo unus et idem est incubus, postea succubus. Vnde daemon aliquando suscipit formam quam ex aere conficit [. . .] Assumit ergo formam alicuius mulieris cum aliquo uiro consuetae et cum illo succubo uir coit putans coire cum muliere cuius formam daemon assumpsit. Cum daemon fit succubans in modum mulieris et recipit sperma quod conseruat. Et factus postea incubus accipiens formam uiri alicui mulieri consueti et secum coiens interdum ipsam impregnat. [. . .] Et hoc modo affirmant doctores fuisse genitos gigantes, quorum maior copia fuit ante diluvium quam post': Giovanni Arcolano, *Practica seu expositio noni libri Almansoris* 15 (Basel, 1540), p. 110. For a detailed study of the development of the theory of demonic generation, see van der Lugt, 'Le ver, le démon et la vierge' (above, n. 1).

be denied' (*nec est negandum*) that the symptoms of *incubus* could be caused by a demon. The intervention of a demon could only be ascertained *a posteriori*: if incantations and exorcisms sufficed to bring an end to the symptoms, the latter were caused by a demon. However, even though Arcolano did allow for the possibility of demons harassing dreamers, sleeping with humans and fathering children, he presented this as a very hypothetical eventuality, for he added that sexual intercourse between demons and humans had occurred mainly in ancient times, before the coming of Christ, an era when demons and mankind still lived in each other's proximity.[71] This idea ran counter to a conviction, common to fifteenth-century demonologists, that in their own times demons were doubling their efforts and closely co-operating with witches to bring humanity to ruin. By contrast, Arcolano, when citing the idea that there were more giants before than after the Flood,[72] presented demonic generation as history. By implication, contemporary witness accounts belonged to the realms of pathology.

The belief in demons who harassed people during sleep was undermined even further by Giovanni Arcolano, through his linking the experience of the supposed victims to their belief system:

> In most cases [the patient suffering from *incubus*] believes that the fantasy [that weighs on him] is a demon, because of the popular belief (*opinio vulgarium*) that demons roam around at night and unite themselves with humans and do them harm. It is in fact that belief that leads him to judge the ailment he feels in such a way. But if no such belief about that kind of demons existed, he would think that it was some other kind of heavy thing.[73]

[71] '[. . .] Quod phantasma homines dormientes secundum plurimum reputant esse daemonem. Quod forte aliquando est verum, sed minus post adventum Christi cum antea, cum hominibus magis conversarentur. [. . .] Causa immediata eius qui per essentiam est oppilatio in priori uentriculo uel in origine nuchae uapore grosso, aut paucissimo humore facile resolubili. [. . .] Aliquando uero fit a frigore extrinseco oppilante originem neruorum attenuatorie, nec est negandum quin potest fieri a daemone. Signa incubi absolute habentur ex relatu aegri. [. . .] Verum difficile esset cognoscere esse demonem, nisi per signum sumptum a conferentibus, ut quia passio recederet per coniurationes et similia quae non pertinent ad medicum': Arcolano, *Practica*, p. 110.

[72] Arcolano attributes this idea to the theologians, but I have not been able to find his source. Augustine argued the contrary, rejecting the idea that the biblical giants had been generated by fallen angels. He said that it was perfectly possible for giants to be born of normal parents, and provided contemporary examples. Augustine, *De civitate Dei* xv.23 (IV, 104–8) and *Quaestionum in heptateuchum* i.3 (pp. 2–3).

[73] '[. . .] Sentit autem homo cum somnum ingreditur phantasma grave cadens super ipsum et comprimens ipsum, quod phantasma secundum plurimum existimat esse daemonem propter opinionem vulgarium, quod daemones de nocte ambulent et cum hominibus coniungantur ipsos laedentes. Illud enim nocumentum perceptum in somno facit hominem sic iudicare. Si vero non esset opinio de huiusmodi daemonibus existimarent esse aliud grave alterius generis': Arcolano, *Practica*,

The way the patient interpreted what was happening to him was conditioned by his convictions, which depended in turn on collective beliefs. In other words, disease has a social dimension. This apparently original idea seriously subverted the reality of demonic harassment.

Conclusion

After tracing the *incubus* from late Antiquity to the end of the Middle Ages, we need to make a few final remarks.

First of all, we have seen that all along physicians and dream theorists defended a physiological explanation of nocturnal suffocation. The *incubus*, they maintained, was nothing but a bad dream. In the mean time, they rejected an alternative 'realist' explanation, according to which nocturnal suffocation was caused by a demon or other evil being who attacked people during sleep. Historians have learned to be suspicious of repetitious denunciations. How do we know that those who condemned the beliefs of others were not just perpetuating literary stereotypes, which merely served to enhance their own position? In the case of *incubus*, however, this seems quite unlikely. The many stories about nocturnal attacks that have come down to us, told by authors like Guibert de Nogent or Benedict of Peterborough, who share the belief in *incubi* themselves, confirm the existence of realist beliefs about *incubi* in wide strata of medieval society. The variety of details in the physicians' descriptions of these beliefs points in the same direction, as do the references made by some physicians to vernacular terminology specific of certain regions: *zobiana* in the work of the north Italian physician Antonio Guaineri, and *calcamara*, a word of Picard origin,[74] in that of Jacques Despars, who spent an important part of his life in Picardy. The belief in nocturnal assailants suffocating people in their sleep was clearly more than a literary cliché.

But if the belief was shared by the clergy and the laity alike, not everyone agreed as to the identity of the nocturnal attacker. Scholastic medicine recognized this divergence of opinion, by distinguishing between popular belief and theology: while theologians regarded the *incubus* as a demon, the common people thought of an animal or more frequently, a malicious old woman, a witch. This opposition between theological theory and popular opinion, which we first encountered in Bernard of Gordon, reflected a distinction already made by William of Auvergne between orthodoxy and superstition. By categorically rejecting the idea that the *lamiae*, who are

p. 110. There are similar remarks in the commentary on Rhazes by one of Giovanni's contemporaries and colleagues at the university of Padua, Cristoforo Barzizza, *Introductorium ad opus practicum medicinae* (Pavia, 1494), fols. 46v–47r.

[74] Cf. *Dictionnaire historique de la langue française*, ed. A. Rey (Paris, 1992), s.v. 'cauchemar'.

believed to kill babies at night-time, were real women, William trod in the footsteps of the famous ninth-century *Canon episcopi*, which characterized as contrary to Christian faith the belief that women really fly through the air at night to do harm to other people.[75]

However, orthodoxy and superstition were never monolithic blocks. Not all medieval clerics defined the border between accepted and disapproved beliefs and practices in exactly the same way; and some were more tolerant of folk-lore than others. We have seen that Gervase of Tilbury, a cleric close to the courts, was far less preoccupied with the orthodoxy of the beliefs he described than was William of Auvergne, a bishop much concerned with pastoral care. Apart from the differences in outlook between individual clerics, the border between the allowed and the condemned could also change over time. Just as certain beliefs and practices, which were once embraced and even propagated by the church, started at some point to be considered as superstitious – the ritual of the humiliation of saints, for example, from the thirteenth century on[76] – other beliefs that were first considered superstitious, were later transformed into accepted doctrine. Ideas about witchcraft are a famous example of the latter development. After rejecting their reality for centuries, theologians started, by the middle of the fifteenth century, to accept the existence of the night witch and of the witches' sabbath, thus paving the way for the great witch-hunt.

Although this fateful conceptual shift is not directly visible in the late medieval medical discussions of *incubus*, these discussions do seem to reflect the rise of the witch-craze in fifteenth-century Western society. The descriptions of the beliefs physicians claimed to naturalize underwent some significant changes. Jacques Despars maintained the distinction between popular belief and theology, but he put the Augustinian sexual *incubus* in the place of the oppressing demon. Giovanni Arcolano (followed by Cristoforo Barzizza) did not mention witches at all, but he combined the sexual and the oppressing demon without distinction. Antonio Guaineri, for his part, attributed both the demonological and the witch version to the common people. This divergence bears witness to the uncertainty among fifteenth-century physicians about the appropriateness of the pattern defined by Bernard of Gordon, while the incorporation of the Augustinian definition of *incubus* into medical debate points to the growing force of the belief in sexual demons at the dawn of the modern period. Giovanni Arcolano's acknowledgement of a possible demonic background to the *incubus* shows even more eloquently that times had changed. With the ever increasing empowerment of the devil, articulated in sermons, confession manuals,

[75] For the *Canon Episcopi* and night flight see W. Tschacher, 'Der Flug durch die Luft zwischen Illusionstheorie und Realitätsbeweis. Studien zum sog. Kanon episcopi und zum Hexenflug', *Zeitschrift der Savigny-Stiftung für Rechtsgeschichte* 116 (1999), 225–76.

[76] Cf. J.-C. Schmitt, 'Les superstitions', in *Histoire de la France religieuse: Des origines au XIVe siècle*, ed. J. Le Goff and R. Rémond (Paris, 1988), p. 513.

treatises and trials, it was no longer possible for physicians to dismiss demonological beliefs as categorically as before. They were led to make concessions to theology, even though they obviously continued to privilege their own naturalistic explanations.

Finally, it must be noted that the integration of the definition of the sexual incubus into medical debate led to certain incongruities, because the symptoms and the causes traditionally associated with the medical incubus corresponded well with the belief in suffocating demons, and much less well with the belief in sexual demons. It may seem surprising that the success of the sexual *incubus* had not led to any modification of the *medical* description of the disease. Would it not have been logical for Despars and Arcolano to associate the *incubus* with the nocturnal pollution that was described in the sections in their treatises devoted to diseases of the genital organs? If they had done this, the accounts of copulation with demons could have been easily explained away as erotic dreams. However, this cross-connection does not seem to have been made. Apart from the inclusion, by Giovanni Arcolano, of the idea that the sleeper had the impression that the demon was sleeping with him, the symptoms described by Jacques Despars and Giovanni Arcolano remained devoid of sexual experiences. Neither Despars nor Arcolano adapted the aetiology of the disease. It may be that, in their opinion, the sexual aspect was secondary to the feeling of oppression and thus did not need to be developed explicitly. But the absence of any cross-connection must also be understood as a consequence of the scholastic method, which consisted first and foremost in the commenting of texts. The mechanism of the commentary is likely to have blocked any association of the *incubus* and the erotic dream. In medical sources, the *incubus* and diseases of the head on the one hand and nocturnal pollution and disorder of the genital organs on the other hand, appeared in different places and gave rise to separate commentaries.

But this incoherence far from nullifies the importance of the physicians' arguments about the *incubus*. Their discussion opened the way to a scientific refutation not only of the belief that witches suffocated people in their sleep and killed babies in their beds, but also of the idea of sexual intercourse between witches and demons. For it was in the works of late medieval physicians that well known early modern critics of the witch-craze, such as Symphorien Champier (who copied Arcolano almost verbatim) or Johannes Wier found the arguments they used to attack the reality of the witches' alleged actions.[77]

[77] Symphorien Champier, *Dialogus in magicarum artium destructionem*, in A. Rijper, 'Symphorien Champier, *Condamnation des sciences occultes*, édition critique du *Dyalogus in magicarum artium destructionem*, avec une traduction française, une introduction et des notes', *Anagrom* 5–6 (1974), 3–54; Johannes Wier, *De praestigiis daemonum et incantantionibus ac ueneficijs libri V*, ii.36 (Basel, 1566), pp. 291–3 (1st edn Basel, 1563).

Medicine and Immortality in Terrestrial Paradise

Joseph Ziegler

A short history of how I was drawn to this topic provides the setting for this paper. As we are dealing with a biblical scene directly connected with the story of creation, let me start this way: In the beginning there was question 18 in the fourth *Disputatio de quolibet* of the Augustinian master James of Viterbo (*c.* 1255–1308).[1] Of the four *disputationes de quolibet* he held in Paris in the years 1293–6, the fourth is packed with questions which show particular interest in the natural sciences. Among them, the following triggered my attention.

If man[2] had not sinned, would the attention of physicians have been useful and would he have needed the aid of the art of medicine? ('Utrum, si homo non pecasset, utilis fuisset consideratio medicorum, et utrum indiguisset adminiculo artis medicine'). As usual, James first starts with *videtur quod non.* Medical attention is needed to restore or maintain health; there was no disease and no loss (*deperditio*) before Sin; hence there would have been no need to restore health and medical attention would have been useless. Furthermore, medical attention is convenient where there is nutrition (*nutritio*). Nutrition is a sort of physical suffering (*passio*). But no *passio* could have existed in prelapsarian man. Therefore the attention of physicians would have been unnecessary if man had not sinned. The argument *contra* also connects nutrition and the necessity of medicine. It cites God's commandment in Genesis 2. 16, 'Of every tree of paradise thou shalt eat', as a proof that man used food before the sin. Consequently, medical attention would have been useful.

James's solution determines that the attention of physicians before sin would have been useful, but not in the same ways as it is useful now. First, medical attention is necessary today for the perfection of the intellect (*ad perfectionem intellectus*) of those who engage in this knowledge. Secondly, it is necessary for the health of the body (*ad salutem corporis* or *corporum sanitatem*).

[1] James of Viterbo, *Disputatio quarta de quolibet*, ed. E. Ypma, Cassiciacum, Supplementband 5 (Würzburg, 1975), pp. 63–6. On James see A. Zumkeller, 'Die Augustinerschule des MA', *Analecta Augustiniana* 27 (1964), 167–262 (pp. 196–9); James of Viterbo, *Disputatio Prima de Quolibet*, ed. E. Ypma, Cassiciacum, Supplementband 1 (Würzburg, 1968), pp. v–vi; D. Gautiérrez, *De B. Iacobi Viterbiensis O.E.S.A.: Vita, operibus et doctrina theologica* (Rome, 1939), pp. 13–21 and 32–4 (on Quodlibet iv).

[2] Throughout this paper I systematically use masculine pronouns (man, he, Adam) because this is how the medieval sources speak. But my text is not gender specific.

Inasmuch as medical attention is useful for the perfection of the soul (*ad perfectionem anime*; James uses *intellectus* and *anima* interchangeably here), it would have had a place before Sin. Man would not have needed medical knowledge (*scientia medicine*) for the care or the cure of his body, but he would have still had to learn to know (*cognoscere*) those things which physicians now examine (*considerant*). He would have had to learn that the nature of man is corruptible and open to diseases; that only through a supernatural gift (*ex supernaturali dono*) had he become immortal and immune to disease. Hence he would have learnt and known about complexions, diseases, therapies, and the other things which the attention of physicians entails. He would have received this knowledge (as well as all knowledge of natural things) directly from God, in a way similar to the angels. His offspring would have received this knowledge by way of purchase and teaching.

As for the usefulness of medicine for the health of the body, the attention of physicians would have been useful in paradise as well. Not being exposed to diseases, man would have needed no medicines for purging the body of harmful humours. The sole medicine conceded by God to man would have been the tree of life, which kept his natural power (*virtus nature*) unharmed; however, knowing and understanding (*cognoscere*) this property of the tree of life in paradise would have been in the purview of medical science (*ad considerationem scientie medicine pertinuisset*). In the State of Innocence knowing medicine thus fulfilled a basic intellectual need: understanding one's place and existence in paradise. By implication, it was necessary for explaining and understanding human existence in this world as well.

But engagement in the medical art would have been convenient also with respect to the consumption of useful food and drink which man would have used for restoring (*restauratio*) the loss (*deperditio*) inflicted by the consuming natural heat. Some food is suitable to mankind, other food is not and may even be poisonous. Man would have needed to have the knowledge to distinguish between suitable and unsuitable food, and to realise the difference (*differentia*) between kinds of food and their properties (*proprietates*). Such knowledge belongs to medical science. Hence, from this point of view, medical attention would have been useful to the first man for preserving health. The first man would have been protected from poisonous food and other physical dangers by medical knowledge rather than by a miraculous reality in which poisons did not poison and thorns did not prick.

This is an interesting debate. First, it openly recognizes the spiritual value of medical knowledge which furthers the perfection of the soul both here and in paradise. Contemplating medicine can promote humility in the face of nature and God – a highly desirable virtue. Secondly, for all those who still believe that the medical art in medieval ecclesiastical imagination was automatically linked to the Fall, here, in a theologian's voice, is a clear view which redeems medicine from this tainted position. Thirdly, almost everything in the terrestrial paradise would have had a rational, natural explanation, even the miraculous properties of the tree of life. Adam's body functioned exactly like ours. He would have liked to understand how the tree of life influenced his body, and for that purpose would have needed access to medical knowledge. James formulated the principles, although he did not burden his discussion (which is probably an edited summary of the longer original debate) with examples. No medical authority is cited in the text. But the fact that he made some use of concepts which echo medical theory (*restauratio, deperditio, calor naturalis, complexio*) stimulated my curiosity to look more closely into the theologians' perception and presentation of Adam's physiology in the State of Innocence. If James was representative of his period and intellectual milieu, I expected to find some medical contribution to the debates concerning Adam's immortality and impassibility.[3] And indeed I did.

Then came Peter Biller's study of the origins of the idea of sex-ratio.[4] Biller did two things which are crucial to our theme. First, he masterfully mapped the way and provided a model for future research for every medievalist willing to cope with scholastic texts (in particular *Sentences* commentaries) as historical sources. Secondly, he showed that the discussions of distinction 20 in Book II of Lombard's *Sentences* were occasionally saturated with high-level natural–philosophical and medical knowledge. Moreover, he drew my attention to the general discussions of paradise extending over distinctions 19 and 20 in these commentaries. More than teaching us about the perception of paradise in a given period, these commentaries divulge valuable information about the contrasting postlapsarian world, the real world. The counterfactual and conditional question of what life and marriage would have been like if the first parents had not sinned allowed the commentators to reconsider (and display their knowledge of) a series of questions related to the human body, its physiology, its generation, its longevity, its appetites. I am following in his footsteps when I explore the commentaries on certain aspects of distinction 19, namely Adam's perfect health and consequent immortality. In limiting myself to this aspect of the physiology of Adam's body, I deliberately ignore the important question of the sexuality of the prelapsarian person, a question which demands a separate study.[5]

[3] E. Cohen, 'Towards a History of European Physical Sensibility: Pain in the Later Middle Ages', *Science in Context* 8.1 (1995), 47–74, (pp. 53–5).

[4] Peter Biller, 'Applying Number to Men and Women in the Thirteenth and Early Fourteenth Centuries: An Inquiry into the Origins of the Idea of "Sex-Ratio"', in *The Work of Jacques Le Goff and the Challenges of Medieval History*, ed. M. Rubin (Woodbridge, 1997), pp. 27–52; 'Confessors' Manuals and the Avoiding of Offspring', in *Handling Sin: Confession in the Middle Ages*, ed. P. Biller and A. J. Minnis, YSMT 2 (Woodbridge, 1998), pp. 165–87 (pp. 178–82); *The Measure of Multitude: Population in Medieval Thought* (Oxford, 2000), pp. 38–9, 89–104.

[5] P. J. Payer, *The Bridling of Desire: Views of Sex in the Later Middle Ages* (Toronto, 1993), esp. ch. 1, pp. 18–41. See also M. Müller, *Die Lehre des HL Augustinus von der Paradiesehe und ihre Auswirkung in der Sexualethik des 12. und 13. Jahrhunderts bis Thomas von Aquin* (Regensburg, 1954).

All this is, of course, tied to my general interest in the interaction between medical knowledge and religious thought in the thirteenth and fourteenth centuries, and to the plea I made in the conclusion of *Medicine and Religion*,[6] that one lacuna in that book – a systematic study of medicine in scholastic theological literature – should be filled one day. A small pilot study of a *quaestio disputata* of Nicholas of Ockham's debate about the assimilation of nutrition to the *Veritas humanae naturae* reinforced my belief in the fertility of this area of study.[7]

The following preliminary contribution will have to be continued, expanded, and perhaps corrected by other scholars. Among the minor themes of future study, but not pursued here, is, for example, theologians' reading of two of Aristotle's *Parva naturalia* which discuss death: *On Length and Shortness of Life* and *On Death*. My method is simple: a chronological study of commentaries on the *Sentences* of Peter the Lombard which I tracked down with the help of Friedrich Stegmüller's *Repertorium* and its updates.[8] For anyone interested in the history of medieval science, the second book of Peter the Lombard's *Sentences*, which discusses issues related to the story of Creation, is the entrance to a veritable gold mine. What I have assembled from commentaries on one *distinctio* alone merely skims its surface.

The Foundations of the Scholastic Discussions

Most Christians do not read the Old Testament for its own sake but with Christ and through Christ. It was St Paul who introduced what became the dominant Christian interpretation of the Fall of Man as a catastrophic change which ruined the close human relationship with God.[9] Wishing to make clear the completeness and finality of Christ's victory over sin, he created the typology of Adam and Christ, by which the total and unqualified gift of

[6] Ziegler, *Medicine and Religion*, p. 275.

[7] Ziegler, '*Ut dicunt medici*'. See also W. H. Principe, '"The Truth of Human Nature" according to Thomas Aquinas: Theology and Science in Interaction', in *Philosophy and the God of Abraham: Essays in Memory of James A. Weisheipl, OP*, ed. R. J. Long, PIMS, Papers in Medieval Studies 12 (Toronto, 1991), pp. 161–77 and Reynolds, *Food and the Body*.

[8] Stegmüller, *Repertorium*; V. Doucet, *Commentaires sur les Sentences: Supplément au Répertoire de M. Frédéric Stegmüller* (Quaracchi, 1954); J. Van Dyk, 'Thirty Years since Stegmüller: A Bibliographical Guide to the Study of Medieval Sentence Commentaries since the Publication of Stegmüller's *Repertorium Commentariorum in Sententias Petri Lombardi, 1947*', *FS* 39 (1979), 255–315; M. L. Colish, *Peter Lombard*, 2 vols., Brill's Studies in Intellectual History 41 (Leiden, New York and Cologne, 1994), I, 2 n. 2.

[9] This paragraph heavily relies on J. Barr, *The Garden of Eden and the Hope of Immortality* (Minneapolis, 1992), pp. 4–6, 16–17. See also J. Ratzinger, '*In the Beginning . . .*': *A Catholic Understanding of the Story of Creation and the Fall* (Edinburgh, 1995).

salvation through Jesus was the reversed image of the equally total and unqualified disaster brought about by Adam. The First Man sinned and transmitted sin to the entire human race. Consequently death followed. This directly led to Christ's death for sin and to his overcoming sin through overcoming death. According to the traditional Christian reading of Genesis 2, the first humans were sinless and free from all threat or reality of death. Through their one act of disobedience they immediately came under the total dominion of sin and became subject to the power of death. This reading is, however, incompatible with the Hebrew Genesis text which nowhere says that Adam, before his disobedience, was immortal.[10] According to the Hebrew text, the problem that Adam's disobedience created was that he brought near to himself the possibility of immortality – a divine property. This is the only reason why he and his wife had to be expelled from the Garden of Eden. This explains why the questions with which Christian theologians and exegetes were preoccupied regarding Adam's body before sin, find little if any echo among their Jewish counterparts.

My presentation of the state of Adam's body before the sin according to post-Lombard theologians must start with a brief look at the Patristic period, which laid the foundation for these discussions throughout the Middle Ages, and then some Carolingian biblical commentaries and several pre-Lombard sources of the twelfth century. In all these debates I shall limit my analysis to the particular medical or natural–philosophical elements which they include in the descriptions and explanations of Adam's body in the State of Innocence.

The pre-Lombard sources[11]

In his commentary on the book of Genesis, Augustine was intrigued by the fact that Adam was created immortal yet received nourishment from every seed-bearing herb and seed-yielding fruit (Genesis 1. 29). If Adam became mortal as a result of sin, surely before that event he did not need such food for his body, which could not be destroyed by starvation. It is difficult to find an answer for this question, complained Augustine, but he hinted at a possible solution. The First Man multiplied before sin. But multiplication cannot take place, so it seems, without coition and the corruption of lust, which characterize mortal bodies. However, it can be said that before sin there was a unique mode of multiplication which did not entail the corruption of lust and which was initiated by dutiful affection (*affectu pietatis*). Augustine thus hints that perhaps one should speak of a different mode of nourishment. But apart from rejecting the necessary consequence – that, through eating,

[10] A possible Hebrew antecedent of Paul is the Wisdom of Solomon 2. 23 which speaks of God who created man for incorruption and made him in the image of his own eternity.

[11] For a survey of some of the pre-Lombard sources on the original condition of man see G. Boas, *Primitivism and Related Ideas in the Middle Ages* (Baltimore and London, 1997), pp. 15–86.

Adam's body was corruptible – Augustine gave no further explanation of this particular mode of consuming food.[12]

Augustine also formulated the three essential questions which would engage theologians discussing the story of creation throughout the Middle Ages. His answers to them remained essentially valid in later periods.

1. Is the animate body (distinguished from the spiritual body) compatible with immortality? (*Quomodo ergo inmortale, si animale?*) Augustine replied that there is no necessary contradiction between the two characteristics of Adam's body: he could be animate before sin. Following a life of absolute justice (as was expected of him) his animate body would become spiritual, hence immortal.[13]

2. What is the nature of his immortality? Augustine decided that Adam's body before Sin could be reckoned at the same time mortal and immortal: mortal, because he *could* die (*quia poterat mori*); immortal, because he *was able* not to die (*quia poterat non mori*). It is one thing not to be able to die (*non posse mori*); it is quite another thing to be able *not* to die. It is by the second mode that Adam had been created, since it was offered to him to eat from the tree of life; this brought about his immortality, which was not part of his natural constitution (*non de constitutione nature*). Adam was mortal as a result of his animate condition (*mortalis erat conditione animalis*), but he was rendered immortal by the help of the creator (*beneficio creatoris*). So he was concomitantly mortal and immortal. Only a spiritual body such as we may have after the resurrection will be purely immortal.[14]

3. How can one define and explain the physical effect of the tree of life? Augustine speaks of the tree as a special corporeal food responsible for the body's long-term and stable health. Its particular power emerges from 'some secret inbreathing of healthiness' (*nonnulla inspiratio salubritatis occulta*).[15] As in the previous cases, Augustine identified the question and formulated the answer, but refrained from detailed biological analysis of the impact of the tree of life on Adam's mortal body. He left ample room for miraculous or divine explanations for the strange behaviour of Adam's body, which was animal, exactly like ours, yet at the same time immortal. Food was available to prevent hunger, drink to prevent thirst, and the tree of life was there to guard against old age and dissolution. There was no trace of decay in the body, or arising from the body, and no risk of disease from within or of injury from without. Man enjoyed perfect health in the body and complete tranquillity in the soul as a result of the divine gift of grace, which was transmitted via the tree of life acting upon the human body in a supernatural way.[16] We shall have

[12] Augustine, *De Genesi ad litteram* III.xxi.33; ed. J. Zycha, p. 88; *La Genèse au sens littéral en douze livres*, ed. and trans. P. Agaësse and A. Solignac, 2 vols., Bibliothèque Augustinenne, Oeuvres de Saint Augustin 7 (Paris, 1972), I, 264–7.

[13] Augustine, *De Genesi ad litteram* VI.xxii.33–xxiii.34; ed. Zycha, pp. 195–6.

[14] Augustine, *De Genesi ad litteram* VI.vi.36; ed. Zycha, p. 197.

[15] Augustine, *De Genesi ad litteram* VIII.v.11; ed. Zycha, pp. 238–9.

[16] Augustine, *De civitate Dei* xiii.20 and 23 (III, 308–10 and 314–22); xiv.26 (III, 456–8).

to wait until the twelfth century for more biologically or medically oriented thinkers who transcended Augustine's general assertions about the hidden (hence miraculous) powers of the tree of life. According to the simple Augustinian story there is no place for a question like that of James of Viterbo. But by determining the animate property of Adam's body, Augustine paved the way for centuries of future discussions.

The Ordinary Gloss on Genesis 2. 9 ('the tree of life also in the midst of paradise'), cites Walafrid Strabo (d. 849) specifically saying that the tree of life had the force (*virtus*) to defend the first man against any kind of disease, anxiety, or the symptoms of old age (both physical and intellectual) in a natural manner (*naturaliter*).[17] As early as the ninth century a natural explanation of the effect of the tree of life on Adam's body was certainly a legitimate possibility for every biblical commentator. However, I know of no real attempt to pick up this point in a systematic way before the end of the twelfth century. The interlinear gloss to the last words of Genesis 3. 22 ('therefore now, lest perhaps he put forth his hand and take also of the tree of life, and eat and live for ever') says: 'this [immortality], is God's action' (*hec dei actio est*) and implies that it was not the tree's natural capacity. In the gloss itself the two conflicting approaches coexisted, the natural and the divine.

In the 1230s, a sharp mind like Grosseteste's was acutely aware of the tension between the 'natural' approach and that of the Augustinian explanation which stressed the supernatural dimension of the story. In his *Hexameron*, Grosseteste quoted almost literally Strabo's words but attributed them to unnamed *expositores*.[18] He then proceeded to hail the miraculous effect of the tree of life which had this power of giving health by 'some secret inbreathing' (*inspiracione salubritatis occulta*), thus introducing the Augustinian terminology. Everyone familiar with the biblical stories about Elijah the prophet who was kept from the need of hunger for forty days by one cake (I Kings 19. 6–8) or about Christ's miraculous effects on oil and flour should not be surprised by this capacity of the tree of life, Grosseteste tells us, and he cites Augustine and Rabanus as his sources; Paschasius Radbertus (*c.* 790 – *c.* 860) was his real source here. There is an apparent contradiction between this and the contention (by Strabo) that the tree had a natural power ('quod videtur contrarium verbis supra dictis quibus dicitur quod hanc vim naturaliter habuit'). Grosseteste solved the problem by suggesting that the biblical and Patristic sources understood the word *naturaliter* in an unusual and distinctive way. The tree did not have this capacity by the nature that it

[17] *Biblia Latina cum glossa ordinaria*, I, 21. See also Hugh of Saint-Cher, *Postilla super Genesim*, in his *Opera omnia in universum vetus et nouum testamentum*, 8 vols. (Lyons, 1645), I, 4va, and Peter of Tarentaise, *In sententias* ii.17 (II, 139F), who quotes Strabo and Bede when he defines the tree of life.

[18] Robert Grosseteste, *Hexaëmeron* XI.iv.1, ed. R. C. Dales and S. Gieben, Auctores Britannici Medii Aevi 6 (Oxford, 1990), pp. 308–9 (English version, in Robert Grosseteste, *On the Six Days of Creation*, trans. C. F. J. Martin [Oxford, 1996], pp. 315–16).

had in common with other trees, nor was this power a specific difference that followed naturally from the general nature of trees. But as Augustine suggests, the tree of life had this power from 'the secret inbreathing of healthfulness', and because this power inhered in an inseparable way (*adherebat inseparabiliter*) it could be said to inhere in that tree *naturaliter*. Grosseteste sensed the problem of grace versus nature in the story of Adam, but was keen to remove it from sight.

In the fourteenth century Nicholas of Lyra (*c.* 1270–1349) would have to supply a much more elaborate explanation for Adam's physical condition. It was no longer sufficient to suggest that Adam as an animal needed food. In his commentary on Genesis 2. 9 ('And the Lord God brought forth of the ground all manner of trees, fair to behold, and pleasant to eat of') Nicholas first devotes some words to explaining why food is needed for the continuous animal life (*vita animalis*) which has been given to Adam.[19] Food is necessary in order to restore the moisture lost by the action of natural heat. But this restoration is not perfect because the new repaired condition was not equal (*non sit secundum equivalentiam*) to the original condition before the loss of moisture. Here Nicholas explicitly refers to Aristotle's water and wine analogy in *De generatione et corruptione* i.5, which compares the gradual weakening of the human flesh to the gradual weakening of wine when mixed with water until its final destruction. Then he moves on to explain what exactly was the contribution of the tree of life to Adam's immortality. Avoiding old age was merely the result of the tree of life's physical action on the body, which would restore its lost moisture to the perfectly balanced former condition before the loss ('ad hoc quod predicta restauratio fieret secundum equivalentiam'). In comparison with the earlier biblical commentaries this is an entirely different discourse. As we shall see, the change reflects the development of the theological debate during the thirteenth century.

The attempt to explain and visualize the biblical story of creation by inserting it into a biological or physiological framework did not start in *Sentences* commentaries. When answering the question why do men die, Adelard of Bath called God 'The Equal One' (*Equalis*), who created the soul in a most balanced manner (*equaliter*) so that it can be duly united with the body as long as the body is elementally balanced.[20] It has already been shown how twelfth-century theologians in their schools became proponents of a new

[19] *Biblia sacra, cum glossa ordinaria . . . et postilla Nicolai Lyrani* (Lyons, 1589), I, 68–70. See also Nicholas's general description of *status innocentie* on p. 67. Unlike angels, Adam was immortal and impassible by distancing himself from the causes of corruption and not by nature or intrinsic physical qualities. This ability was given to him directly by divine providence or through the intermediary of the powers of the soul. One of the external corruptive forces is the environment; this was mended by divine providence which created paradise characterized by temperate air and physical pleasantness.

[20] Adelard of Bath, *Questiones naturales* 43, in *Adelard of Bath, Conversations with his Nephew*, ed. C. S. F. Burnett, Cambridge Medieval Classics 9 (Cambridge, 1998), p. 172.

balance between grace and nature. Cistercian mystics like Willam of St Thierry and philosophers like William of Conches gave physiological and anatomical basis and substance to their discussions of spiritual matter and of the soul. Biblical commentators like Andrew of St Victor came to express the role of nature in the story of creation more boldly than before.[21]

The visionary writings of Hildegard of Bingen present us with one such earlier attempt. They suggest that the abbess, in her own peculiar way, assimilated into her analysis of the story of creation and Adam's sin the principles of Arabic Galenism recently introduced to the Latin West by Constantine the African.[22] Hildegard visualized Adam's body with the aid of rudimentary humoral theory. And though her account is not as sophisticated as the thirteenth-century explanation, she shows that the attempt to understand with the aid of medical concepts the story of creation – and in particular of Adam's prelapsarian and postlapsarian body – was already there in the twelfth century. In *Causae et curae* she described the effect of Adam's sin as the stripping of physical perfection and purity from his body. The Fall modified his pure blood to such an extent that instead of purity he started emitting the foam of his poisonous semen. Adam before Sin did not have superfluous phlegmatic humours which are the cause of many diseases today. Hence his flesh remained flawless as long as he did not sin. After the Fall, the humours became unbalanced, the melancholy temperament predominated, and diseases arose.[23]

Along the Augustinian lines, most twelfth-century theologians agreed that Adam was mortal by his nature, but conditionally immortal. To this belief they attached the conviction that his body performed all the physiological and metabolic functions (internal and external) that characterize an ordinary human body today. Though he suffered no physical pain, disease, hunger, or thirst, his body needed food for sustenance.[24] Had he not sinned he could have become a spiritual being, but 'the body of Adam before Sin was animal, that is mortal . . . Hence everyone who in order to live needs food and such things is said to be animal.'[25] It is in this period that the term *complexio* begins

[21] M.-D. Chenu, 'Nature and Man: The Renaissance of the Twelfth Century', in *Nature, Man, and Society in the Twelfth Century: Essays on New Theological Perspectives in the Latin West*, ed. and trans. J. Taylor and L. K. Little (Chicago and London, 1968), pp. 1–48 (pp. 16–18, 34–5); B. Smalley, *The Study of the Bible in the Middle Ages* (Notre Dame, 1970), p. 144.

[22] D. Jacquart, 'Hildegard et la physiologie de son temps', in *Hildegard of Bingen: The Context of her Thought and Art*, ed. C. S. F. Burnett and P. Dronke, Warburg Institute Colloquia (London, 1998), pp. 121–34; Boase, *Primitivism*, pp. 75–7.

[23] Hildegard of Bingen, *Causae et curae*, ed. P. Kaiser (Leipzig, 1903), pp. 33, 36 (chapters on Adam's fall and on diseases).

[24] Lottin, *Psychologie et morale*, IV.1, 15–16 (for Anselm of Laon), 21–2 (for William of Champeaux). For Anselm of Laon see also F. P. Bliemetzrieder, 'Trente-trois pièces inédites de l'oeuvre théologique d'Anselme de Laon', *Recherches de théologie ancienne et médiévale* 2 (1930), 54–79 (p. 55).

[25] 'Corpus Adae ante peccatum erat animale, id est mortale . . . Unde et animale dicitur omne quod, ut uiuat, cibis et talibus indiget': Anselm of Laon, *Liber pancrisis*, in

to be employed to describe the physical transformation which Adam underwent due to Sin. Thus according to Anselm of Laon (d. 1117), in his *Sententie divine pagine*, Adam's transgression of the divine command resulted in weakening and corruption of his complexion as a punishment.[26]

Position 51 in Abelard's *Sic et non* is entitled 'That the first parents were created mortal and that they were not' (*Quod primi parentes sint creati mortales et non*) and it summarizes the main questions twelfth-century theologians asked about the physique of the prelapsarian person. It reflects the powerful impact of the Augustinian approach, which marginalized the natural interpretation of the story of the terrestrial paradise.[27] Abelard ascribes to Augustine the notion that Adam's body was not indestructible and that only the eating from the tree of life prevented its corruption. But in what way did he have an immortal body, if this body was sustained by food? For he who is immortal needs neither food nor drink. Abelard's reply is entirely Augustinian: the immortality was not natural; it was brought about by the tree of life which acted as a medicine preventing bodily corruption. He introduces other passages from Augustine supporting the idea that the first man ate (albeit not meat), that his body, which was of earth, was *animale* (and hence was mortal), and that had he not sinned his body would have turned into a spiritual body (*in corpus fuerat spirituale mutandus*) allowing him to assume a mode of incorruptibility, which is the privilege of the saints and the faithful (like Enoch and Elijah) before the resurrection. Under such circumstances, Adam would not age. He ate from the leaves of trees to sustain his body and from the tree of life to prevent senescence. He was therefore mortal by virtue of the condition of the animal body that he possessed, but immortal by virtue of divine favour. The explanation is entirely Augustinian, and so is the lack of any real attempt to weave into the debate natural philosophical concepts or arguments.

Peter the Lombard

Like their predecessors, most of the theologians of Peter the Lombard's time gave pride of place to the soul of prelapsarian man, its faculties, and its attributes. They had far less to say about the human body. This is indicative of their strongly hierarchical assumption about the human constitution. Dismissing the claim that the investigation of human nature before the fall is a matter of vain curiosity, Peter the Lombard concurred with the idea that human sexuality was the chief topic to be considered under the heading of

Lottin, *Psychologie et morale*, V, p. 37 no. 41. See also pp. 26 no. 24 and 37 no. 39 for more references to the behaviour of Adam's body.

26 'Adam transgressus est mandatum dei, ex illa transgressione complexio fuit debilitata et corrupta in pena peccati et omnes partes eius debilitate sunt': F. P. Bliemetzrieder, *Anselms von Laon Systematische Sentenzen*, BGPTM 18. 2–3 (Münster, 1919), p. 33; Lottin, *Psychologie et morale*, IV.1, pp. 35–6 n. 4.

27 Peter Abailard, *Sic et Non: A Critical Edition*, ed. B. Boyer and R. McKeon (Chicago, 1976–7), pp. 226–8. See also his *Expositio in hexaemeron*, in *PL* 178, 776–7.

man's physical nature. Agreeing that prelapsarian man had the capacity to die or not to die and the ordinary functions of life in his body, such as the need to eat and drink, he placed human sexuality in the same naturalistic perspective. For Peter the conception, gestation, birth, and growth of offspring, together with all of man's other natural processes (eating, drinking, sexuality), are a good and essential part of the creation, not punishment for Sin. Just as the body itself is not a defect or a consequence of Sin, so the natural physical functions and processes are not a defect.[28]

Let us briefly examine the Lombard's discussion in distinction 19.[29] After explaining in chapter 2 that the phrase according to which man has been made a living soul means that he had *corpus animale* that needed food, the Lombard discusses in chapter 4 whether immortality was a natural condition or the result of divine grace ('Utrum immortalitas quam habuit ante peccatum esset de conditione naturae an ex gratiae beneficio?').[30] The wholly Augustinian reply is that insofar as man could die (*posse mori*) he was a natural being and had a natural body. But as regards not being able to die (*non posse mori*) this quality was in him from the tree of life, namely from the gift of grace ('ex ligno vitae, scilicet ex dono gratie').

The Lombard then asks in chapter 5, 'if Adam had not been commanded to eat from the tree of life and from other trees and if he had not eaten from them, would he have been able not to die?'[31] Some say, the Lombard tells us, that even without eating he would have lived forever, but it seems to others that the tree of life was the cause of his immortality. The tree of life, which he has described earlier as a source of divine grace, represents for him the supernatural option. The Lombard unfolds the two conflicting approaches but makes no decision, and leaves the doubt as to the exact source of the immortality unresolved.

Chapter 6 summarizes the opinions concerning Adam's immortality.[32] The Lombard attributes the question and the solution to Augustine. But the real source in this case is Bede, who described the process by which man would reach (by food) the size and the numbers allotted to him by God and then would need no more food. Thus it seems that the flesh of man had *in se* the quality of immortality which would be maintained by the sustenance of food until he was transferred to a better status, when he would eat from the tree of life and become entirely immortal (*omnino immortalis*). Hence some (*aliqui*) say that he had immortality *a natura* (by which he had the potentiality not to

[28] Colish, *Peter Lombard*, I, 355–6, 368; II, 731.

[29] Peter the Lombard, *Sententiae*, ii.19; I, 421–7. See also distinction 17, ch. 4 (I, 414–15), where the Lombard gives a short explanation (based on Bede and Strabo as they appear in the Ordinary Gloss).

[30] Peter the Lombard, *Sententiae* II.xix.4; I, 424.

[31] Peter the Lombard, *Sententiae* II.xix.5; I, 424–5: 'queritur si non esset preceptum ut de ligno vite ederet, et aliis et non illo vesceretur, numquid posset non mori?'

[32] Peter the Lombard, *Sententiae* II.xix.6; I, 425–7: 'De hac vero hominis immortalitate, qualis fuerit . . .?'

die – *poterat non mori*), which was conserved by eating from the other trees but which could not be completed (*consummari*) without eating from the tree of life. Food in general could sustain the body (*corpus sustentare*) but the tree of life would strengthen it with unfailing health. The Lombard's conclusion is ambiguous: 'as in his nature he had some mortality, that is, an aptitude to die, so he had some sort of immortality in his nature, that is, an aptitude by which with the help of food he could not die; but had he persisted [in his obedience] there would have been in him a perfect immortality from the tree of life'.[33]

A certain quality of immortality was naturally built into Adam from creation. But the Lombard makes no attempt to elaborate what this meant for the body's natural composition, disposition, and function, and he uses no concepts taken from medical theory or natural philosophy. The tree of life only completed the natural quality of immortality. But at the end of his commentary the Lombard adds the following warning: those who transmit this opinion should carefully inquire how they do not contradict Augustine, who had said that the first man was immortal from the tree of life ('quod erat immortalis ex ligno vite'). The question is thus left unsolved: was immortality natural or supernatural? Was Adam created 95 per cent immortal and did the tree of life serve only to make him *omnino immortalis*? Or was the tree of life the sole or main cause of his potential immortality? Although the Lombard only partially supported a natural explanation for the physical reality of the State of Innocence, his ambiguity launched a long debate about the natural element in Adam's immortality. From then on, Lombard would represent in many discussions of the topic those who stressed the natural explanation and minimized the supernatural explanation that attributed everything to grace through the tree of life. Nature has been introduced to the story of the State of Innocence, and it was now up to the Lombard's commentators to elaborate more in this direction.

The early post-Lombard discussions

In the last third of the twelfth century the famous and successful master at the cathedral school in Paris, Simon of Tournai (d. *c.* 1201), twice discussed in his *Disputationes* questions related to our topic. *Disputatio* X starts with the following question: Was the immortality of Adam before sin given or a gift, that is, was it conferred by nature or grace? ('Utrum immortalitas Adae quam habuit ante peccatum fuerit datum vel donum, id est naturale vel gratuitum'). Two quotations from Peter the Lombard (which support the notion that Adam's immortality was natural) and one from Augustine (which supports the notion that grace rather than nature was the source of

[33] 'Ex quo consequi videtur quod, sicut in natura sui habuit mortalitatem quandam, scilicet aptitudinem moriendi ita aliquam immortalitatem in natura sui habuit, id est aptidutinem qua poterat non mori, cibis adiutus; sed si perstitisset, immortalitatis perfectio esset ei de ligno vitae': Peter the Lombard, *Sententiae* II.xix.6; I, 426–7.

Adam's immortality) reveal at the outset the dialectical reality, according to Simon.

Simon's answer – that Adam's immortality was both natural and by grace – uses the concept of a fully balanced complexion (*complexio equalis*) in which Adam was made and which Simon equates with Adam's immortality, since it prevented him from dying. This complexion was in him by nature, but was insufficient on its own to assure immortality. It provided the starting point on the way to immortality, but it needed to be maintained and this maintenance was provided by the tree of life. The punishment for sin was not robbing Adam of his natural qualities, but rendering his complexion imbalanced (*complexio inequalis*).[34]

Parallel to Simon or perhaps a few years earlier Alain of Lille (d. 1203), in his Summa *Quoniam homines* (compiled *c.* 1160), used the same concept of *complexio equalis* to describe Adam's body before the Fall and to stress nature's role in providing him with perfect health. He also used the concept when explaining the particular influence of the tree of life on Adam's body.[35] To my knowledge this is the first time that this concept of a fully balanced complexion appears in theologians' discussions of the State of Innocence. It is impossible to determine with certainty from which source Alain or Simon drew the term. Was it their own original invention, some kind of refinement or improvement of the use of the term *complexio* in theological debates (use of which I found starting at the beginning of the century in the school of Laon)?[36] Or was it drawn from some medical source with which they had

[34] 'Adam creatus fuit in complexione equali. Complexio vero equalis dicta fuit eius immortalitas, quia ea aptus natus erat ad non moriendum. Hec autem equalis complexio naturalis erat ei. Quod enim dicit auctoritas: *Adam fuisse immortalem non de conditione nature, sed de ligno vite* [Augustine, *De Genesi ad litteram* VI.xxv.36], sic concipitur: non conditione nature tantum, sed ligno vite cooperante. De conditione enim nature tantum habuit complexionem equalem, sed usu ligni vite complexio corroboranda erat in sua equalitate, nisi pecasset Adam; sed merito peccati homo ipsi relictus est, Deo qui dederat equalem complexionem non conservante eam in sua equalitate. Merito ergo peccati complexio Adae facta est inequalis, ingruentibus molestiis nimii caloris, nimii frigoris, et aliis. Non ergo per peccatum privatus est naturali, sed in eo vulneratus, quandoquidem complexio non est sublata, sed inequalis facta': J. Warichez, *Les "Disputationes" de Simon de Tournai: Texte inédit*, Spicilegium sacrum Lovaniense 12 (Louvain, 1932), p. 41. See also *Disputatio* 49 (pp. 141–5), which concerns *status innocentie* and introduces a medical analogy (a comparison between the seriousness of leprosy and acute fever) to explain his distinction between *gravis in se* and *gravis pernicie.*

[35] P. Glorieux, 'La Somme "Quoniam homines" d'Alain de Lille', *AHDLMA* 28 (1953), 113–364 (pp. 290, ch. 151, and 294, ch. 154). See also Alexander Neckam (1157–1217), *De naturis rerum* ii. 156, ed. T. Wright, RS 34 (London, 1863), p. 250, who speaks of Adam's most temperate complexion (*complexio temperatissima*) which was responsible for his health and longevity.

[36] Theologians were already familiar with the concept of equal complexion as a fully balanced condition in the 1120s. See for example William of Saint-Thierry (*c.* 1085–1148), *De natura corporis et animae*, in *PL* 180, 696–7: 'Itaque in corpore animali sua propria est complexio prima et naturalis in ipso elementorum conjunctio: quae si

become familiar? Here I particularly refer to Haly Abbas's medical compendium translated under the title *Pantegni* by Constantine the African (died before 1098/9).[37] For Simon *complexio equalis* is equal to immortality. As we shall see shortly, this notion was absolutely incompatible with the medical understanding of the concept as formulated by the physicians. Furthermore, beyond the introduction of the concept itself into the narrative, there is no indication that Alain or Simon borrowed anything from Avicenna's detailed discussion of equal complexion.[38] Be this as it may, from the last third of the twelfth century the concept of *complexio equalis* was introduced into debates about immortality as an explanatory tool for those wishing to stress the natural elements in Adam's immortality. Within two generations or so it would force some theologians to remove the apparent contradiction between their way of understanding the concept and the physicians'.

Commentators from the first third of the thirteenth century contributed little to the 'medicalization' of the debate about Adam's immortality. Stephen Langton[39] (d. 1228), William of Auxerre[40] (who composed his *Summa aurea* after 1215 and before 1229 and died in 1231), Philip the Chancellor[41] (who died in 1236, and whose *Summa,* which was one of the sources for Alexander of Hales's *Glossulae,* was composed possibly between 1225 and 1228), Roland of Cremona OP[42] (who composed his commentary in 1234 and was very much influenced by Hugh of Saint-Cher), Hugh of Saint-Cher OP[43] (who read the *Sentences* in 1230–5, composed his commentary in 1230–2 and died in 1264) all asked various questions about the nature of Adam's immortality and impassibility and about the tree of life, but did not provide a description or explanation substantially different from Peter the Lombard's. When discussing the nature and quality of original sin, they occasionally used the concept of *complexio* as an accident which affects the behaviour of the soul. In considering the uniqueness of original sin with respect to other sins they all

aequalis est et bene composita ut contraria non impugnentur vel destruantur a contrariis, sed calida temperentur a frigidis, frigida a calidis, sicque de reliquiis, bona fit complexio et consentiente natura fit eucrasia, bona scilicet temperantia quatuor qualitatum.'

37 Haly Abbas, *Pantegni*: *Theorica* i.7 (*De divisione complexionum*), in *Omnia opera ysaac* (Lyons, 1515), fol. 2rb–va.

38 Avicenna, *Canon* I.i.3.2; fol. 3rb–va.

39 *Der Sentenzenkommentar des Kardinals Stephan Langton*, ed. A. M. Landgraf, BGPTM 37.1 (Münster, 1952, repr. 1995), pp. 88–9.

40 William of Auxerre, *Summa Aurea*, ed. J. Ribaillier, 4 vols. in 5, SB 16–20 (1980–7), II.1, 244–50. On the *Summa*, see the *Introduction générale* in this edition's last part, SB 20.

41 Philip the Chancellor, *Summa de Bono*, ed. N. Wicki, 2 vols., Corpus philosophorum Medii Aevi 2, Opera philosophica Mediae Aetatis selecta (Bern, 1985), I, 299–314.

42 Paris, Bibliothèque Mazarine, MS 795, fol. 54rb ('De corruptione carnis'). His commentary includes no question on *Distinctio* 19. When he discusses the corruption of Adam's body he uses the term *armonia* (not *complexio*); Lottin, *Psychologie et morale*, VI, 171–80.

43 Paris, BnF, MS lat. 3073, fols. 43ra–44ra; Stegmüller, *Repertorium*, I, 174–5.

came up against this puzzling question: if original sin is one and equal among all humans, why are some more prone to sin than others? All inclinations to sin are equal among all people, Hugh of Saint-Cher tells us, yet one person is more prone to sin than another. This is due to an accidental variable (*propter adiuuans annexum*) which is the individual complexion of each person. A person of sanguine complexion, for example, is more inclined to the sin of lust than a choleric person.[44] Complexion became important in explaining varied inclination to sin.

The Turning Point of the 1240s–60s

Two theologians among those active in the 1220s and 1230s should be noted, the first, William of Auvergne (*c.* 1180–1249), because of his highly original views, and the second, Alexander of Hales (*c.* 1186–1245), for his introduction into the discussion of hitherto unknown medical arguments.

William of Auvergne did all he could to demystify paradise and the tree of life. When discussing in *De universo*[45] the capacity of the tree of life to conserve life and endow the person with immunity from death, he posed two questions which allowed him to discuss the natural aspects of the tree of life.

First he asks: If someone said that all healthy food has this vital power to preserve life (*virtus vitalis vite conservativa*), I would say this is true, but it (the other food) does this only partially and temporarily and not perpetually. Death would occur at the end of *status innocentie* but would come not as a punishment but as a blessing because it would allow the passage (*translatio*) from terrestrial to celestial paradise.

He goes on to warn his readers of the fables and fantasies of the Jews (*fabulis et deliramentis Hebreorum*) concerning the tree of life. According to William, their description of the tree involved its legendary huge size (more than the size of the whole earth), its extraordinary loftiness, which reached the distance of a journey of five hundred years, and its tendency to move around (*dicunt quod arborem vite ambulasse*).[46] By so doing, he implied that

[44] 'Omnes pronitates, quantum est de se, sunt equales in omnibus, tamen unus pronior est ad peccandum alio, sed hoc est propter adiuuans annexum, ut sanguineus colerico cuius complexio inclinat ad coitum magis . . .': Lottin, *Psychologie et morale*, IV.1, 128. For a similar view by Roland of Cremona see p. 133. See also p. 135 for a similar view (based on William of Auxerre) of an anonymous *Summa*, and pp. 139–40 n. 2 for the definition of *pronitas peccati* made by Guerric of Saint-Quentin.

[45] William of Auvergne, *De universo* 1.i.59 'De ligno vite, quod est creatum in medio paradisi scilicet propter quid lignum vite dicatur', in *Opera omnia* I, 676; see also *De sacramento eucharistie*, in *Opera omnia* I, 440, col. 1F.

[46] For the Hebrew Agada which was the source for William of Auvergne's critique see L. Ginzberg, *The Legends of the Jews*, 7 vols. (Philadelphia, 1954), I, 70, 131–2 and the Talmudic references cited there. This Agada is quoted in Maimonides, *The Guide of*

the tree of life was more like all other fruit-bearing trees than a supernatural giant tree, except that the salubrious efficacy of eating its fruit is perpetual or at least long-lasting. The fact that he introduced death to the State of Innocence is also unique and difficult to reconcile with the common Christain exegesis of Scripture. To us however it is important to emphasize that such views reinforce the natural approach to Adam's existence in the State of Innocence. The tree of life is not only a vehicle for divine grace, it is first a natural tool for the prolongation of life. This is reiterated in the second question which William introduced in his discussion of the tree of life.

If someone asks how (*qualiter*) it could have such power to protect both innocent people and sinners from death, he should know that myrrh, aloe, balsam, salt, and many other things prevent corpses from putrefaction for a long time after death; many medicines prolong life, whether by preserving the natural moisture (*naturalis humiditas*) and the life-bringing heat (*vitalis calor*) or by purging or restraining those things which expose the body to the dangers of death. Other medicines have the effect of renewal (*renovatio*) and are not only preventive. Thus the flesh of serpents, which is called *thir* (theriac), has such power and 'this you can know by experience' (*experimento istud cognoscere potes*). William himself testifies that he has personally heard of such cases. Therefore, 'it is not marvellous if the tree of life or its fruit had the power to preserve human life' ('non est igitur mirabile si arbor vite vel fructus ejus virtutem habebat conservativam vite humane'). The reduction of the marvellous to a necessary minimum is patent. Over two centuries later Denis the Carthusian (d. 1471) would cite these lines almost word for word in his commentary on the *Sentences*.[47]

Alexander of Hales is the second theologian active in the 1220s and 1230s who in his commentary on the *Sentences* made a significant new contribution

the Perplexed ii.30, which may have been the partial source of William's words. On William's use of Maimonides see J. Guttmann, *Die Scholastik des dreizehnten Jahrhunderts in ihren Beziehungen zum Judenthum und zur jüdischen Literatur* (Breslau, 1902), pp. 15–17, and Ch. Merchavia, *The Church versus Talmudic and Midrashic Literature [500–1248]* (Jerusalem, 1970), p. 352 [in Hebrew]. I am grateful to Charles de Miramon for this reference. Notes 35, 36 and 47 benefited from his advice as well.

47 Denis the Carthusian, *In IV libros sententiarum*, in his *Opera omnia*, 44 vols. in 42 (Montreuil-sur-Mer, Tournai and Parkminster, 1896–1935), XXII, 157. At p. 191, when he discusses the question, 'Utrum homo in statu innocentie potuit tolerare aliquod malum poene?', he speaks of the concurrence of the *virtuositas complexionis* of Adam, the virtuosity of the tree of life, and the virtuosity of original justice as the key to the soul's ability to prevent the loss of radical humour as well as the weakening of the natural heat. He attributes this opinion to Thomas of Strasbourg and to a certain Richardus (Middleton?). For an early twelfth-century echo of the same approach that calls people not to marvel at the special power of the tree of life, when the bible tells of mandragora that cured Rachel of sterility and the medical books of the gentiles report that Asclepius cured and revived his patients by means of herbal medicine, see Rupert of Deutz, *De trinitate et operibus ejus libri xlii – in Genesim* iii.30, ed. H. Haacke, CCCM 21 (1971), p. 271.

to the style of the debate.[48] Most of the following discussion is based on the treatise *De corpore humano* which is appended to the *Summa Theologica* attributed to Alexander. Today we know that he was responsible only for part of the *Summa* which was continued and edited by his disciples at the Franciscan *Studium* in Paris in the late 1240s. *De corpore humano* may have been added to the text as late as the 1260s.[49] When I cite Alexander of Hales as the source of the following discussion, I mean the school of Alexander of Hales.

Alexander devotes a whole *titulus* to discussing whether and in what way Adam's body was composed of equally balanced mixed elements (*ex elementis mixtis secundum equalitatem*). There are three kinds of equality, by mass or weight (*molis vel ponderis*, quantitative), by power (*virtutis*, qualitative), and by justice (*iustitie*), and accordingly he divides his discussion into three respective parts, each of which analyses one of these. I shall adhere to the original structure of Alexander's discussion.

He starts by discussing the existence of *equalitas molis*. Let us look at one argument from this debate. The premise of the third argument *Contra* (which asserts the existence of *equalitas molis*) is the notion that Adam's body was created in a way that was suitably adapted to receive the rational soul. According to al-Ghazali, the more perfectly balanced an elemental combination is the more it is suitably adapted to receive and sustain the rational soul. According to Constantine in *Pantegni,* an elemental combination is balanced (*equalis*) when it contains equally quantities and qualities of the constituent elements. Fusion of the two authorities produces the conclusion that Adam's body was *equalis secundum molem*.[50] Haly Abbas's *Pantegni* (translated by Constantine the African) was thus part of the pool of sources available to theologians who dipped into it at their discretion to support this or that argument.

Alexander's solution determines that there are two kinds of complexional balance (*duplex est equalitas complexionis*). The first, which exists only in thought (*secundum rationem*) and not in reality and hence never existed in Adam, involves a perfect quantitative and qualitative balance of constitutive

[48] Alexander of Hales, *Glossa in quatuor libros sententiarum petri Lombardi*, 4 vols., BFSMA 12 (1951–7), II, 165–74; Alexander of Hales, *Summa* II, 528–43, 686–91.

[49] V. Doucet, 'The History of the Problem of the Authenticity of the *Summa*', *FS* 7 (1947), 26–41, 274–312 (pp. 310–11).

[50] 'Item ut habetur ab Algazel, "cum commixtio elementorum fuerit pulcrioris et perfectioris equalitatis" etc., tunc est corpus aptum ad susceptionem anime rationalis; sed constat quod corpus Adae fuit aptum ad susceptionem anime rationalis; ergo in illo erat commixtio elementorum in perfectiori equalitate; sed, ut habetur a Constantino, in *Pantechni*, equalis est commixtio elementorum que continet equaliter quantitates et qualitates elementorum. ergo etc': Alexander of Hales, *Summa* II, 529. Alexander later removed Constantine from the debate by saying that Constantine had expressed himself there 'secundum rationem quam secundum rei existentiam': Alexander of Hales, *Summa* II, 530; cf. Haly Abbas, *Pantegni*: *Theorica* i.7, in *Omnia opera ysaac*, fol. 2rb–va.

elements in addition to a perfect level of temperance in each individual element. The second kind of balance is that which may present qualitative excess, but an excess which still does not surpass the limit of the second degree, up to which, according to the *physici*, a perfectly balanced complexion is said to be safe.[51] This is *equalitas a iustitia*, which was in Adam's body. But by *equalitas a iustitia*, says Alexander, we do not mean the same thing as the *physici* do ('Non tamen intendimus de equalitate a iustitia hoc modo, hoc est in sensu quo utuntur physici sed alio modo'). Alexander will return to this point when he discusses separately *equalitas a iustitia*.[52]

Then he moves on to investigate whether the elements in Adam's body were equally balanced *secundum virtutem qualitatum*. The *Quod sic* arguments start with a specific reference to Constantine's definition of equal complexion which represents equality of elemental qualities. Equality of elemental qualities represents equality of power. But since an equal complexion was in his body, it was equally balanced *secundum virtutem qualitatum*.[53]

Among the arguments *Contra* one finds the following. If there had been such a balance in Adam he would have been able to live without food. Why then was he ordered to eat? Alexander solves the problem by distinguishing two sorts of equality of powers (*equalitates virtutum*). The first, which does not exist in mixed bodies, is absolute equality of elemental powers which are rooted in the elements themselves. The second equality of powers, which existed in Adam's body and contributed to his optimal complexion and most perfect health (*optima complexio et perfectissima sanitas*), is measured in relation to contrary elements in the mixed body which normally spark a continuous process of action and passion that weakens the body. This process was neutralized in Adam's body, but it was not the entire cause of his longevity, which required the fodder of the fruit of paradise.[54]

Alexander then discusses two separate questions, first whether heaviness and lightness were equally present in Adam's body, and then whether heaviness was predominant in his body. Here another medical authority is used to back the notion that some bodies are composed of matter where

[51] 'alia est equalitas, in qua, licet qualitatis vel qualitatum sit excessus, non tamen ultra metam secundi gradus extenditur, secundum quod dicunt physici quod complexio equalis dicitur incolumis usque ad secundum gradum': Alexander of Hales, *Summa* II, 529; cf. Avicenna, *Canon* I.i.3.1 (fols. 2–3). I did not find such an expression in Avicenna. But the general discussion and the distinction between two sorts of equal complexion is Avicennan.

[52] See p. 220 below.

[53] 'Complexio equalis ponit equalitatem qualitatum elementarium, ut habetur a Constantino, equalitas qualitatum elementarium ponit equalitatem virtutis; in Adam autem fuit equalis complexio; ergo etc. Equalis autem complexio est que qualitates elementares equaliter continet in se vel quando cum moderatione ducitur corpus incolume': Alexander of Hales, *Summa* II, 531.

[54] For an interesting discussion of whether the first parents or anything else could be incorruptible by virtue of *equalitas secundum virtutem* see Nicholas of Ockham, *Quaestiones*, q. 3, pp. 107–44.

heavy elements like earth and water are predominant, others are composed of matter where light elements like air and fire are predominant, and still further others are composed of matter where the four elements are equally present and hence are equally light and heavy. All this is attributed to Isaac's *De dietis universalibus*. Those who support the idea that Adam's body was neither light nor heavy combine Isaac's distinction with two notions: first, the belief that a complexion whose harmony is situated at a middle point is better than one whose harmony is situated towards one of the extreme points, and secondly, the conviction that Adam had the best possible complexion. They reach the logical conclusion that heaviness and lightness were equally present in his body.[55] According to Alexander, *ratio medii,* which leads to equality between heaviness and lightness, should be criticized (*vituperabilis*) because it automatically implies the existence of *equalitas mollis,* hence a qualitative imbalance, which could not be the case in Adam's body. He then gives a detailed explanation of Isaac's words (including a further citation from the text) to show that Isaac was interested in explaining the varied tendencies of living bodies to be stable (for example, trees and plants), to be highly mobile, or to move with great difficulty (the case of the turtle). Isaac's words are thus irrelevant in the particular context of the debate about the equal complexion.

According to Alexander the quality of heaviness dominated Adam's body. One of the arguments in favour of the opposite position is that human life is maintained by vital heat and moisture. They dominated Adam's body and assured his life; but they are light elements, so lightness was the dominant quality. Alexander – who states that the matter from which the body is composed (earth and water in the case of Adam) is the determinant factor, which renders heaviness dominant in Adam – has to refute this argument. He asserts that the heaviness which predominates in Adam is an expression of divine wisdom; if it were lightness, this would mean the predominance of heat in his complexion, and excess heat would cause the swift destruction of the body.[56]

[55] '*Utrum gravitas et leuitas erant in corpore Adae secundum equalitatem.* De primo sic: 1. Ut habetur a Philosopho, scilicet Isaac, in *Dietis universalibus* quedam sunt que componuntur ex materia cui dominantur elementa gravia, scilicet terra et aqua; quedam que componuntur ex materia cui dominantur elementa levia, scilicet aer et ignis; quedam que componuntur ex materia cui equaliter dominantur quatuor elementa, et hec sunt equaliter gravia et levia . . . Illa autem complexio que tenet proportionem et harmoniam in ratione medii, melior est illa que tenet harmoniam et proportionem in ratione extremi . . .; igitur, cum primi hominis erat complexio optima, erat in equalitate gravitatis et levitatis': Alexander of Hales, *Summa* II, 533; cf. Isaac Israeli, *De diaetis universalibus* 29, in *Omnia opera ysaac*, fol. 63ra.

[56] He adds to his refutation the following remark: 'Nota tamen hic quod secundum physicos duplex est caliditas naturalis: una elementaris, et ista non est medium in participatione vite; alia est que resultat ex oppositione elementorum ad invicem et ex confractione qualitatum, sicut ex commixtione elementorum resultat mixtum'; Alexander of Hales, *Summa* II, 535–6.

Alexander then moves to discuss *equalitas a iustitia*, which he had only mentioned in the beginning of his discussion. He opens with a direct reference to physicians and tries to differentiate their way of understanding and using the concept of *equalitas a justitia* from the theologians' way. His declaration is accompanied by a direct quotation from Avicenna's *Liber canonis*. 'We are not concerned here with the same equality with which physicians are concerned. [The medical equality] is observed in respect of the measure of elements with their quantities and qualities being in the optimal proportion that human nature should have. Of [this equality] Avicenna says . . .'. Here Alexander introduces a literal citation from Avicenna's definition of *equalitas iustitie* from the *Canon's* chapter 'On the complexions of the organs', where Avicenna rejected the possibility of the natural existence of a perfectly balanced complexion.[57]

Let us first look at the medical understanding of *equalitas iustitie* and then proceed with Alexander. According to Avicenna, though human complexion is the most temperate among all animals (the skin, especially that of the hand at the tip of the index finger, is the most temperate organ in the body), it can never be measured with respect to an ideal value of a humoral balance. God gave this complexion (or complexions) to man and his organs, as he did to all other animals, but it is measured by comparison with other organs, with the normally healthy state of an individual body and not against an ideal, quantitatively measurable value of balance. No complexion is absolutely temperate as such, but only temperate with respect to something comparable. A temperate medicine, Avicenna tells us, is not really temperate, for such a thing is impossible.[58]

So what is complexion according to medical theory? Complexion is the result of the action and passion of the constitutive particles of a certain elemental combination. The friction between the particles which put their forces (*virtutes*) and qualities into operation is a sum balance which is the

[57] Avicenna, *Canon*, I.i.3.2, fol. 3rb ('De complexionibus membrorum'); Arnau de Vilanova, *Speculum medicine*, ch. 3 'De complexionibus', in *Opera* (Lyons, 1520), fol. 2ra. On the idea of a perfect complexion in learned medicine see Michael McVaugh's discussion in *Aphorismi de gradibus*, ed. M. R. McVaugh, *AVOMO* 2 (1975), pp. 20–2, and Jacquart, *Médecine médiévale*, pp. 391–402; see p. 393 and n. 167 on the Galenic origins of the distinction between *equalitas ponderis* and *equalitas iustitie* (Galen *De complexionibus* i.6, in *Burgundio of Pisa's Translation of Galen's "De complexionibus"*, ed. R. J. Durling [Berlin and New York, 1976], p. 30). The concept of *iustitia* as a fully balanced, healthy condition has Hippocratic roots in the noun *dike* and the adjective *dikaios* (for example see Hippocrates, *On Fractures* 1, in *Hippocrates with an English Translation*, Loeb edn [Cambridge, MA, and London, 1923–], III, 94–5, which speaks of restoring a fractured bone *hypo tes dikaies physios* [according to the right nature]; I am grateful to Orna Harari for this reference).

[58] 'Debes autem scire ultra hoc quod sciuisti quod cum dicimus de medicina quod est temperata nolumus dicere quod sit temperata certe, quoniam illud est impossibile; neque volumus dicere quod temperamento humano in sua complexione sit temperata': Avicenna, *Canon* I.i.3.1, fol. 2vb.

complexion of the combination.[59] The complexion, which is measured according to the same prime powers of the elements (i.e. hot, cold, wet, dry), can be logically divided into two kinds: first, *complexio equalis,* which I translate as a perfectly balanced or uniform complexion, such that the quantities of the contrasting qualities are fully balanced so that none dominates the others nor is it dominated by any other. The fully balanced complexion is a quality exactly in the middle of these contrasting qualities.[60] Second, a complexion which tends to one of the extreme ends of the registers cold to hot or wet to dry. That is, an absolutely hot complexion, or cold, or dry, or wet, or any possible combination of the four. But according to Avicenna, these two kinds of complexion have nothing to do with what medical teaching understands by *equalis complexio*. In fact, here the physician must believe the natural philosopher, that it is impossible to find such complexions, particularly in humans or their organs.[61]

Physicians do not speak of quantitative balance which has absolute values but of qualitative balance which has proportional values. In a well balanced body or a single organ the elements which compose it are expected to be in that proportioned quantity and combined quality required by human nature to allow it (the whole body or a specific organ) to have an optimal disposition, hence to function properly as expected. This complexion may well be near the ideal point of the *equalis complexio* mentioned above, but it will never be identical to it.[62]

Alexander of Hales knew the medical opinion about balanced complexion and *equalitas a iusticia,* and added to it a clear distinction between the medical and the theological ways of understanding it. Wishing to make it clear that he was not talking about the same *complexio a iustitia* which physicians used as a key concept when they were studying and treating their patients, he specifically stressed, 'But we are concerned with that equality which was in Adam by divine justice before Sin.'[63] Whilst physicians look for natural

[59] 'summa qualitas in toto earum similis que est complexio': Avicenna, *Canon* I.i.3.1, fol. 2ra.

[60] 'Quorum unus est ut sit complexio equalis: ita ut quantitates qualitatum contrariarum in complexionato sint equales, non superantes neque superate; et sit complexio qualitas in medio earum vere': Avicenna, *Canon* I.i.3.1, fol. 2ra.

[61] 'Quod autem in doctrina medicine consideratur equale aut extra equalitatem non est hoc neque illud; sed medicus physico credere debet quod equale secundum hanc intentionem quam diximus impossibile est aliquo modo inueniri quanto magis ut sit hominis complexio aut membri humani': Avicenna, *Canon* I.i.3.1, fol. 2ra.

[62] 'Debes autem scire quod equale de quo medici in suis inquisitionibus tractant, non est denominatum ab equalitate in qua equalitas cum pondere equaliter existit; sed denominatur a iusticia in diuisione; et hoc est quod in complexionato in primis attenditur, siue sit corpus totum siue membrum unum, ut sit in eo de elementis cum suis quantitatibus et qualitatibus mensura, quam humana natura habere debet secundum meliorem proportionis et diuisionis equalitatem': Avicenna, *Canon* I.i.3.1, fol. 2ra–b.

[63] 'Et non intendimus hic de huiusmodi equalitate, secundum quod physici intendunt, que attenditur penes mensuram elementorum cum suis quantitatibus

equality, he is after divine equality, or equality bestowed upon Adam by divine justice before he sinned. God is called *justitia* because he distributes things to everyone in due order with respect to measure, quantity, and beauty.[64] Alexander freely uses a term borrowed from medical theory. Though he understands it perfectly well and even accurately cites its medical source, he adapts it to the theological context and clearly differentiates between the medical and the theological ways of employing it.

Alexander's discussion of Adam's immortality includes the standard questions whether Adam was mortal or not and whether his immortality was from nature or grace.[65] The debate includes a curious incidental discussion of whether wild beasts, had they eaten from the tree of life, would have gained immortality as well. The answer to this question, which reminds one of similar eleventh-century doubts concerning the Real Presence in the Eucharist, is of course negative. Here Alexander adheres to the opinion that grace, not nature, is responsible for Adam's immortality. When he refutes those who suggest that the immortality was natural, because Adam from creation had a body in perfect equality and levelled qualities ('in perfecta equalitate et optima libratione qualitatum'), he cites three internal causes for death and the specific remedies for each. I shall mention only the first, because in discussing it Alexander introduces for the first time in this context the concept of radical and nutrimental moistures. Against the consumption of internal moisture, Adam ate from the trees of paradise. 'For the consumption of moisture is double, that is radical and nutrimental. The consumption of radical moisture was hindered by eating from the tree of life, which received its name because it increased that moisture in which life is rooted. The consumption of the nutrimental moisture was hindered by eating from the other trees of paradise.'[66] To the complexion given to man naturally should be added the pure soul given to him by divine grace and the

et qualitatibus in optima proportione quam debet habere natura humana, de qua dicit Avicenna: "Debes scire quod 'equale' de quo medici in suis inquisitionibus tractant, non est denominatum ab equalitate, in qua equalitas cum pondere equaliter existit, sed denominatur a iustitia in divisione: et hoc est quod complexionatum in primis attenditur, sive sit corpus totum sive sit membrum unum, ut sit in eo de elementis cum suis quantitatibus et qualitatibus mensura, quam humana natura habere debet secundum meliorem proportionis et divisionis equitatem".' Sed intendimus de illa equalitate que fuit in corpore Adae a divina iustitia ante peccatum': Alexander of Hales, *Summa* II, 536; cf. Avicenna, *Canon* I.i.3.1, fol. 2ra–b.

[64] 'Divina iustitia est omnium commensuratio et ordinatio': Alexander of Hales, *Summa* II, 537.

[65] Alexander of Hales, *Summa* II, 686–91.

[66] 'Prima causa removebatur ab Adam per esum lignorum: nam duplex est consumptio humidi, scilicet radicalis et nutrimentalis. Consumptio humidi radicalis impediebatur propter esum ligni vite, quod ideo lignum vite dicebatur, quia per illud vegetabatur illud humidum in quo radicatur vita; consumptio vero humidi nutrimentalis impediebatur per esum aliorum lignorum paradisi . . .': Alexander of Hales, *Summa* II, 689.

tree of life, which together assured his immortality. The role of pure soul was more important than optimal complexion.

The detailed discussion of equal complexion (with direct reference to Avicenna) and the link between the tree of life and radical moisture are the two great contributions of the school of Alexander of Hales to the debate about Adam's immortality. From now on these two key terms in medical theory, complexion and radical moisture, would become standard in theologians' discussion of the topic.[67] Their introduction did not shatter the traditional arguments about the State of Innocence, but they created a more refined and exact picture of paradise and engulfed the debate in a medical and natural aura that rendered paradise and the life there less miraculous and more natural.

These medical categories had to be adapted to the traditional story, which accorded an important role to grace in assuring Adam's immortality. This 'medicalization' suggests a narrowing of the space devoted to miraculous explanations. The miraculous is not denied as such; it only loses some ground to natural explanations. This suits well the recent masterly treatment of attitudes to the marvellous by Lorraine Daston and Katharine Park.[68] Thirteenth-century theologians and natural philosophers were ambivalent if not occasionally hostile to unexplained natural wonders. Wonder became for them a taboo passion, a mark of ignorance, a characteristic of the old woman or the empiric. Consequently they tried to minimize and marginalize the marvellous or the supernatural. If this was done with natural *mirabilia*, it could be done with scriptural *mirabilia* as well, as is patent from the discussion of the State of Innocence.

The period of the introduction of these terms, the 1240s-60s, coincides perfectly with the time of the assimilation of Avicenna's *Liber canonis* into the academic medical milieu in the West. It suggests that theologians began to use the book at the same time as physicians, or shortly after, for their own purposes.

According to the general opinion of physicians in the thirteenth century, the art of maintaining health is not one that makes us immune from death; neither does it defend the body against external harm or grant bodies the greatest longevity. It can do two things: prevent putrefaction and defend the moisture against too rapid consumption. The purpose of all this is to allow a

[67] On the emergence of radical moisture as a key concept in theoretical medicine in the thirteenth century see McVaugh, '*Humidum Radicale*'; García-Ballester, '*Artifex factivus sanitatis*', pp. 131–3; Reynolds, *Food and the Body*, pp. 105–19; Ziegler, '*Ut dicunt medici*', pp. 217, 221.

[68] L. Daston and K. Park, *Wonders and the Order of Nature 1150–1750* (New York, 1998), esp. pp. 109–33. See also A. Boureau, *Théologie, science et censure au xiiie siècle: le cas de Jean Peckham* (Paris, 1999), esp. pp. 241–44, 257–87, 338–40, and 'La preuve par le cadavre qui saigne au xiiie siècle, entre expérience commune et savoir scolastique', *Micrologus* 7 (1999), 247–81 (pp. 256–71) for the infiltration of natural explanations concerning the phenomenon of the cadaver bleeding in the presence of the murderer.

person to live as long as has been predetermined by his complexion.[69] All this was highly useful for theologians trying to explain in a natural way Adam's immortality and the impact of the tree of life on his body. On the basis of this natural description and explanation, theologians could then use the same medical knowledge to allot grace its due place in the story. Adam was immortal partly because of his physical complexion and the physical effects of the food he ate. But all this did not and could not suffice to assure his immortality, which needed the supernatural touch. Physicians denied the natural possibility of immortality, but medical theory could account for extremely long life. Medicine could serve both those upholding the role of grace (and rejecting natural immortality) and those upholding the role of nature (and defending the biological explanation of the impact of the tree of life on Adam's body).

The Medicalized Story

The medicalized story of the State of Innocence after Alexander of Hales revolved around three topics: the balanced complexion, a detailed discussion of the causes of death according to the physicians, and a natural explanation of the efficacy of the tree of life with recourse to the concepts of radical and nutrimental moistures. It usually appeared in the commentaries on distinction 19 of Peter the Lombard's *Sentences* as part of the article treating the creation of Adam's body.[70] I now proceed to a thematic survey of the story of Adam's existence in paradise in order to uncover the scope of the medical input into the debate.

Adam's complexion

Usually a separate question specifically asked whether Adam's body had been constituted from elements which had been in a state of equal complexion and composition. The negative (or partially negative) reply relied very much on a medical authority, namely Avicenna. Adam was created with a fully balanced complexion (*complexio equalis*) or had an optimally complexioned body (*corpus optime complexionatum*). This elemental equality was not quantitative (*equalitas ponderis,* in Avicenna's words) but according to the equality of justice (*secundum equalitatem iustitie*), namely natural justice as it is exhibited by the ordered nature of creation. The theologians happily endorsed the medical and natural philosophical view that *equalitas a pondere* cannot be detected in nature, and consequently they decided that it could not

[69] Avicenna, *Canon* i.3, c. *Singulare,* fol. 53ra.

[70] For the rough sketch of the story I mainly use the *Sentences* commentaries of the Dominican Peter of Tarentaise, later Pope Innocent V, from the late 1250s, *In sententias* ii.17 (II, 145) and ii.19 (II, 158–62), and the Franciscan Bonaventure, *In sententias* ii.17 (II, 424–6) and ii.19 (II, 464–74), also found in his *Opera theologica selecta,* 5 vols. (Quaracchi, 1934–65), II, 436–9, 477–87.

have been found in Adam. They accepted the medical definition of *equalitas a iustitia* which is measured in terms of scope (*latitudo*) and degree (*gradus*), and not in terms of a single, ideal point of balance (*equalitas punctalis*). The distinction was sometimes attributed to unnamed natural philosophers and physicians ('sicut distinguunt naturales et medici') or specifically to Avicenna. Towards the end of the thirteenth century there were theologians who gave a specific reference which included the fen number ('fen' was the name of a 'part' of the *Canon*) and sometimes chapter number.

One of the clearest examples of this tendency is the Franciscan William de la Mare, a disciple of Bonaventure; a Regent Master in Paris in 1275, he died in 1298. He begins his reply to the standard question (whether the elements in Adam's body were in a state of equal complexion) thus: 'I answer according to Avicenna, in his book *On medicine,* book 1, Sentence 1 doctrine 3, chapter one, that equality is double . . .'. He then lays out the Avicennan idea of what is complexion *a pondere* and *a iustitia* along the lines of Bonaventure, and he ends his discourse with Avicenna's words from the second chapter about complexions: 'God gave man the most temperate complexion which is possible in this world.'[71] William's subsequent reply, that there was no equal complexion in Adam because there is no such thing in nature, relied entirely on Avicenna, who became a theological source.

To reject the acceptance of a simple complexional equality in Adam (a belief which most theologians wished to refute), some theologians introduced into the debate the notions, specifically attributed to physicians, that heat and moisture are the principles of life, and that in Adam's body, exactly as in a normally functioning body, certain organs are particularly hot (the heart and liver) and others are dominated by specific humours. The heart and the spirits are the beginning of life and both are excessively hot. Furthermore, moisture is the basis of growth.[72] The body cannot be an

[71] 'Respondeo secundum Avicennam, libro suo *De medicina* li. 1., sent. 1., doctrinae 3. ca. 1., quod duplex est aequalitas, scilicet a pondere et a iustitia . . . Aequalitas autem complexionis a iustitia secundum Avicennam est ut complexionatum "sive totum corpus sive membrum corporis sit de elementis cum suis quantitatibus et qualitatibus mensura quam humana natura habere debet, scilicet meliorem proportionis aequalitatem", et hoc "cum homo eam habuerit vere aequalitati est vere propinqua", et infra: "Donavit autem Deus homini complexionem temperatiorem quam in hoc mundo possibile est esse." Haec verba sunt Avicennae': William de la Mare, *Scriptum in secundum librum sententiarum* xvii.5, ed. H. Kraml, Veröffentlichungen der Kommission für die Herausgabe ungedruckter Texte aus der mittelalterlichen Geisteswelt 18 (Munich, 1995), pp. 224–5; cf. Avicenna, *Canon,* I.i.3.2, fol. 3rb. See also the anonymous commentary in Paris, Bibliothèque Mazarine, MS 925, fol. 27v (ascribed to Nicholas of Ockham).

[72] See for example: 'Vita est per calidum et humidum, et omnis operatio animae in corpore est per calorem, sicut dicunt naturales et medici; sed in corpore Adae anima habebat expeditas operationes: ergo magna erat ibi abundantia caloris: ergo praedominabatur calidum; et si hoc, ergo non erat perfecta aequalitas complexionis. Item, etsi complexio hominis est deteriorata, tamen non est totaliter corrupta; sed nos videmus quod cor per naturam est calidissimum et hepar similiter; et quaedam

ideal middle point of elemental qualities for it must be hot and moist more than cold and dry.[73]

The theologians who adopted the medical concept of *equalitas a iustitia* for their explanation of Adam's physique probably understood the term *iustitia* differently from the physicians. While for physicians like Avicenna it was a purely natural concept (meaning the order of nature by which every combination is composed in a specific balance according to the due proportion and the requirement of the introduced form), the theologians added to the concept *iustitia* a supernatural dimension by linking it to the biblical context, as did Anselm of Canterbury. Anselm, who was quoted by Bonaventure in his commentary on distinction 19, equated *iustitia originalis* with *donum gratie,* which was the opposite of everything existing *a natura.*[74]

The fact that Adam did not have a perfect complexion (*equalitas perfecta*) meant that some inter-elemental activity had taken place. This, however, was problematic because action immediately entails passion; and passion can theologically be perceived only as a postlapsarian punishment. Here too a medical authority was of help. In an anonymous commentary, which may possibly be ascribed to the Franciscan Nicholas of Ockham (*c.* 1242 – *c.* 1320), the author asserts that not every elemental activity in a compound is a punishment ('non omnis accio elementorum in mixto est pena') but only that which is felt by the senses (*sensibilis;* its by-product is pain). One of the authorities he cites in this context is Avicenna's discussion in the first book of the *Canon* in a chapter entitled 'On pain'.[75]

According to Richard Fishacre (d. 1248), the first Dominican Master in Oxford whose *Sentences* commentary was compiled between 1241 and 1245, a

sunt alia membra in quibus regnat phlegma et melancholia: et tunc ita erat: Si ergo in corpore Adae erat praedominatio humorum, pari ratione et qualitatum elementarium: ergo non erat ibi perfecta adaequatio miscibilium': Bonaventure, *In sententias* (II, 424b, or *Opera theologica selecta* II, 437); cf. Avicenna, *Canon* I.i.3.1, fol. 2rb–va: 'Vite et enim principium sunt cor et spiritus; que quidem ambo vehementer calida existunt ad superfluitatem declinantia; et vita quidem existit per caliditatem et augmentum per humiditatem; et etiam caliditas in humiditate existit et ab ea nutritur.'

73 Richard Middleton mentioned the Avicennan principle and attached to it the biblical verse about the soul which is in the blood thus fortifying a biological definition of life with a biblical reference: 'Sicut enim supra dist. 17 ostensum est, qualitates elementares in corpore Adae non fuerunt in punctali equalitate equiparantie; quia ad hoc quod corpus sit animabile, maxime tam nobili anima sicut est rationalis, oportet quod caliditas et humiditas plus possint in corpore quam frigiditas et siccitas: quia vita hominis principaliter in calido et humido radicatur: unde quia sanguis inter humores calidus et humidus dicitur Levit. 17[.11] quod anima omnis carnis in sanguine est et accipitur ibi anima pro vita': *Super quatuor libros sententiarum* ii.19; 4 vols. (Brescia, 1591), II, 245.

74 Bonaventure, *In sententias* II.xix.3; II, 470.

75 'sicut patet in febribus unde dam. liber 2 c. 21 passio non facit dolorem sed passionis sensus. hoc idem dicit avicenna primo canonis c. de dolore': Paris, Bibliothèque Mazarine, MS 925, fol. 27r. Cf. Avicenna, *Canon* I.ii.1.19, fol. 38rb ('De causis doloris absolute'): 'Dicemus igitur quod dolor est sensibilitas rei contrarie.'

perfect complexional balance (*equalitas perfecta*) would exist in the State of Glory. An intermediate degree of complexional balance existed in the intermediate State of Innocence, namely a harmonious combination which, with some internal (soul governing the body) and external (eating) aid, prevented all elemental discord. Potentially this balanced complexion could be destabilized and destroyed, but *in actu* this could not happen as long as Adam remained obedient. Since not every loss is penal, acknowledging that Adam suffered some physical loss was not contradicting biblical truth that punishment came only after the sin. Richard Fishacre suggested that the effect of constant change of the flesh through eating is similar to the effect of constant change of air in the body through breathing: neither is penal.[76]

Some theologians were happy to show off in their debates their knowledge of other concepts taken from medical theory. When discussing Adam's potential corruption in *status innocentie*, an anonymous late thirteenth-century theologian (possibly Nicholas of Ockham) declared that he could preserve himself from the corrupting elemental battle; he could do it by the gift of natural justice, and he knew how to do it by acquiring and maintaining a suitable, harmonious mixture of natural things like food, drink, sleep, and the like.[77] Nicholas (or more possibly the scribe, since later on in the text he correctly uses the term *res nonnaturales*) made here an error in talking about *res naturales* when he should have been talking about *res nonnaturales* (namely the six nonnaturals which were the physiological, psychological, and environmental conditions held to affect health: air, exercise and rest, sleep and waking, food and drink, repletion and excretion, and accidents of the soul). But he implies what James of Viterbo openly acknowledged: that for his survival Adam needed medical knowledge of the correct regimen.

Despite its superior (though imperfect) complexion, Adam's body was identical in species and nature to our bodies. It underwent some loss (*deperditio*), for Adam ate, digested, and copulated. He even produced waste matter which would be excreted, but God would have provided against any offensiveness (*indecentia*) resulting from this necessity. But because of his complexion this loss was moderate and did not lead to the corruption of the whole body. Furthermore, not every local loss (*deperditio*

[76] 'non omnis deperdicio est penalis. Sicut retinere semper eundem aerem esset penale, renouacio vero per exspiracionem et inspiracionem delectabilis est, sic semper manere eandem carnem ex alimento et ipsam fluendo non renouari penale esset': Paris, BnF, MS lat. 15754, fol. 106ra.

[77] 'non sola contrarietas nec pugna est causa dissolutionis sed victoria unius contrariorum per aliquid excitans vel soluens prohibens et educens unum miscibilium magis ad actum quam alterum; ipse autem potuit et sciuit se preseruare ab illa victoria; potuit quidem per donum originalis iusticie et sciuit per contemperationem rerum naturalium ut cibi, potus, sompni et huiusmodi': Paris, Bibliothèque Mazarine, MS 925, fol. 30r.

particularis) is a cause for the corruption of the whole body (*deperditio universalis*).[78] Nevertheless, because of this loss Adam constantly had the potentiality of dying, a potentiality which was not activated until he had sinned.

Although theologians used medical authority to fortify their arguments, occasionally they were forced to go onto the defensive and clarify the difference between their use of the concept and the medical use. Thus for example, Richard Fishacre determined that Adam's body was an unusual elemental combination whose constitutive elements were fully balanced and at peace ('elementorum mixtio in qua nullum eorum agit in reliquum sed erit pax'). He based his discussion on a specific reference to Avicenna's *Liber canonis* where complexions were discussed.[79] But Fishacre did not feel at ease using a medical concept which Avicenna suggested could not be found in humans. He solved the problem by suggesting that Avicenna denied the natural possibility of having a perfectly balanced complexion because he had written his definitions regardless or ignorant of the state of paradise or the heavens.[80]

The causes of corruption/death

The story of the State of Innocence included a detailed discussion of the causes of death according to the physicians.[81] Physical corruption is intro-

78 Paris, Bibliothèque Mazarine, MS 925, fol. 30r.

79 'Unde dicit Avicenna libro 1: Complexio est duobus modis: unus est ut sit complexio equalis ita ut equalitates contrariarum sint non superantes nec superate et sic complexio est qualitas in medio earum nature; aliter est modus ut ad unam magis declinet extremitatum aut in contrarietatem que est inter caliditatem et frigiditatem aut in contrarietatem que est inter humiditatem et siccitatem aut inter utraque. Videlicet medicus phisico credere debet quod equale secundum hanc intentionem impossibile est aliquo modo inueniri sed complexio huic propinquissima est complexio optima humana': Paris, BnF, MS lat. 15754, fol. 106va; cf. Avicenna, *Canon* I.i.3.1, fol. 2ra.

80 Paris, BnF MS lat. 15754, fol. 106va. Adam's balanced complexion became such an essential explanatory tool that when medical opinion seemed to undermine it, theologians had to exercise all their wit and knowledge in order to save it. See, for example, the third *questio disputata* on human nature by Nicholas of Ockham from the academic year 1287/8 where he becomes a commentator of Haly's discussion in *Pantegni* of temperate and lapsed complexions. Nicholas of Ockham, *Quaestiones*, pp. 110, 125–7.

81 Peter of Tarentaise, *In sententias* II.xix.3; II, 64a. See also Giles of Rome who in the commentary on the second book of the *Sentences* (from 1308/9) used as a starting point for the discussion of Adam's immortality the physicians' and Aristotle's explanation of death. His explanation includes the lamp metaphor so popular in theoretical medicine for describing the process of dying. ' . . .vel si volumus assignare causam mortis sicut assignant medici et etiam sicut innuit Philosophus in *De generatione* quia fit continua deperditio in corporibus animalium, quia vita consistit in calido et humido et semper calidum depascit humidum et consumpto humido extinguatur, et moriatur animal sicut ignis in lucerna consumit humiditatem olei et consumpto oleo extinguitur lucerna. Secundum hunc autem modum

duced into our bodies by four biological causes: (1) inequality of primary complexion; (2) a slow failure of the radical moisture by the action of natural heat; (3) a weakening of natural heat due to the consumption of radical moisture and the constant admixture of nutrimental moisture;[82] (4) the inclination of contrary elements to fight each other and to separate to opposite regions. Adam's body, which was very well complexioned ('valde bene complexionatum erat'), was nevertheless exposed to these dangers. Against the first cause of death Adam enjoyed the greatest complexional equality. Against the second he ate food. Against the third he ate from the tree of life which strengthened and repaired the natural heat. The grace of innocence in the soul protected him against the fourth cause of death.

Here, however, there was some variety. According to Thomas, there were only two failures (*defectus*) threatening his body.[83] Against the first – the loss of moisture by the action of natural heat (*deperditio humidi per actionem caloris naturalis*) – man was sustained by eating of the other trees of paradise, exactly like us today. Against the second – the gradual decline of the *virtus activa speciei*, which after growth (*augmentum*) and full restoration of its losses (*restauratio deperditi*), causes shrinkage, and ultimately the natural dissolution of the body – the tree of life would sustain man. For it had the power to fortify the *virtus speciei* (the specific vital propensity of the body) against the weakness resulting from the admixture of extraneous matter.

According to another recurrent (Franciscan?) version there was one external cause for physical corruption – by external harm – against which Adam had angelic protection. But there were also three internal causes for death. Against the first – the action of the elements (*actio elementorum*) – Adam had the necessary knowledge to regulate to a full balance all things non-natural. Against the second – the consumption of the radical and nutrimental moistures by heat – he ate from the tree of life and the other trees of paradise respectively. Against the third – the weakening of the digestive power (*virtus digestiva*) – he had the tree of life as a remedy.[84]

The tree of life

Thirteenth- and fourteenth-century theologians tried to gain a better understanding of the function and the actual impact of the tree of life on the human body. They were no longer satisfied by the Augustinian explanation that the particular power of the tree emerged from a hidden cause like the 'secret

mortis loquitur Philosophus cum dicit quod carens colera est longeuum': Giles of Rome, *In sententias* ii.19; pp. 130–44 (p. 130).

82 Here the theologians regularly introduced the Aristotelian analogy of water added to wine. At first the water becomes vinous fluid, but as more and more water is added, it diminishes the strength of the wine until the wine becomes watery and is destroyed. Aristotle, *De generatione et corruptione* i.5, 322a10.

83 Aquinas, *Summa theologiae* Ia, qu. 97, art. 4; XIII, 144–9.

84 Paris, Bibliothèque Mazarine, MS 925, fol. 30v (possibly Nicholas of Ockham); William de la Mare, *Scriptum in secundum librum sententiarum*, pp. 249–50.

inbreathing of healthiness'. Some philosophers were puzzled how a perishable thing like the fruit of the tree of life could be responsible for causing imperishability, for nothing can act against its own *species* and a result can never exceed its cause.[85] But despite their reluctance to attribute to the tree of life a certain natural capacity to prolong life, thirteenth- and fourteenth-century theologians saw no harm in investigating the tree of life's natural dimension, and while engaged in this enquiry they made use of a variety of medical and natural philosophical concepts.

Some theologians suggested that the tree of life preserved the radical moisture from being consumed.[86] Others gave it a double role in restoring the consumed radical moisture and preventing the weakening of the digestive or transformatory power (*virtus digestiva* or *virtus convertendi*).[87] Some suggested that it rendered the nutritive power able to produce moisture which was identical to the radical moisture and was thus able to prevent the weakening of natural heat rooted in the radical moisture.[88] Several suggested that the tree of life was given not specifically as food, but as a nourishing agent for the digestive power, which by divine force was strengthened to such an extent that it could convert the nutrimental moisture to a moisture which was equal in its purity to radical moisture.[89] They all medicalized the explanation. But there were those who stuck to the ancient description and suggested that the tree of life gave the body the material disposition that removed from it all causes of old age, stifling of the organs,

[85] Paolo Cortese (Paulus Cortesius, 1465–1510; Stegmüller, *Repertorium*, I, 298–9) heavily criticized this 'Pseudo-Aristotelian group which attracts flocks of adherents like jackdaws that are attracted to a tower': *Libri iiii. in quibus . . . Magister sententiarum et eius loci reliqui habent* ii.6, De homine ante peccatum (Basel, 1504), pp. 45–7 (p. 45).

[86] Bonaventure, *In sententias* II.xix.3.1 (II, 470): 'Sed quia humidum radicale paulative consumitur nec potest reparari per quodcumque alimentum, ideo data est virtus specialis cuidam ligno, quod dictum est lignum vitae, per cuius sumtionem repararetur humidum radicale.' On the tree of life and radical moisture see Reynolds, *Food and the Body*, pp. 331–4.

[87] Paris, Bibliothèque Mazarine, MS 925, fol. 30v; Peter of John Olivi, *Quaestiones in secundum librum sententiarum*, ed. B. Jansen, 3 vols., BFSMA 4–6 (1922–6), II, 228–9. On Olivi's discussion of the topic see Reynolds, *Food and the Body*, pp. 432–4.

[88] '. . . poterat anima prohibere ne fieret tanta consumptio in radicali humido nec tanta debilitatio in naturali calido que restaurari non posset. Per efficaciam ligni vite cuius virtus erat tanta quod de illo poterat virtus nutritiua ipsius Adae cum adiutorio originalis iustitie generari humidum ita virtuosum ad conseruationem calidi naturalis sicut est humidum radicale': Richard Middleton, *Super quatuor libros sententiarum* II.xix.2; II, 245.

[89] 'ideo prouidit Deus de ligno vite que prohibebat impuritatem illam per hoc, quod modo mirabili confortabat et vigorabat digestiuam, unde non dabatur proprie in alimentum, sed etiam in nutrimentum virtutis digestiue quam Dei virtute vigorabat quod potest alimentum conuertere in humidum cibale aeque purum sicut humidum radicale': Peter Aureoli (OFM; d. 1322), *Commentariorum in primum (-quartum) librum sententiarum pars prima (-quarta)*, ed. C. Boccafuoco, 2 vols. (Rome, 1596–1605), II, 245B.

and putrefaction of the humours.[90] Yet even those who supplied a natural description of the impact of the tree of life on the body admitted that its efficacy was not purely natural; it was linked to the moral perfection of the eater and to divine will. Hence it would not have the same efficacy in the state of sin and would certainly not have created immortality in a sinner's body. Eating from the tree of life was natural (*per naturam*); however, the power impressed on it was supernatural, and occasionally it was compared to a sacrament because God's grace was inherent in it.[91]

In most discussions the radical moisture played a key role in explaining the efficacy of the tree of life. Occasionally it also assumed a role in explaining the physical results of sin. In his questions on the second book of the Lombard's *Sentences* Richard Kildwarby OP (d. 1279) determined that sin destroyed the material disposition in the radical moisture where human nature *secundum speciem* dwells and which created a potentiality for perpetuating the life. The primary agent of Adam's immortality was the particular disposition of his radical moisture which enabled the tree of life fully to restore it.[92]

All theologians I have examined allotted some role to grace as a variable in explaining Adam's immortality. But some turned grace into the core of their argument. According to Thomas Aquinas, Adam had no natural or formal imperishability and was said to be imperishable only on the part of the efficient cause (*ex parte cause efficientis*). His body possessed no particular force of immortality (*vigor immortalitatis*) which rendered it indestructible; but he was given in a supernatural way a force of the soul (*vis anime quedam supernaturaliter divinitus data*) which inhered in him as long as he remained obedient to the Lord and which was responsible for preserving his body from corruption. This force was given by divine grace.[93] Thomas does not mention radical moisture in this context. The power (*virtus*) to preserve the body would not be derived from the tree of life, which could not endow the body with a disposition of immortality either. Since the virtue of any body is finite, the virtue of the tree of life could preserve life for a certain length of time sufficient for the first man to survive intact until he either was transported to the spiritual state or needed to take another dose of the tree of life.

90 Albertus Magnus, *Commentarii in ii sententiarum*, in his *Opera omnia*, ed. A. Borgnet, 38 vols. (Paris, 1890–9), XXVII, 326–38 (pp. 333–5). See also pp. 489–90.

91 For example, 'aptitudinem habuit a natura ut semper uiueret, complectionem tamen habuisset a gratia': Paris, Bibliothèque Mazarine, MS 925, fol. 30r; Peter of John Olivi, *Quaestiones in secundum librum sententiarum*, II, 229.

92 Robert Kilwardby, *Quaestiones in librum secundum sententiarum*, ed. G. Leibhold, Veröffentlichungen der Kommission für die Herausgabe ungedruckter Texte aus der mittelalterlichen Geisteswelt 16 (Munich, 1992), p. 253. See also questions 84 (pp. 236–7), 89–90 (pp. 246–51).

93 Aquinas, *Summa theologie* Ia, qu. 97 ('De statu primi hominis quantum ad conservationem individui'), vol. 13, pp. 137–49. See also his *Scriptum super libros sententiarum magistri petri lombardi*, dist. xix, qu. 1, art. 2–4, in *Opera omnia* (Parma, 1856), VI, 556–9; J. B. Kors, *La justice primitive et le péché originel d'après Thomas* (Le Saulchoir, 1922), pp. 66, 84–94, 128–46; Reynolds, *Food and the Body*, p. 359.

In the first *Quodlibet* from Lent 1270, John Pecham OFM (d.1292) identified in the first parents' bodies a certain *habitus* which was responsible for their immortality. The tree of life did restore the radical moisture and maintain the natural heat, but this could not prevent corruption which was inherent in every mixed body by nature since nature never exceeds its own faculties. The supernatural *habitus*, which was added to Adam's vivifying soul and health, was given in order to bind the constitutive elements in due proportion.[94] Sin did not change man's nature but only deprived him of the *habitus* given to him by divine grace.

Conclusions

Peter the Lombard left the question of Adam's immortality open. The debate that then developed attempted to fill that lacuna. It had two areas. In the first the question was asked in what way (*quomodo*) Adam was immortal and tried to decipher the *conditio nature* which gave Adam a uniquely strong and healthy body. It stressed the natural setting for Adam's immortality and struggled with its limits. In the second there was analysis of the impact of the tree of life on Adam's body and apparent immortality, which was alien to his animal body. The standard debate fused both question and analysis into one explanation. Both approaches freely employed concepts borrowed from medical theory (equal complexion, radical and nutrimental moisture). In both approaches a natural or a supernatural emphasis was possible. But whilst the natural emphasis was marginal until *c.* 1200, thirteenth-century theologians seem to have been increasingly attracted to the natural causation of Adam's immortality, without denying the important role of grace. The rudimentary beginning of the introduction of some of the medical concepts into the discussions of the State of Innocence can be detected as early as the beginning of the twelfth century. But it was in the second third of the thirteenth century that medical theory was fully introduced into these debates.

A group of leading thirteenth-century theologians starting from Alexander of Hales and Richard Fishacre embarked upon an attempt to provide a

[94] 'Quia calor naturalis, qui est instrumentum anime, continue depascit humidum in quo est vita, et per consequens ipse calor depascitur et minuitur. Isti autem speciali modo corruptionis providebatur homini duplici via. Primo per esum lignorum communium paradisi quo restaurabatur deperditio humoris, sicut in nobis fit restauratio per cibos. Sed per lignum vite fiebat restauratio ipsius humidi radicalis et calor ipse vitalis fovebatur. . . . Sed quia corruptio ipsa corpori mixto est naturalis, maxime quia qualitates elementares sunt in maiori actualitate in ipso quam in aliis, ideo impossibile est quod virtute aliqua naturali perpetuitas daretur illi corpori, quoniam natura non excedit propriam facultatem. Et ideo supra vivacitatem anime et sanitatem eius habebat donum supernaturale et habitum aliquem quo poterat elementa in proportione debita continere . . .': John Pecham, *Quodlibeta quatuor*, ed. G. J. Etzkorn, BFSMA 25 (1989), pp. 37–40, (pp. 38–9).

natural description and, to a certain extent, an explanation of the reality of the State of Innocence and in particular Adam's immortality. This group included theologians from all religious orders as well as secular masters, but it is my impression that the Franciscan element was particularly strong. With the exception of Richard Fishacre, the great thirteenth-century Dominican theologians from Hugh of Saint-Cher through Albertus Magnus to Thomas were not particularly keen on this approach. On the standard question of whether Adam's immortality was natural the general reply was negative. But the description and detailed explanation of the miracle, which was described as a divine gift or supernatural benefice, was natural or according to nature (*secundum naturam*). It was linked to natural philosophical and medical concepts about the causes of death and healthy longevity. In the end, the efficacy of the miracle could be explained largely within the frame of the known natural order. Nevertheless, the primary causation of the effect of the tree of life was not natural or solely by nature (*a natura* or *per naturam*).[95]

Giles of Rome (d. 1316), for example, described meticulously the effect of food in general and the tree of life in particular on Adam's physical well-being, but determined that all this just looked to us as if it were natural (*quasi per naturalia*). Adam's immortality had a significant natural aspect, but at the same time for its perfection it needed a supernatural aid. To explain this, Giles brought to bear his extensive knowledge of embryology. A complexion pathologically imbalanced (*malitia complexionis*) in a way which prevents the person from living for a long time can occur either by the unfitness of matter, a defect of the natural principal agent, or the inordinate superiority of a certain contrary element. That is, when the seed does not find the menses well disposed, or when the seed itself is so defective that its weakness prevents it from overcoming the menses. This will create a defective foetus which will not have an equal balance, and consequently will not live long. The overabundance of heat can create a foetus so choleric that it will certainly not survive. All this one knows from nature. God, however, created Adam's body from the dust of the earth with none of these potential flaws but with a complexion that is most naturally geared to long life. Furthermore, he equipped Adam with natural instincts and impulses by which he knew when and what to eat so as to protect the capacity for immortality which had been installed in him. This complexion, however, did not suffice to ensure immortality, and Adam cannot be regarded as simply immortal by nature. It merely prepared Adam's capacity (*habilitas*) to receive the divine gift of immortality like those who have fine natural properties (*habentes bona naturalia*) and tend more easily to follow God's calling.[96] There is, according to Giles, a natural infrastructure for hearing and following the divine calling.

[95] On this distinction between *secundum naturam* and *a natura* see William de la Mare, *Scriptum in secundum librum sententiarum*, p. 250.

[96] Giles of Rome, *In sententias*, pp. 136–7.

Similarly, the Dominican John of Paris (Quidort), who commented on the *Sentences* between 1292 and 1296 as a bachelor of theology and regent master in Paris in 1304, determined that the *ordo originalis iustitie* contributed to the perfection of immortality. But most of his explanation of Adam's immortality is natural, consisting in an analysis of the effect of the tree of life on the humoral balance and the natural heat.[97]

Reading between the lines in some *Sentences* commentaries we can discern the dissatisfaction of physicians with any belief in naturally caused unlimited immortality. This medical notion served the theologians' cause for they could not reject the supernatural causation for Adam's immortality. The Franciscan Hugo of Novocastro (d. after 1322), who lectured on the *Sentences* in Paris between 1307 and 1317, devoted two questions to distinction 19. In the first he determined that Adam in himself was corruptible and could be corrupted (*simpliciter ex se corruptibile et poterat corrumpi*). The second question was whether Adam in terrestrial paradise could have lived forever. One of the two arguments which refute immortality is patently a medical opinion. It is certain (says Hugo), *secundum medicos,* that part of the radical moisture is always lost and that the lost part can never be fully restored by food which, *ut dicunt medici,* can only restore the nutrimental moisture, which slightly helps radical moisture. Hence it is impossible that from the power of the fruit of the tree of life, however frequently it is consumed, the life of the eater will be perpetuated.[98] The other argument in Hugo's commentary used the mixture of water and wine as an analogy for explaining the inevitable weakening of the power to convert food into the bodily nature in the act of conversion itself. Hugo's avowal is interesting indeed. He does not talk of *equalis complexio* in the State of Innocence, but pleads for recognition that man in that status could be kept alive for an extremely long time ('homo remanens in statu innocentie poterat tempore prolixissimo conservari'), surely longer than the long age of the first generations of mankind, as the Bible reports. Tough complexion (*fortis complexio*) accompanied by healthy food (*sanior cibus*) and temperate air were responsible for man's longevity. His particular complexion was responsible for the difference between him and the next generations, which lived for a long time, but not as long as he would have lived. Yet however extended his life span would have been, it would have had an end.[99] So his natural and biological properties would be only partially responsible

[97] 'Et in remedium huius datus fuit ei esus ligni vite, scilicet ad confortationem humidi radicalis et calidi. Perfectio autem immortalitatis erat ab intra, scilicet ex ordine originalis iustitie . . .': John of Paris (Quidort), *Commentaire sur les Sentences*, ed. J.-P. Muller, 2 vols., Studia Anselmiana philosophica theologica 47 and 52 (Rome, 1961–4), II, 151–2 (p. 152).

[98] Paris, BnF, MS lat. 15865, fols. 75vb–77va at 76va–b; Stegmüller, *Repertorium*, I, 170–2; R. Sharpe, *A Handlist of the Latin Writers of Great Britain and Ireland before 1540*, Publications of the Journal of Medieval Latin 1 (Turnhout, 1997), pp. 189–90.

[99] 'quantumcumque posset diu vivere tamen virtute huius loci et virtute fructus vita haberet terminum et peryodum . . .': BnF, MS lat. 15865, fol. 76vb.

for his immortality. The argument *contra*, which supports the immortality of Adam, discusses those noble places whose environment is such that they enhance longevity. Specifically he mentions islands in Ireland where death and the corruption of bodies were nonexistent.[100]

The infiltration of medical knowledge and opinion may account for the tendency of fourteenth-century theologians like Hugo of Novocastro to give up on the idea of proving Adam's immortality.[101] For if immortality is medically impossible, it is useless to try to explain or prove it. Instead, they suggested that he was merely given the natural disposition and was protected by divine providence to live long enough for him to be transferred to celestial paradise.

The Franciscan William of Nottingham (d. 1336) provides us with a good example of this tendency (though he certainly was not the first to think in such a manner).[102] William was a lector at the Oxford convent *c.* 1312 – *c.* 1314 before becoming Provincial Master (1316 – *c.* 1330).[103] Quoting Augustine's Genesis commentary, he suggested that 'some people add that some supernatural force (*virtus supernaturalis*) was given to the tree and endowed it with the power to cause such an effect'. William does not deny this view; he could not have done so (and in the third *questio* in this debate he does acknowledge that the tree of life had its efficacy 'non ex sua virtute naturali sed ex speciali divina virtute'). But by not overtly joining these *aliqui* here, and by suggesting that the fruit of the tree of life was eaten *frequenter* and not *ad hoc*, he seems to be making a real effort to reduce to a minimum the supernatural characteristic of the tree of life. Its influence was gradual, accumulative, and continuous, and it exerted effects which could be scientifically described and perhaps even partly explained. Its role was to enable man to survive until he was transferred to the *status glorie*. This immortality was thus only temporary and was not *simpliciter naturalis*; rather than immortality, it can be described as a substantial delay in the causes of death. Death and *status innocentie* dwelt

100 On the legendary islands off Ireland, see also Nicholas of Ockham, *Quaestiones*, pp. 115, 134–6, and Pierre de la Palud in Paris, Bibliothèque Mazarine, MS 899, fol. 134vb. Cf. Gerald of Wales, *Topographia Hiberniae* ii. 4, trans. J. J. O'Meara (Harmondsworth, 1982), p. 60; A. Graf, *Miti, leggende e superstizioni del medio evo* (Bologna, 1980), I, 23–4.

101 See also the discussion of the topic by the Franciscan John of Bassoles in his *In secundum sententiarum questiones . . .* (Paris, 1516), fol. 117vb. John explained that, *secundum medicos*, radical moisture can never be restored and hence he was adamant that Adam would have died in the State of Innocence if he had not been transferred on time to the celestial paradise. See also fol. 118rb and Duns Scotus, *Opera omnia*, ed. C. Balic et al. (Vatican City, 1950–), XIX, 181–6 (pp. 183–5).

102 See for example Giles of Rome (*In sententias*, p. 137), who determined that the tree of life could only prolong life, but without a supernatural gift could not confer immortality on Adam.

103 *BRUO*, pp. 1377–8; B. Smalley, 'Which William of Nottingham?', *Mediaeval and Renaissance Studies* 3 (1954), 200–38; M. Schmaus, 'Neue Mitteilungen zum Sentenzenkommentar Wilhelms von Nottingham', *Franziskanische Studien* 19 (1932), 195–223. Cambridge, Gonville and Caius, MS 300, fols. 147va–149ra at 148vb.

together, but never coincided de facto. The first man was exposed to the internal causes of death. God would have transferred Adam to the State of Glory before the necessary death which is the punishment for sin and hence would not be part of human life before Adam's Sin.[104]

This change in the perception of Adam's immortality led some theologians in the fourteenth century to deny the thirteenth-century commonplace that the tree of life had the natural capacity to convert food to the originally pure bodily substance. If it were true that the tree of life had such a nature as some allege, claims the Dominican Durand of Saint-Pourçain (d. 1334), nothing would have prevented this immortality from being natural and lasting forever.[105]

The scholastic urge to use the sciences of the trivium and quadrivium to push back the frontiers of mystery and enlarge the area of intelligibility emerged in the late 1050s, during the controversy between Lanfranc of Bec and Berengar of Tours over the explanation of the real presence of the body and blood of Christ in the Eucharist.[106] Lanfranc's argument was one of the first successfully to give full scope to the operations of the natural world. It satisfied a most powerful urge of his period: to improve the explanations of the mysteries of faith. Over the next two centuries the use of the sciences to clarify theological problems was to have many triumphs, one of which has been described in this essay.

It is necessary to stress that the surge of natural reasoning documented in this paper cannot and should not be simplistically interpreted as the triumph of reason over superstition. The attempt to recruit scientific knowledge concerning nature in order to prove the truth of holy texts is characteristic of some fundamentalist groups in a variety of religions today. It is not necesarily a sign of their rationality; on the contrary, it can be the sign of naive, rigid, and even manipulative reading of the texts. The medicalization of the descriptions of the State of Innocence in the thirteenth century did not amount to a rejection of the Augustinian insights into the story. The theologians of the thirteenth century introduced no dramatic theological innovations to the interpretation of the story of paradise. But they added

[104] Duns Scotus, *Opera omnia* XIX, 185: 'Unde dico quod possibile est quod simul stent innocentia et mors in primo homine, ita quod fuisset mors in statu innocentie; tamen de facto numquam simul stetissent'; John of Bassoles, *In secundum sententiarum questiones*, fol. 118r. Gabriel Biel (d. 1495, one of the founders of the University of Tübingen where he taught between 1484 and 1491) rejected this opinion and alleged that the tree of life had the power perpetually to preserve human life in the State of Innocence. Experience (*per experientiam*) drawn from the physical behaviour of ill and healthy people proves his opinion: *Collectorium circa quattuor libros Sententiarum*, ed. W. Werbeck and U. Hofmann (Tübingen, 1973–), II, 417–24 (pp. 420–2).

[105] Durand de Saint-Pourçain, *In quattuor sententiarum libros questionum plurimarum resolutiones* II.xix.1 (Paris, 1508), fol. 183rb. See also his discussion of impassibility in Adam at fols. 182rb–184ra.

[106] R. W. Southern, *Saint Anselm: A Portrait in a Landscape* (Cambridge, 1990), pp. 44–50.

scientific depth to it and reflected the intellectual needs of a milieu which was no longer satisfied with simple, general, and wholly supernatural explanations.

Here I would like to reiterate a remark I made in an earlier study where I drew attention to an apparent 'English connection' in the phenomenon of theologians who incorporated medical knowledge into theological debates.[107] The above presentation invites the same remark. The Englishmen Alexander of Hales, Richard Fishacre, William de la Mare, Nicholas of Ockham, Richard Middleton (possibly), and William of Nottingham all stand at the forefront of theologians whose discussions of the State of Innocence were saturated with high level medical knowledge and exact citations and references from medical texts. But is the English origin of these theologians a significant variable, or is it just a coincidence? Would not their stay in Paris for studies or teaching be more significant? At this stage I must leave these questions unanswered.

The biological approach in describing the State of Innocence infiltrated other domains of religious discourse. This makes an independent study pertinent. One short example taken from the sermon literature can illustrate this. Giovanni da San Gimignano OP (d. 1333) stressed before his clerical audience in Siena that the human body in the State of Innocence would not have been exempt from the laws of nature. In the terrestrial paradise, various types of people would have been born, depending on the changing disposition of the air and the variable astral constellations. Uniformity would not be its characteristic. Some people would be stronger, bigger, more beautiful, or with a better complexion than others. But the variety could never amount to a defect which would damage either body or soul.[108]

Another fruitful area of inquiry for those interested in the infiltration of medical and biological concepts into theological debates is the discussion of the functioning of Christ's body and the perception which often appears, that he had a perfectly balanced complexion. Here I will only summarize a question that appears in John Pecham's third *quodlibet*, possibly in the

[107] Ziegler, '*Ut dicunt medici*', pp. 234–5; Reynolds, *Food and the Body*, pp. 213–14. Cf. R.W. Southern, *Robert Grosseteste: The Growth of an English Mind in Medieval Europe*, 2nd edn (Oxford, 1992), pp. xxxiv–xxxix, on a distinctive twelfth to early thirteenth century 'English scientific tradition'.

[108] 'Preterea etiam corpus humanum non fuisset ita exemptum a legibus nature, quin ab exterioribus agentibus aliquod commodum aut auxilium reciperet magis vel minus. Cum etiam cibus eorum vita substentaretur. Et sic nichil prohiberet dicere quin secundum diuersam dispositionem aeris et diuersum situm stellarum, aliqui robustiores corpore generarentur quam alii et maiores et pulchriores et melius complexionati; ita tamen quod illis qui excederentur nullus esset defectus vel peccatum siue circa animam siue circa corpus': Giovanni da San Gimignano, *Opusculum . . . de quibusdam materiis predicabilibus de operibus sex dierum predicatum ab eo in adventu domini in conuentu senarum*, sermo 17, De productione hominis et complemento operis vi diei (Paris, 1512), fol. 53ra.

Advent of 1270. It is asked concerning the blood that Christ emitted as sweat when 'being in an agony, he prayed the longer' (Luke 22. 43): was this sweat natural? Seemingly it was not. For the cause of a sweat of blood, according to Aristotle, is natural, namely a complexional flaw or humoral residue (*defectus complexionis vel excessus*). But there was in Christ an utmost equality (*summa equalitas*), so it could not be natural in his case. The counter-argument determines that one of the forces in Christ's soul was able to expel every humoral superfluity. But in Christ's body there was an aggregation of superfluity because he used food in the most perfect way. Hence his sweat was natural. It was not the result of an imbalanced complexion but of an ideal mechanism of digestion. Pecham's solution – that the sweat of blood in Christ was natural – describes in a quite scientific way the physiological effects of Christ's passion. His agony affected the humoral constitution of his heart and led to the concentration of blood around it. This blood was consequently dispersed to the other organs through the action of the heat and emitted in the form of a sweat which was mixed with blood. Secondly, Christ imagined the forthcoming bloodshed and according to the physical law that imagination moves the humours, his blood, moved by his imagination, was dispersed outside the body in the form of sweat. And thirdly, his most noble complexion was highly refined and delicate, and consequently was particularly disposed to efficient evaporation of residual humours.[109]

The *Sentences*-commentary was the key literary genre for theologians well into the sixteenth century. For the infiltration of medical knowledge into theological debates it is thus a historical source of long duration. I have mainly looked at the thirteenth century, the period in which the questions, the key arguments, and the patterns of using medical concepts and authorities were formed. Someone else will perhaps one day look more systematically at the later commentaries.[110] I shall close this paper with one fascinating early sixteenth-century example. It shows better than all the commentaries since Alexander of Hales how far theologians were incorporating medical terms, theories, authorities, even daily experience to substantiate their arguments.

The commentary is that composed between 1509 and 1517 in Paris by the Scottish-born John Major (Mair) (*c.* 1469–1550).[111] John Major, a philosopher

[109] John Pecham, *Quodlibeta quatuor*, Quodlibet iii.4 , pp. 139–40 (cf. Roger Marston, Quodlibet iv.12, in *Quodlibeta quatuor*, ed. G. F. Etzkorn and I. C. Brady, BFSMA 26 [1968], p. 390); see also Quodlibet iv.41, pp. 263–6 (from early 1277): 'Utrum corpus Christi descendat in stomachum.' See also the question, 'Would Christ have died of old age if he had lived long enough and had not been violently killed?', in Dietrich von Freiberg, *Opera omnia*, ed. K. Flasch et al. (Hamburg, 1977–), III, 365–6. On the debates about Christ's body after the crucifixion see Boureau, *Théologie, science et censure*, pp. 87–136.

[110] Few natural explanations survive in seventeenth-century descriptions of paradise. See P. C. Almond, *Adam and Eve in Seventeenth-Century Thought* (Cambridge, 1999), pp. 42–4, 190–1.

[111] John Major, *In sententias* ii.19 (fols. 54vb–56ra); Stegmüller, *Repertorium*, I, 226; *The*

and theologian, is regarded as one of the last exponents of scholastic philosophy. He concluded his arts course in Paris in 1496 and became Doctor of Divinity in 1505. After a teaching period in Paris he returned in 1518 to Scotland to take up the post of principal of the university of Glasgow before transferring briefly to St Andrews. After a further short period in Paris, he returned to St Andrews *c.* 1531, and became Provost of St Salvator's College. His discussion of Adam's immortality entails many minor additions to the arguments we have already met. He rejects the analogy of the mixture of water and wine and the debilitating effect of the water on the wine, an analogy which was so frequently used by those describing the gradual weakening of natural heat and other bodily substances and powers as a result of nutrition. Nutrition should be compared to adding fire to existing fire so it does not automatically weaken the body. He compares the tree of life to good food which generates good *chyme*. He explains that though Adam ate no meat and drank no wine (both dietary essentials for longevity because they generate good blood), the fruit and water of paradise were different in terms of nutritional value from our fruit and water nowadays and more nourishing than the meat we eat today.

The geographical setting of paradise (closeness to the sun and good air quality) enhanced the superior quality of the fruit. The proof for this is the well known fact that the side of the apple which faces the sun ripens more quickly, and the side of trees facing the sun is easily recognizable in the woods. Citrus trees (*mala aurea*) grow more easily in hot regions, and oranges (*mala punica*) from Egypt are much better than those from the countries of the West (Italy or Spain). In paradise there were two temperate summers and two temperate winters; hence fruit of some kind was ripening there on the trees around the year. Neither vines nor oranges grow in Britain as they do in Spain, Italy, and Marseilles; other good fruits come from Africa and none of the Western countries have them. John Major teaches us something about the Scottish image of paradise in the shape of Mediterranean orchards in springtime.

John Major recruits St Jerome's longevity, as well as that of sylvan people who live in second, third, or fourth climates and drink with the king's horses and eat wild herbs, to show the natural possibility of extreme longevity. He dismisses the argument of those who deny the ability of the fruit of paradise to assure extreme longevity and assert (on the basis of current medical knowledge) that meat and good wine generate better blood than the fruit and water which constituted Adam's essential diet. Citing an aphorism attributed to Hippocrates, that gluttony kills more people than the

Dictionary of National Biography, ed. L. Stephen and S. Lee, 22 vols. (London, 1917), 12, 830–2; J. Durkan, 'John Major: After 400 Years', *The Innes Review* 1 (1950), 131–9; A Broadie, *The Circle of John Mair: Logic and Logicians in Pre-Reformation Scotland* (Oxford, 1985), pp. 2–3, and *The Shadow of Scotus: Philosophy and Faith in Pre-Reformation Scotland* (Edinburgh, 1995), pp. 5–6.

sword, he declares that what generates good blood is complexion and moderation in the consumption of food. The same food will generate better blood in a person with a sanguine complexion than in a melancholic, in a person of temperate sanguine complexion than in a fat person with a bulging belly.[112]

Adam was exempt from all the symptoms of old age (baldness, for example). He remained biologically in the stage of youth (*iuuentus*), which meant that throughout his life he had the intense and pure natural heat of a well complexioned sanguine person in his thirtieth year.[113] Biblical examples (Caleb in Joshua 14. 11 who was eighty-five years old but felt as young as he was forty years earlier) fortify John's argument that despite the Avicennan division of age periods, age should not necessarily be measured by the number of years, and old age does not always start at forty.

The rest of his debate is devoted to proving that children's radical moisture is not more pure than the radical moisture of youths, nor is their natural heat more intense. This was necessary in order to prove that no physical decline took place in the passage from childhood to adulthood, as Adam was believed to have the supreme complexion of someone in his thirtieth year. The detailed discussion refers to Galen's *Tegni* and commentary on Hippocrates's *Aphorisms*. To those who insist that the heat of the child and the youth differ because the one causes growth vertically ('magis extendit, rarefacit corpus'), the other horizontally (*in latitudine*), John replies that the heat of the child and the youth are the same, and that had not man reached his ultimate size, the *calor iuuenilis* would have had the same effect as the *calor pueri*. Furthermore, the heat of the *iuuenis* is used for other purposes, generation, for example, and hence it is not weaker. Adam, according to John Major, had food at will and wisdom which exceeded that of Galen or Hippocrates. If he had not used the appropriate medicine (that is, eaten from the trees of paradise according to due regimen) he would have sinned. Adam possessed medical knowledge and made use of it, precisely as James of Viterbo determined two hundred years earlier.[114]

[112] 'Complexio cum cibo multum facit ad boni sanguinis generationem et temperies cibi: secundum illud vulgare hippocratis plures occidit gula quam gladius. intemperantia corpus indisponit. Melior sanguis generabitur ex eodem cibo in sanguineo quam melancholico: temperato sanguineo quam in obeso abdomine referto': John Major, *In sententias*, fol. 55rb.

[113] '. . . habuisset calorem naturalem ita intensum et ita purum tota vita sicut in trigesimo anno habet sanguineus bene complexionatus, licet calor naturalis in humido radicali nutriatur: sicut candela ardens in oleo ad cuius consumptionem candela extinguitur sic ad consumptionem humidi radicalis calor radicalis consumitur sed per humidum cibale purum foueri potest calor naturalis sicut in humido radicali': John Major, *In sententias*, fol. 55va.

[114] 'Cibum habuit Adam ad nutum: et prudentiam longe superiorem quam Galenus vel Hippocrates . si non adhibuisset remedium conueniens pecasset et sic non fuisset in statu innocentie: et eodem modo omnibus aliis': John Major, *In sententias*, fol. 56ra.

Furthermore, the quality of air in paradise was most pleasing and consequently did not encourage corruption in his body. 'For we see air in some places or periods which contracts accidents that are the reason why man does not survive long enough. This is the case in intemperate regions in terms of heat and cold, in the time of the epidemic these days which the French call the "Naples Disease" because there a French soldier first contracted a disease by which the body was infected by the worst scab like Job's disease.' John, who wrote this towards the end of the first generation of the Great Pox, testifies to having seen such a case a few years before. As a theologian he combined here the lay perception of the disease as a divinely inflicted Job's disease and an early medical explanation (one of several before the emergence of the contagion explanation) that the pox was one of those diseases which was derived from a warm and humid intemperance of the air.[115] Poor air-quality was responsible, according to John, for the reality in which few did not suffer from some cough and catarrh that could last for only eight days but could sometimes last longer or shorter. This happened all over Europe, but caused comparatively few deaths. It had not happened in previous periods, and perhaps these infections were dispersed by heavenly influences. Adam never experienced such air troubles. But after Sin death entered the world.[116]

So commentaries on the *Sentences* of Peter the Lombard reveal the actual dissemination of medical knowledge and texts beyond the medical milieu. They show that in thirteenth-century natural theology, medicine and natural philosophy became part of the logical proof and did not merely serve as a rhetorical illustration.[117] Their study shows that an examination of medical texts and issues only in the context of the narrow medical scene gives the historian only partial understanding of the impact of medicine on society and

[115] J. Arrizabalaga, J. Henderson and R. French, *The Great Pox: The French Disease in Renaissance Europe* (New Haven, 1997), pp. 52–4, 73.

[116] 'Aerem habuit paradisus amenissimum et per consequens non Adae corruptiuum. Videmus aerem in locis aliquibus vel temporibus accidentia contrahere ratione quorum parum durat homo: ut in regionibus distemperatis in calore et frigore tempore epidimie nostri temporis paradigmata attulere tempore morbi quen Neapolitanum dicunt Galli eo quod Francus miles primo illic morbum contraxit quo corpus pessima scabie in modum morbi Job inficiebatur non longe dissimile a paucis annis preteritis vidimus: paucissimi enim erant qui non laborarent quadam tussi et catarrho qui aliquibus durauit viii diebus solum aliis magis aliis minus, et hoc in omni regione Europe. Pauci tamen comparatiue mortui sunt. Alio tempore ista non contingunt. Fortasse celitus he infectiones dilabuntur. has aeris erumnas non expertus fuisset Adam. Post peccatum Adae in mundum intrauit mors . . .': John Major, *In sententias*, fol. 56ra.

[117] For the significant contribution of insights from natural sciences like mathematics, medicine, and optics for the natural theology and apologetics of the fourth-century Cappadocians (Gregory of Nazianzus, Basil of Caesarea, Gregory of Nyssa, and Macrina) see J. Pelikan, *Christianity and Classical Culture: The Metamorphosis of Natural Theology in the Christian Encounter with Hellenism* (New Haven and London, 1993), pp. 99–106.

culture. The commentaries may even deepen our knowledge of the concrete medical reality in a given period. Anyone who one day undertakes the important project of writing the history of the introduction and assimilation of the concept of complexion into Latin medieval culture will have to explore these texts as well.

INDEX

Medieval writers are listed by their first names. These names and the titles of works have not been standardised to one language.

YORK MEDIEVAL PRESS: PUBLICATIONS

God's Words, Women's Voices: The Discernment of Spirits in the Writing of Late-Medieval Women Visionaries, Rosalynn Voaden (1999)

Pilgrimage Explored, ed. J. Stopford (1999)

Piety, Fraternity and Power: Religious Gilds in Late Medieval Yorkshire 1389–1547, David J. F. Crouch (2000)

Courts and Regions in Medieval Europe, ed. Sarah Rees Jones, Richard Marks and A. J. Minnis (2000)

Treasure in the Medieval West, ed. Elizabeth M. Tyler (2000)

Nunneries, Learning and Spirituality in Late Medieval English Society: The Dominican Priory of Dartford, Paul Lee (2000)

Prophecy and Public Affairs in Later Medieval England, Lesley A. Coote (2000)

The Problem of Labour in Fourteenth-Century England, ed. James Bothwell, P. J. P. Goldberg and W. M. Ormrod (2000)

New Directions in Later Medieval Manuscript Studies: Essays from the 1998 Harvard Conference, ed. Derek Pearsall (2000)

Cistercians, Heresy and Crusade in Occitania, 1145–1229: Preaching in the Lord's Vineyard, Beverly Mayne Kienzle (2001)

Guilds and the Parish Community in Late Medieval East Anglia, c. 1470–1550, Ken Farnhill (2001)

The Age of Edward III, ed. J. S. Bothwell (2001)

York Studies in Medieval Theology

I *Medieval Theology and the Natural Body*, ed. Peter Biller and A. J. Minnis (1997)

II *Handling Sin: Confession in the Middle Ages*, ed. Peter Biller and A. J. Minnis (1998)

York Manuscripts Conferences

Manuscripts and Readers in Fifteenth-Century England: The Literary Implications of Manuscript Study, ed. Derek Pearsall (1983) [Proceedings of the 1981 York Manuscripts Conference]

Manuscripts and Texts: Editorial Problems in Later Middle English Literature, ed. Derek Pearsall (1987) [Proceedings of the 1985 York Manuscripts Conference]

Latin and Vernacular: Studies in Late-Medieval Texts and Manuscripts, ed. A. J. Minnis (1989) [Proceedings of the 1987 York Manuscripts Conference]

Regionalism in Late-Medieval Manuscripts and Texts: Essays celebrating the publication of 'A Linguistic Atlas of Late Mediaeval English', ed. Felicity Riddy (1991) [Proceedings of the 1989 York Manuscripts Conference]

Late-Medieval Religious Texts and their Transmission: Essays in Honour of A. I. Doyle, ed. A. J. Minnis (1994) [Proceedings of the 1991 York Manuscripts Conference]

Prestige, Authority and Power in Late Medieval Manuscripts and Texts, ed. Felicity Riddy (2000) [Proceedings of the 1994 York Manuscripts Conference]

Middle English Poetry: Texts and Traditions. Essays in Honour of Derek Pearsall, ed. A. J. Minnis (2001) [Proceedings of the 1996 York Manuscripts Conference]

Lightning Source UK Ltd.
Milton Keynes UK
UKHW021819201022
410828UK00003B/128

9 781903 153079